T0297037

A Generation at Risk

A Generation at Risk brings up-to-date and insightful perspectives from experienced practitioners and researchers on how a better future can be secured for the millions of children who are being orphaned or made vulnerable by HIV/AIDS. The current situation of these children is grim, and while there has been significant action in the last few years by governments, international organizations, religious bodies, and nongovernmental organizations, the vast majority of children made vulnerable by AIDS have not benefited from any assistance beyond their own extended family and community. *A Generation at Risk* explains in straightforward terms what is required to fill this gap. The book addresses what needs to be done in the areas of education, community mobilization and capacity building, economic strengthening at household and community levels, psychosocial support, and the protection of children and the fulfillment of their rights.

Dr. Geoff Foster trained in medicine in London and took up an appointment in 1985 as a specialist pediatrician with the government of Zimbabwe. In 1987 he started seeing increasing numbers of children with AIDS, and founded Family AIDS Caring Trust (FACT), a faith-based nongovernmental organization and one of Africa's first AIDS service organizations. During the 1990s, FACT pioneered HIV/AIDS care, prevention, and training programs including a widely replicated community-based model supporting orphans and vulnerable children. He has conducted research around issues related to children affected by AIDS. He is a board member of the Firelight Foundation and FACT, and he is on the editorial board of *AIDS Care*.

Carol Levine is currently director of the Families and Health Care Project at the United Hospital Fund in New York City. She also directs The Orphan Project: Families and Children in the HIV Epidemic, which she founded in 1991. She was director of the Citizens Commission on AIDS in New York City from 1987 to 1991. In 1993, she was awarded a MacArthur Foundation Fellowship for her work in AIDS policy and ethics. She was co-convener with Geoff Foster of the White Oak Conference on HIV/AIDS and orphans and vulnerable children in 1998. She has a master's degree in public law and government from Columbia University.

John Williamson is the senior technical advisor for the Displaced Children and Orphans Fund (DCOF) of the U.S. Agency for International Development (USAID), supporting programming for children affected by armed conflict, street children, and children affected by AIDS. Since 1994, he has written or contributed to publications concerning children orphaned or otherwise made vulnerable by HIV/AIDS, including the *Children on the Brink* series. He is one of the organizers of the Global Network for Better Care, the Children and Youth Economic Strengthening Network, and the Washington Network for Children and Armed Conflict. He has worked as a consultant and been on the staff of the Christian Children's Fund and the United Nations High Commissioner for Refugees. He has a master's degree in social welfare from the University of California at Berkeley.

A Generation at Risk

The Global Impact of HIV/AIDS on Orphans and Vulnerable Children

Edited by

GEOFF FOSTER
Mutare Provincial Hospital, Zimbabwe

CAROL LEVINE
United Hospital Fund, New York

JOHN WILLIAMSON
Displaced Children and Orphans Fund, USAID

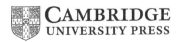

CAMBRIDGE
UNIVERSITY PRESS

CAMBRIDGE
UNIVERSITY PRESS

32 Avenue of the Americas, New York NY 10013-2473, USA

Cambridge University Press is part of the University of Cambridge.

It furthers the University's mission by disseminating knowledge in the pursuit of
education, learning and research at the highest international levels of excellence.

www.cambridge.org
Information on this title: www.cambridge.org/9780521696166

© Cambridge University Press 2005

First published 2005
First paperback edition 2006

A catalogue record for this publication is available from the British Library

Library of Congress Cataloguing in Publication data

A generation at risk : the global impact of HIV/AIDS on orphans and vulnerable
children / edited by Geoff Foster, Carol Levine, and John Williamson.
  p. ; cm.
Includes bibliographical references and index.
ISBN-13: 978-0-521-65264-3 (hardcover)
ISBN-10: 0-521-65264-2 (hardcover)
1. Children of AIDS patients.   2. AIDS (disease) in children.   3. Orphans – Services for.
4. Children's rights.
[DNLM: 1. HIV Infections – Child.   2. Child Advocacy.   3. Child Health Services.
4. Needs Assessment. WC 503.7 G326 2005]   I. Foster, Geoff.   II. Levine, Carol.
III. Williamson, John, 1948 Jan. 1–   IV. Title.
RA643.8.G46   2005
362.196´9792´0083 – dc22   2005010719

ISBN 978-0-521-65264-3 Hardback
ISBN 978-0-521-69616-6 Paperback

Contents

Foreword

It has been said a day is coming when the progress of nations will not be judged by their economic power or military prowess, or by the splendor of their capital cities and public buildings. Instead, the measure of a nation's humanity, and the strength of its civilization, will be based upon the provision it made for its vulnerable and disadvantaged people and the protection that it afforded to the growing minds and bodies of its children.

Children are disproportionate casualties of all sorts of disasters. It is difficult to forget the heart-rending scenes of children swept away from their mothers by the tsunami of December 2004. But in respect to its impact on children, the HIV/AIDS disaster is different. The daily consequences of the global pandemic on millions of children that live with dying parents or have been orphaned lie under the radar of most governments and agencies. The unfolding tragedy is barely visible.

This is a story of painful loss and silent grief, and one that can only be inadequately told. No one who has not experienced the loss of their father and mother can understand its depths. And those that do know first hand are often unable to tell – because of their young age, premature death, their poverty and the insulating layers of discrimination that surround AIDS-related death and disease. *A Generation at Risk: The Global Impact of HIV/AIDS on Orphans and Vulnerable Children* helps to tell this story through chapters that deal with social, economic, and psychological impacts and responses by governments, agencies, faith-based organizations, communities, families, and the children themselves. It is a story of resilience, compassion, and innovation in the face of loss and destitution.

AIDS is not only taking away our children's present, it also has the potential to subtract from their future. Politicians, decision makers, religious and business leaders may neglect the fountain of youth at their peril and allow AIDS to wreak havoc on households and unravel whole societies. Alternatively, we can invest in the reconstruction of devastated families and strengthening of overburdened communities to ensure that adequate provision is made for vulnerable children in our midst for both now and the future. In the battle against apartheid, the solidarity of people from around the world strengthened us in some of our darkest moments. Now, as we seek to counter the ravages of HIV/AIDS on all continents upon our sons and daughters, we need the same solidarity, the same passion, the same commitment and energy.

Desmond Tutu, Archbishop Emeritus
Milnerton, Cape Town, South Africa
May 2005

Preface

In July 1992 at the VIII International Conference on AIDS in Amsterdam, two of this book's editors, Geoff Foster and Carol Levine, were among the few participants with poster presentations devoted to children, either HIV-infected or orphaned. The ways that children were being affected by the emerging pandemic were neither widely recognized nor understood. Geoff, a pediatrician from Zimbabwe, had a presentation on the Family and AIDS Caring Trust (FACT), an organization he founded, and Carol, a health policy and medical ethics specialist from New York City, was presenting the Orphan Project's efforts to respond to the needs of children and families affected by the epidemic. There were no child-related plenary sessions at the conference, no workshops, no oral presentations. The sparse number of poster presentations was equaled by the meager number of people who stopped by to read them and talk to us and other presenters. Since the posters were placed at the outer edge of the vast conference hall ("on the Belgian border," we joked), some of those few visitors were people who were lost. This paucity of interest gave us time to share information about Africa and the United States.

We met again in 1996 at the XI International Conference in Vancouver, and this time we were somewhat closer to the center of the action, although there were still few opportunities at the conference for discussion of children affected by HIV/AIDS. At this conference Geoff suggested that we two join our particular areas of interest and develop a book that would bring together the perspectives of both resource-poor and resource-rich countries dealing with the epidemic. We both felt strongly that the world was not paying attention to the growing crisis of AIDS among women and children and that, in particular, the needs of orphaned children were not being addressed. He then approached the Cambridge University Press representative at the conference and a collaboration was conceived.

Conceived but not born until now. The details of the various delays are of interest only to the editors, the publisher, and the patient authors who had signed on early in the process. Suffice it to say that only when we invited John Williamson, a colleague with much experience and many contacts around the world through his work with the Displaced Children and Orphans Fund (a fund managed by the United States Agency for International Development), to join us as a co-editor did we begin in earnest to bring the book to life.

One intervening event was also critical. In October 1998, The Orphan Project brought together experts from many countries at the White Oak Conference Center in Yulee, Florida, to discuss ways to build international support for children affected by AIDS. That three-day retreat crystallized for us not only the urgency of the issue, but also the benefit of broad collaboration among practitioners, researchers, and funders. Several individual and group collaborations were formed at this meeting, and "The White Oak Report," published by The Orphan Project in 2000, remains a seminal document in the field.

Since then international AIDS conferences have given much more attention to children, although more is needed. Media attention has grown. In particular, since the advent of effective treatment for HIV infection, global concern has been raised about the urgency and the difficulties of providing appropriate care in poor countries. Although we generally no longer have to explain why AIDS is profoundly affecting children, we still have far to go before the appropriate local, national, and international responses are in place. The authors in this volume do not downplay the immensity of the problem and the barriers to action, but they share a commitment to families and children and to a future where children are nurtured, protected, and encouraged to develop to the fullest of their potential. Creating family- and community-centered, child-focused solutions is essential not just for humanitarian reasons but also for each country's future economic, political, and social development.

The examples provided in the book are not endorsements of particular programs but are intended to demonstrate the diversity and energy of local responses that are so often missed when seeing only the vast scope of the problem. Like every other aspect of AIDS, the issues involving children touch deeply held professional and personal beliefs. Each author, it should be clear, is responsible only for the views and examples in his or her own chapter.

We wish to acknowledge, with gratitude, the financial support of The Orphan Project by the Norman and Rosita Winston Foundation, and the administrative support of the Fund for the City of New York.

At various points in the development of the book Karyn Feiden and Debby Stuart Smith provided skillful editing services.

Finally, we also wish to acknowledge, though we cannot do so by name, the legions of unheralded community residents and agency workers throughout the world whose efforts on behalf of children and families have done so much to demonstrate how to create stability out of fragility and strength out of loss.

Carol Levine, New York City
Geoff Foster, Mutare, Zimbabwe
John Williamson, Richmond, Virginia
May 2005

Contributors

Laurie J. Bauman received her PhD in sociology from Columbia University in 1984. She worked at the Bureau of Applied Social Research and the Center for Social Research at Columbia University and then moved to Memorial Sloan-Kettering Cancer Center, where she worked on childhood bereavement and HIV/AIDS prevention in gay men. In 1987, she became co-director of the Preventive Intervention Research Center at the Albert Einstein College of Medicine, Department of Pediatrics. There she conducted multiple studies and randomized trials that applied sociological theory to the prevention of mental health problems secondary to physical conditions in children and their parents. She is currently principal investigator of four randomized trials. Project Care is a succession-planning and disclosure intervention for mothers with late-stage HIV/AIDS. Project Safe is a three-group randomized trial that aims to reduce unsafe sexual behavior among high-risk teenagers aged fourteen to seventeen. StaySafe, also a three-group randomized trial, targets lower-risk teenagers through programs addressing how gender norms increase risk for HIV and STDs. It Takes Two is a two-group randomized trial that addresses how being in a serious relationship can interfere with safe sex practices. She is also co-directing a study of child caregivers (children under age sixteen who are caring for their ill mothers with HIV/AIDS) in New York City and (with Geoff Foster) in Mutare, Zimbabwe.

Tim Brown is a senior Fellow in population and health studies at the East–West Center. He serves as a co-director of the East–West Center/Thai Red Cross Society Collaboration on HIV/AIDS Modeling, Analysis, and Policy in Bangkok. He is currently working with UNAIDS (the Joint United Nations Programme on HIV/AIDS), Family Health International, and other regional partners to develop estimation and projection tools and methodologies for global and Asia-specific application, to implement more comprehensive integrated analysis of Asian HIV epidemics and responses, and to support the development of second-generation surveillance systems in Asia and the Pacific. His research interests include HIV and children, infectious disease epidemiology, HIV-related behaviors, modeling and projection of HIV and its impacts, and public policy for HIV/AIDS prevention and coping. He holds a PhD in physics (high-energy theory) from the University of Hawaii.

Jill Donahue is a microenterprise development specialist whose experience includes project design, management, and evaluation. She has expertise in analyzing household economics and the role of microenterprise services to improve the ability of families and communities to cope with the impact of HIV/AIDS, and she is skilled in mobilizing community concern about, and participation in, activities benefiting children affected by the epidemic. She was a Peace Corps volunteer in Burkina Faso from 1981 to 1983. After working in the United States as a supervisor for a market research firm, she joined the Peace Corps again, with her husband, this time in Sierra Leone from 1986 to 1988. She then served as associate Peace Corps director for small enterprise development in Mali from 1988 to 1991, and in Botswana from 1991 to 1993. She continued with the Peace Corps as an expert consultant for the Office of Training and Program Support based in Washington, DC, from 1994 to 1997. She also provided consulting services to a variety of organizations from 1994 to 2001, including USAID's Displaced Children and Orphan's Fund (DCOF) and Volunteers in Technical Assistance (VITA). In 2001, Donahue and two other consultants conducted a study on HIV/AIDS among microfinance clients in Kenya and Uganda, and then she joined Catholic Relief Services as a regional technical advisor for the Southern Africa regions. Currently she is a freelance consultant, based in Jeffreys Bay, South Africa.

Barbara Draimin is the founding director of The Family Center, which provides in-home legal and social services to families throughout New York City who are dealing with life-threatening illnesses. Before she created this agency in 1993, she was director of planning for six years at the Department of Social Services AIDS Division, and associate to the commissioner of the Department for the Aging for eight years. At The Family Center, she heads a team of more than forty-five who work with families affected by serious illness, primarily AIDS. The legal services provided to families include wills, power of attorney, court-appointed guardianship, custody, and adoption. Additional social services include mentoring and buddy programs for children, family camping, and mental health counseling. The Family Center also conducts research, evaluating services provided by the center and assessing the changing needs of families affected by illness. Draimin, who holds a doctorate in social work from Hunter College of the City University of New York, has written three books for children affected by AIDS, including *Coping When a Parent Has AIDS* (Rosen Publishing, 1994), and numerous articles for professional and academic publications.

Geoff Foster is a consultant in pediatrics and child health in Mutare, Zimbabwe. He holds MB, BS, and MRCP (Paeds.) degrees. He started treating children with AIDS in 1987. He was instrumental in the formation of the Family AIDS Caring Trust (FACT), one of the first HIV/AIDS service organizations in Africa. During the 1990s, FACT pioneered HIV/AIDS programming, including a widely replicated community-based model supporting orphans and vulnerable children. After helping FACT develop a regional role as a technical support organization, he resigned as director and now works as a consultant on international responses to the orphan crisis. He has written extensively and has conducted research around responses to children affected by AIDS, including a multicountry study documenting the role of faith-based organizations in response to orphans. In 2003, he received the Order of the British Empire from Her Majesty Queen Elizabeth II for his work with FACT.

Stefan Germann has been working for twelve years in the field of HIV/AIDS and development with the Salvation Army in Southern Africa, with a main focus on Southern Zimbabwe. For the past ten years he has focused on orphans and children affected by AIDS in rural and urban communities. In 1998, he started the Masiye Camp program that provides psychosocial support for children affected by AIDS, as well as household management camps for child-headed households. Since 2001 he has been part of the Salvation Army Africa Regional Facilitation team on HIV/AIDS, Health, and Development as focal person on children, youth, and AIDS. He is also on the World Council for Religion and Peace task force on orphans and vulnerable children. In 2002 he started as an adviser for the Regional Psychosocial Support Initiative (REPSSI) in Southern Africa, which aims to scale up psychosocial support to children affected by HIV/AIDS in the region. Germann has published several articles and reports on children and youth affected by HIV/AIDS. In September 2002 he was invited by Nelson Mandela to participate in the African Leaders Consultation on Children and AIDS.

Sofia Gruskin, who holds degrees in law and international affairs, is an associate professor of health and human rights in the Department of Population and International Health at the Harvard School of Public Health. She is the director of the Program on International Health and Human Rights at the Harvard-based François-Xavier Bagnoud Center for Health and Human Rights. She is editor of *Health and Human Rights* and an associate editor of the *American Journal of Public Health*. The emphasis of her work concerns the implications of linking health to human rights, with particular attention to women, children, gender issues, and vulnerable populations in the context of HIV/AIDS.

Michael J. Kelly is a Jesuit priest and formerly a professor of education at the University of Zambia, Lusaka. He currently works as a consultant in the field of HIV/AIDS and education. He is a member of the Mobile Task Team, a virtual organization of experts from Southern Africa who respond to requests from education ministries to provide technical assistance in the field of HIV/AIDS and education. He is also a member of the reference group that advises the Swedish-Norwegian AIDS Team for Africa. He has participated in numerous HIV/AIDS-related conferences and workshops in Africa, Asia, Europe, and the Caribbean and has written many books and articles. His most recent book, *Education and HIV/AIDS in the Caribbean*, was published by the International Institute for Educational Planning, Paris, in October 2003.

Carol Levine is currently director of the Families and Health Care Project at the United Hospital Fund in New York City. This project focuses on developing partnerships between health care professionals and family caregivers who provide most of the long-term and chronic care to elderly, seriously ill, or disabled relatives. She also directs The Orphan Project: Families and Children in the HIV Epidemic, which she founded in 1991. She was director of the Citizens Commission on AIDS in New York City from 1987 to 1991. As a senior staff associate of The Hastings Center, she edited the *Hastings Center Report*. In 1993 she was awarded a MacArthur Foundation Fellowship for her work in AIDS policy and ethics. She was co-convener with Geoff Foster of the White Oak Conference on HIV/AIDS and orphans and vulnerable children in 1998 and co-editor of the report from that conference. She has published extensively on HIV/AIDS, medical ethics, and family caregiving. Her most recent books are *The Cultures of Caregiving: Conflict and Common Ground among Families, Professionals, and Policy Makers* (co-edited with Thomas H. Murray, The Johns Hopkins University Press, 2004) and the second edition of *Always on Call: When Illness Turns Families into Caregivers* (Vanderbilt University Press, 2004). She is also editor of the 11th edition of *Taking Sides: Controversial Bioethical Issues* (McGraw-Hill Dushkin, 2005). She has a master's degree in public law and government from Columbia University.

Stanley Ngalazu Phiri is regional project officer for children orphaned and made vulnerable by HIV/AIDS in UNICEF's Eastern and Southern Africa Regional Office. As a director of Malawi's Community-based Options for Protection and Empowerment (COPE) program, he facilitated the development of community coalitions to address the needs of children either orphaned or otherwise made vulnerable by HIV/AIDS, and he worked with government and other partners at district and national levels to capacitate the response and influence and inform the policies that address these issues. He was national coordinator of Malawi's Children at Risk Committee and coordinator of the Children and War program for Mozambican refugee children. He received a master's degree in international development policy from Duke University.

Warren A. Reich received a PhD in social psychology from Rutgers University in 1994. He joined The Family Center in 2003, where he serves as its research and evaluation manager. His current projects include an analysis of predictors of HIV-positive clients' progress through The Family Center's program of services and the design of a methodology for assessing the impact of Family Center psychoeducational programs on individual families. He has published studies on personal identity, conflict style, and methodology and has taught a variety of undergraduate and graduate psychology courses at Rutgers University and the University of Toledo, Ohio.

Werasit Sittitrai, a Thai national, is Director of the Department of Programme Development, Coordination and UN System Relations at the Joint United Nations Programme on HIV/AIDS (UNAIDS), Geneva, Switzerland. He is responsible for mobilizing and strengthening the expanded UN response to AIDS through the United Nations' governance mechanisms, interagency Unified Budget and Workplan, and mainstreaming HIV/AIDS into the development agenda and programs of UN agencies. He started his career as an assistant professor at Chulalongkorn University in 1979, where he conducted pioneering research and published several articles on family planning, rural development, sexual behavior surveys, condoms, health issues, and support systems for the elderly. He then joined the Office of the Prime Minister in the early 1990s to coordinate the National AIDS program and the AIDS plans of all ministries. Before he joined UNAIDS in 1996, he was the deputy director of the Thai Red Cross Society Program on AIDS and co-founded the Thai Red Cross Anonymous Counselling and Testing Centre on HIV and STD. He provided technical support to several Asian countries including Cambodia, Myanmar, Pakistan, Laos and Singapore on HIV/AIDS prevention and care programs. From 1996 to 2001 he was Associate Director of Policy, Strategy and Research at UNAIDS, responsible for UNAIDS Best Practice publications and for overseeing the policy and technical strategy for prevention and care. From 2001 to 2003, he headed the Asia/Pacific Middle East and North Africa Division at UNAIDS. He is co-author of Candles of Hope (United Nations Development Program, 1994), co-editor of *Impact of HIV/AIDS on Children in Thailand* (Thai Red Cross Society, Save the Children Fund UK, and Program on Population, East-West Center, 1995), co-author of chapters in King Holmes et al., eds., *Sexually Transmitted Diseases*, 3rd edition, 1999, and in Philip Pizzo and Catherine Wilfert, *Pediatric AIDS*, 3rd edition, 1998 and the author of other articles and reports.

Daniel J. M. Tarantola received his medical degree from the Paris University Medical School. He pursued his clinical postdoctoral training in nephrology and, later, his public health training with a focus on childhood infectious diseases prevention and control and epidemiology. He had a long career with the World Health Organization devoted to large-scale international health programmes, including the eradication of smallpox, the launching of the Expanded Programme on Immunization, the development of diarrhoeal disease and acute respiratory infection control programmes, and the WHO Global programme on HIV/AIDS. In 1991, Dr. Tarantola joined the Harvard School of Public Health where he taught, conducted research and published over a period of eight years. In 1993, he took part in founding the François-Xavier Bagnoud Center for Health and Human Rights at the Harvard School of Public Health. In 1998, he rejoined the World Health Organization where, until 2004, he assumed the dual functions of Senior Policy Adviser to the Director General and Director, Immunization, Vaccines and Biologicals. He is currently a New South Global Professor in Health and Human Rights at the University of New South Wales, Sydney, Australia, and a Senior Associate of the Harvard-based François-Xavier Bagnoud Center for Health and Human Rights.

David Tolfree originally trained as a social worker and worked with children and families in fieldwork and residential and day-care settings in the United Kingdom and other countries. As a researcher he has been interested mainly in issues concerning separated and orphaned children and children in situations of armed conflict and forced migration. He has published several books, including *Roofs and Roots: The Care of Separated Children in the Developing World* (Ashgate, 1995), *Restoring Playfulness: Different Approaches to Assisting Children Who Are Psychologically Affected by War and Displacement* (Save the Children Sweden, 1996), and *Whose Children? Separated Children's Protection and Participation in Emergencies* (Save the Children Sweden, 2003), as well as numerous articles and reports. He is currently working for Save the Children UK to prepare the first two volumes in the "First Resort" series.

Desmond Mpilo Tutu, Archbishop Emeritus, received his Licentiate in Theology in 1960 from St. Peter's Theological College, Johannesburg, and was ordained to the Anglican priesthood in Johannesburg in 1961. Not long after his ordination, Tutu obtained his Bachelor of Divinity Honors and Master of Theology degrees from King's College, University of London, England.

From 1967 to 1978 he served in a number of increasingly prominent positions, including lecturer at the Federal Theological Seminary at Alice, South

Africa, and chaplain at the University of Fort Hare; lecturer in the Department of Theology at the University of Botswana, Lesotho, and Swaziland; Associate Director of the Theological Education Fund of the World Council of Churches, in Kent, United Kingdom; Dean of St. Mary's Cathedral, Johannesburg; and finally Bishop of Lesotho.

By 1978, in the wake of the 1976 Soweto uprising Bishop Tutu was persuaded to take up the post of General Secretary of the South African Council of Churches (SACC). Justice and reconciliation and an end to apartheid were the SACC's priorities, and as General Secretary, Bishop Tutu pursued these goals with vigor and commitment. Under his guidance, the SACC became an important institution in South African spiritual and political life, challenging white society and the government and affording assistance to the victims of apartheid.

Inevitably, Bishop Tutu became heavily embroiled in controversy as he spoke out against the injustices of the apartheid system. For several years he was denied a passport to travel abroad. He became a prominent leader in the crusade for justice and racial conciliation in South Africa. In 1984 he received a Nobel Peace Prize in recognition of his extraordinary contributions to that cause. In 1985 he was elected Bishop of Johannesburg.

In 1986 Bishop Tutu was elevated to Archbishop of Cape Town, and in this capacity he did much to bridge the chasm between black and white Anglicans in South Africa. And as Archbishop, Tutu became a principal mediator and conciliator in the transition to democracy in South Africa.

In 1995 President Nelson Mandela appointed him Chairman of the Truth and Reconciliation Commission, a body set up to probe gross human rights violations that occurred under apartheid. In 1996, shortly after his retirement from office as Archbishop of Cape Town, Tutu was granted the honorary title of Archbishop Emeritus.

Archbishop Tutu has held several distinguished academic and world leadership posts. In recent years Tutu has turned his attention to a different cause: the campaign against HIV/AIDS. The Archbishop has made appearances around the globe to help raise awareness of the disease and its tragic consequences in human lives and suffering.

Archbishop Tutu holds honorary degrees from well over one hundred universities, including Harvard, Oxford, Cambridge, Columbia, Yale, Emory, the Ruhr, Kent, Aberdeen, Sydney, Fribourg (Switzerland), Cape Town, Witwatersrand, and the University of South Africa.

He has received many prizes and awards in addition to the Nobel Peace Prize, most notably the Order of Meritorious Service Award (Gold) presented by President Mandela; the Archbishop of Canterbury's Award of Outstanding Service to the Anglican Communion; the Prix d'Athene (Onassis Foundation); the Family of Man Gold Medal Award; the Mexican Order of the Aztec Medal (Insignia Grade); the Martin Luther King Jr. Non-Violent Peace Prize; and the Sydney Peace Prize.

His writings include *No Future Without Forgiveness* (2000), and *God Has a Dream* (2004).

Douglas Webb is a social scientist currently based at the Eastern and Southern Africa Regional Office of the UNICEF office in Nairobi, Kenya. He obtained his PhD in human geography from Royal Holloway, University of London, in 1995, where he examined the social responses to HIV/AIDS in South Africa and Namibia. He then spent three years with UNICEF Zambia, working on HIV/AIDS responses and researching the impacts of HIV/AIDS on children. From 1998 to 2004 he worked with Save the Children UK in London, most recently as the policy adviser on HIV/AIDS. He is the author of *HIV/AIDS in Africa* (New Africa Books, in association with University of Natal Press, 2002) and numerous other publications on HIV/AIDS, children, and young people.

John Williamson is the senior technical advisor for the Displaced Children and Orphans Fund (DCOF) of the U.S. Agency for International Development (USAID), which supports programs for children affected by armed conflict, street children, and children affected by AIDS. He has been engaged with assessing and responding to the impacts of AIDS on children and families since 1991 and since 1994 has written or contributed to a number of publications in this area. These include: *Action for Children Affected by AIDS* (WHO and UNICEF, 1994), the *Children on the Brink* series (USAID, 1997 and 2000; USAID, UNICEF, and UNAIDS, 2002 and 2004), and *Conducting a Situation Analysis of Orphans and Vulnerable Children Affected by HIV/AIDS* (USAID, 2004). He is one of the organizers of the Global Network for Better Care, the Children and Youth Economic Strengthening Network, and the Washington Network for Children and Armed Conflict. He has worked as a consultant and been on the staff of the Christian Children's Fund and the United Nations High Commissioner for Refugees (UNHCR). While with UNHCR, he wrote the *Handbook for Social Services* (1984), edited the *Guidelines of Refugee Children* (1988), and chaired the Working Group of Refugee Children. He has a masters degree in social welfare from the University of California at Berkeley.

Introduction

HIV/AIDS and Its Long-Term Impact on Children

Carol Levine, Geoff Foster, and John Williamson

HIV/AIDS has changed the world in profound and still-evolving ways. The last children born before HIV/AIDS[1] emerged in the late 1970s and early 1980s are now in their mid-twenties, many with children of their own. All children born in the foreseeable future – at least for the next several decades – will be living in a world where the epidemic persists, albeit with variable consequences for each of them. Children, among the most vulnerable members of society, are bellwethers of adult leaders' willingness and capacity to respond to economic, health, and social challenges. What happens to children and adolescents now will determine not only their futures but also the futures of their families, communities, and societies.

In the first years of the HIV/AIDS epidemic, though, there was relatively little direct focus on children, particularly children who were not themselves HIV-infected but were nevertheless significantly affected by the disease. In the past decade or so the massive and growing number of orphans in Africa has received periodic media attention and many program responses. To be sure, in developed countries in North America and Europe, pediatric HIV/AIDS has become a highly sophisticated medical specialty. Treatments to reduce mother-to-child HIV transmission have succeeded extraordinarily well in these countries and are being introduced slowly in poor countries where the need is greatest. In every country affected by the epidemic, dedicated individuals and groups – most with very meager resources – serve children and families and advocate for more attention to their needs. (See the Chronology of Important Events in this volume for some key developments.) On the whole, however, the more

---

[1] The human immune deficiency virus (HIV) and the acquired immune deficiency syndrome (AIDS) are commonly linked by the term HIV/AIDS; infection with the virus is the initial stage of a disease that ends with the more serious complications and opportunistic infections that define AIDS.

1

general impact on children has been a lower priority on policymakers' and international agendas than are adult problems.

There are many reasons for this. Biomedical responses – scientific inquiry, basic epidemiology, and initial prevention and care efforts – were understandably at the top of the priority list. Even these responses were complicated and constrained in many places by widespread official and informal denial that a problem existed. Families with ill and dying adults also struggled to take care of surviving children as they had always done – on their own. By the time the multiple, cascading impacts of HIV/AIDS on families and children became more apparent, the scope of the problem seemed too huge to tackle. Furthermore, children are generally powerless in society and have no political voice. But the silence about HIV/AIDS has now been broken, and the number of orphans is too massive to ignore. It is essential to understand that loss of parents is only the most obvious impact of the epidemic on children, and that other vulnerabilities must be recognized and addressed as well. Nevertheless, solutions proposed in haste or based on inaccurate or incomplete data will not achieve their goals, and may even have negative effects.

This book brings together in a multidisciplinary and multifaceted way what is now known, what must be learned, and (most important) what must be done to address children's needs effectively. Each chapter vividly illustrates that all the aspects of children's lives – economic, educational, medical, psychosocial, legal, and spiritual – are intertwined (see especially Chapters 3 and 4). Solutions must take into account each society's cultural, political, social, and economic infrastructure. The book's emphasis on Africa reflects the preponderance of research and experience in the field and the advanced state of the epidemic on that continent. Two chapters, however – one on Asia and the Pacific region (Chapter 7) and one on the United States (Chapter 8) – present different paradigms, and wherever possible, information from non-African contexts has been added.

PARADOXES AND DILEMMAS

Researchers, practitioners, and advocates engaged with children's issues and HIV/AIDS find themselves facing some unsettling paradoxes. For example, the realities of the epidemic's scope are surely daunting – yet they ought not be interpreted so negatively that any intervention seems pointless. In the past it has been seen as necessary to emphasize only the worst in order to gain any attention at all. Now that there is at least a beginning of support, it is important to point out the positive side – that there are indeed many interventions, some requiring incredibly modest resources by American or European standards, that can make a substantial difference in children's lives. As in so many other areas, focusing on children's issues lays bare a society's problems but also reveals its strengths.

Another paradox is that while families are children's natural protectors (and in most cases do their best under extraordinarily difficult circumstances) it is also true that some households exploit and abuse children in their care. But some instances that appear to be – and may well be – exploitative (children taken out of school to work in fields, for example) might be the only means available for that family's survival. Other instances, such as the sexual exploitation of children, are clearly abusive and unconscionable. Families should not be romanticized, nor should they be demonized. The vast majority of children orphaned or otherwise made vulnerable by AIDS are living within families. The balance here is to find ways to support families so that they can more adequately meet children's needs, but also to protect children from being pressured into activities that contravene their best interests or subject them to outright abuse and exploitation.

Still other quandaries arise about language and definitions. Even "child" is defined differently in various contexts and for different reasons. This book is concerned with all children and young people below the legal age of majority. The term "AIDS orphan" still appears occasionally in the popular media, but it has become anathema to most professionals addressing the impacts of HIV/AIDS on children. This book avoids the term because it is stigmatizing, and suggests to some that children who have lost a parent are themselves "victims" (another unacceptable term) of AIDS, although most are not HIV-infected.

Even the term "orphan," despite its long religious associations (see Chapter 6) and its epidemiologic neutrality, is problematic because its meaning varies among cultures and is potentially stigmatizing. Focusing solely on children who have lost a parent fails to take account of those who are in similar or even greater need. It can result in the inappropriate categorization and labeling of children, and it may generate conflicts over resources and priorities at community and household levels. While orphans are often referred to in this book, this designation is not advocated as a criterion for individual eligibility for assistance. The unfortunate reality, though, is that some donors do tie funding to orphans, or specifically to orphans whose parents have died of HIV/AIDS. Programs often walk a fine line between telling donors what they want to hear and implementing services that serve other vulnerable children as well.

One of the solutions to this dilemma is the targeting of resources in two stages: first, to geographic areas seriously affected by HIV/AIDS; and second, to the most vulnerable children identified by communities in these areas (described in Chapter 10). Attempting to find another solution, many programs and national-level policymaking and planning agencies have begun to focus on "orphans and vulnerable children." Some donors and programs understand this specifically as children orphaned or otherwise made vulnerable by HIV/AIDS. Others, though, take the term at face value, recognizing that the number of orphans and vulnerable children has been greatly increased by AIDS in countries with high HIV prevalence, but that other factors also contribute. Consequently, different people and agencies use the term "orphans and vulnerable children" to mean somewhat different things. In this book, the phrase is generally used to mean all children who are orphaned or are otherwise vulnerable in countries where the epidemic is having significant impacts.

"Orphans and vulnerable children" becomes problematic in another way when it is contracted to the label "OVC." Similar problems arise with the acronym "CABA", which stands for "children affected by AIDS." Those who use OVC or CABA as convenient shorthand in technical documents certainly do not intend any ill effects. Because these labels have been used frequently in official documents, however, people at the local level have begun to use them as well to show organizations with resources that they understand and share their commitments. The unfortunate result has been that one can now visit communities where particular children are identified (at least to visitors) using such labels. The debates on terminology issues undoubtedly will take new turns in the coming years. For this book, we have chosen to avoid the terms AIDS orphans, OVC, and CABA, except in quotations or organizational names, but we have not imposed a single terminology, thus acknowledging the fluidity of the discussion and the different contexts being described.

THE HIV/AIDS EPIDEMIC: SCOPE AND TRENDS

Statistics cannot convey the individual human suffering created by the HIV/AIDS epidemic, but they are necessary to portray its cumulative effect. As the epidemic has evolved, so too have better methods of data collection and interpretation. Still, there are many gaps (see Chapter 9). In a report published in July 2004, the Joint United Nations Programme on HIV/AIDS (UNAIDS) estimated that about 38 million people around the globe were living with HIV/AIDS, 2.5 million of them children under the age of fifteen (UNAIDS 2004). Around 5 million people became newly infected with HIV in 2003 (4.2 million adults and 700,000 children), (and in that year an estimated 3 million people died (2.5 million adults and 500,000 children).

The epidemic is most severe where it emerged earliest – in sub-Saharan Africa, which has between 25 million and 28.2 million people living with the disease, with about 3 million newly infected in 2003. Over 2 million adults and children died due to AIDS in 2003 (UNICEF 2003). Beyond these hardest-hit countries, Thailand (where the epidemic is well established) is being joined by other Asian countries where HIV infection is spreading rapidly (particularly India, China, Indonesia, and Vietnam). HIV/AIDS is also growing in Eastern Europe and Central Asia among the countries of the former Soviet Union (Field 2004). In Latin America the epidemic is entrenched in parts of the Caribbean (the Bahamas, Haiti, and Trinidad and Tobago) and in Brazil and Guyana. In the developed world – which has benefited from the advent of multidrug treatments called HAART (highly active antiretroviral therapy) – mortality has declined but new infections continue. In the United States this is particularly true among African American and Latino young women and men. Only a few countries, notably Senegal and Uganda, have succeeded in slowing the epidemic by early and large-scale prevention efforts.

In this global pandemic, each regional or local epidemic has a specific time frame, pattern, primary mode of transmission, and availability of resources. Injecting-drug use in Asia and Eastern Europe is a common mode of transmission but is much less prevalent in Africa. Heterosexual transmission occurs everywhere but is the primary mode of transmission in Africa and, increasingly, in the United States.

This is the broad picture. Three-quarters of the people living with HIV/AIDS are in sub-Saharan Africa, and the epidemic's impact on children follows the adult epidemic. In 1990, fewer than 1 million children in that region under the age of fifteen had lost one or both parents to HIV/AIDS (UNICEF 2003). By the end of 2001 the number had reached over 11 million children, according to the joint estimate of UNICEF, UNAIDS, and the U.S. Agency for International Development (USAID). By 2010 that number is expected to grow to 20 million. About 5.7 percent of all children in sub-Saharan Africa will be orphaned by AIDS by 2010 (USAID et al. 2002). The most recent estimates extend the age of "child" to eighteen, bringing the statistics in line with international definitions and recognizing that children of different ages have different problems and needs (USAID, et al. 2004). In fact, more than half of the orphans in sub-Saharan Africa, Asia, and Latin America and the Caribbean are aged twelve to seventeen, and a third are aged six to eleven.

According to UNICEF (2003), "The worst is yet to come." As increasing numbers of young adults with HIV infection progress to AIDS and die, they will leave ever larger numbers of orphaned children (see Figure 1.1). Because there is such a long lag time between infection and illness, even if there were no new infections the numbers of affected children would still increase. Better access to treatment will delay but not stop this inexorable process. Prolonging the lives of HIV-infected parents and giving them a good quality of life will improve the educational, economic, and psychosocial outcomes for their children.

Ironically, however, the most effective medical methods of preventing transmission to newborns – the administration of antiretroviral therapy during pregnancy and delivery and then to the neonate through Prevention of Mother-to-Child Transmission programs (PMTCT) – can lead to an

Epidemic Curves, HIV/AIDS, and Orphans

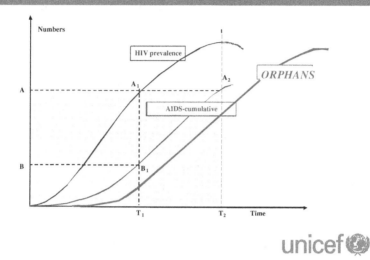

FIGURE I.1. The worst is yet to come. (Reprinted from UNICEF 2001, 27.)

increase in orphans. HIV-positive women in PMTCT programs are more likely to have uninfected babies. If they do not receive drug therapy themselves after giving birth, however, they are more likely to sicken and die, leaving their children as orphans. Some agencies are establishing "PMTCT-plus" initiatives to provide life-prolonging interventions to HIV-positive parents identified through these programs. Programs to provide antiretroviral treatment to HIV-infected children in developing countries are still in their infancy, with some agencies targeting HIV-infected orphans. As important as these programs are for reducing child mortality, they will have only a minimal effect on reducing the number of orphans because more children will survive the death of a parent. Preliminary estimates suggest that the number of orphans may be reduced by about 3 percent if anti-retroviral treatment and PMTC+ are fully implemented (Neff Walker, personal communication, April 2005).

Just as HIV/AIDS is a dynamic pandemic, its impacts on children, families, and households unfolds gradually and in many directions. Beginning with a parent's HIV infection, and then through the more serious illnesses of AIDS and ultimately death, children's lives are increasingly circumscribed by the economic problems that beset the family, by their lost or limited educational opportunities, and by psychosocial distress and other

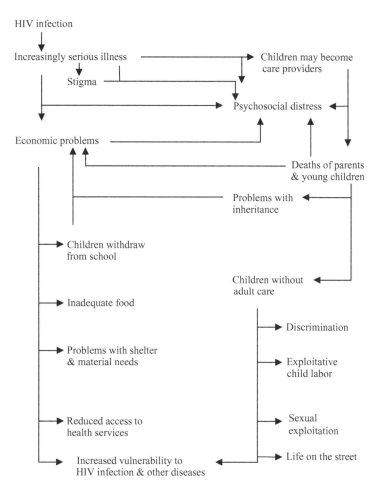

FIGURE I.2. The cascading impacts of HIV/AIDS on children.

difficulties that can ultimately lead to the worst outcomes. (See Figure I.2 for a schematic presentation of this downward spiral, and see Chapter 2 for more details.)

The staggering level of suffering that HIV/AIDS is causing should be sufficient to motivate an adequate collective response to this situation. Moreover, the almost universally agreed upon rights of children defined in the United Nations Convention on the Rights of the Child (see Chapter 5) should be sufficient to generate the action needed. However, to date such considerations have been insufficient motivators of national and international agencies. Perhaps the additional stimulus needed can come from greater attention to the consequences of failing to make an adequate response.

Clearly, the number of children and families made vulnerable by HIV/AIDS is massive and will remain so for decades. AIDS is causing unprecedented child and family welfare problems, but the collective response in every country seriously affected by the pandemic falls far short of what is needed. What affected children and their families require, and what their own countries and the international community owe them, is a combination of efforts, large and small, that together match the scale and duration of the problems that AIDS is causing. Only a small minority of children and families affected by HIV/AIDS are currently benefiting significantly from assistance coming from outside their extended family and neighbors (USAID et al. 2004). While there are many effective programs and funding has increased, the gap between the impacts of these initiatives and what needs to be done remains huge (World Vision 2005). More resources are desperately needed, but there is no solid consensus on just where this might come from, how it can be sustained for decades, or how it should be applied (see Chapter 10).

BUILDING AN EFFECTIVE RESPONSE

The way a problem is understood influences what is done about it. The starting point for developing effective responses to the impacts of the pandemic on children is recognizing that families and communities are the first line of response (see Chapter 1). Whether or not outside bodies intervene, families and communities will be dealing with the impacts of AIDS, often with great difficulty. Consequently, governments, international organizations, nongovernmental organizations (NGOs), religious bodies, and others will have significant, sustainable impacts on children's safety and well-being to the extent that they strengthen the ongoing capacities of affected families and communities to protect and care for their vulnerable children. Special efforts are needed for the care and protection of children on the street or in child-headed households.

A global consensus has emerged on the necessity of a collaborative international response of building family and community capacities, ensuring that children benefit from essential services, and establishing appropriate and meaningful governmental and societal responses. This consensus is reflected in a recent and very important document: *The Framework for the Protection, Care, and Support of Orphans and Vulnerable Children Living in a World with HIV and AIDS* (2004). The *Framework* was developed through an extensive global consultation process and reflects a broad, international consensus on the actions needed to address the needs and rights of orphans and vulnerable children. By July 2004, when it was released, it had been endorsed by twenty-three international, governmental, and nongovernmental organizations. While UNICEF took the lead in developing the document, the *Framework* incorporates the contributions of many organizations. It was issued by all the endorsing organizations, rather than any specific one.

Developing programs that significantly improve the lives of individual children and families affected by HIV/AIDS would be relatively easy if there were enough resources, organizational capacity, and political will. Vulnerable children and households can be identified, health services provided, school expenses paid, food distributed, and supportive counseling provided. The reality, however, is that the funding either currently or likely to become available will be too limited to sustain such an intensive direct service delivery approach for the duration required. The challenge, then, is to implement approaches that:

- improve substantially the safety and well-being of vulnerable children and families,
- make maximum use of all available resources,
- match the massive scale of the impacts of AIDS, and
- can be sustained for decades.

Creating an adequate response will require careful consideration of the spectrum of the epidemic's impacts. On the one hand, it is necessary to recognize the problems on a human scale – what happens to parents, children, and orphans' guardians. This perspective by itself, though, is inadequate to guide the scaling up of responses to these problems. Thus on the other hand, it is also essential to keep in mind the magnitude and duration of the HIV/AIDS pandemic and its collective impacts. The authors in this volume provide not only essential information and perspectives, but also critical recommendations for action that, taken together, point a way forward.

References

Field, M. 2004. HIV and AIDS in the former Soviet bloc. *New England Journal of Medicine* 351 (2): 117–20.

The framework for the protection, care, and support of orphans and vulnerable children living in a world with HIV and AIDS. 2004. Prepared by the Global Partners Forum for Orphans and Vulnerable Children, convened and led by UNICEF, July. Available at http://www.unicef.org

UNAIDS. 2004. *2004 Report on the global AIDS epidemic*. Geneva: UNAIDS, July. http://www.unaids.org/bangkok2004/report.html.

UNICEF. 2003. *Africa's orphaned generations*. New York: November. http://www.unicef.org/publications/index_16271.html.

USAID, UNAIDS, WHO, UNICEF, and the Policy Project. 2004. *Coverage of selected services for HIV/AIDS prevention, care and support in low and middle income countries in 2003*. June, 84 pages. http://www.policyproject.com/pubs/generalreport/CoverageSurveyReport.pdf

USAID, UNICEF, and UNAIDS. 2002. *Children on the Brink 2002: A joint report on orphan estimates and program strategies*. Washington, DC: TvT Associates/The Synergy Project, USAID. http://www.unicef.org/publications/pub_children_on_the_brink_en.pdf

―――. 2004. *Children on the Brink 2004: A joint report of new orphan estimates and a framework for action*. New York: UNICEF. Available at http://www.unicef.org/publications/index_22212.html.

World Vision UK. 2005. *More than words? Action for Orphans and Vulnerable Children in Africa. Monitoring Progress toward the UN Declaration of Commitment on HIV/AIDS*. World Vision UK: Milton Keynes. 64 pp. Available at www.worldvision.org.uk.

1

Family- and Community-Based Care for Children Affected by HIV/AIDS

Strengthening the Front Line Response

Stanley Ngalazu Phiri and David Tolfree

The overwhelming majority of children orphaned or affected by HIV/ AIDS in sub-Saharan Africa are currently being cared for within their immediate and extended families. For most of these children, no option is as good as living with healthy parents; where this is not possible (given the realities of the HIV/AIDS epidemic), family- and community-based sources of care are the most child-centered – and the only practical – means of responding to the scale of the problem. Considerations of both child rights and child development unequivocally support family-based care, with the responsibility for it located firmly in local communities.

Achieving a strong and reliable system of family-based care, however, requires a systematic approach to strengthening family and community capacities by mobilizing communities. Mobilizing communities in turn requires the support of national and local policy. Steps also need to be taken to provide appropriate care for those children who have slipped through family and community safety nets. This care is likely to consist of various forms of fostering (by which we mean the care of children by unrelated adults, whether informally or with agency involvement) or adoption. Both approaches need to be adapted according to cultural considerations.

This chapter has three main sections. The first section critiques the practice of offering institutional forms of care as a benevolent and efficient response. The second provides a detailed examination of the need for strategies to support families and communities in their attempts to provide care for children who require it, with examples drawn from various African contexts. The final section examines fostering, adoption, and other alternative care arrangements for children whose care and protection cannot be met within their own families and communities.

THE CASE AGAINST INSTITUTIONAL CARE

As the HIV/AIDS epidemic tightens its grip on communities already weakened by endemic poverty, traditional family systems to care for parentless children have been forced to change. Examples of this kind of change are care by maternal rather than paternal kin where the latter is more traditional (Foster et al. 1995), more widespread care of children by grandparents, or the emergence of a new form of coping with care provided by child-headed households (Ali 1998; Foster et al. 1996).

In some situations, residential institutions have been created or expanded by governmental or religious organizations (Harber 1998). Although hard data are elusive because many institutions are not registered or regulated, in six Southern African countries there was a 35 percent increase in institutions between 1999 and 2003, even though the predominant response from faith-based organizations was community-based (Foster 2004b). The countries in which faith-based institutional responses were most common are Mozambique, Kenya, Swaziland, and Malawi, and among Muslim, Pentecostal, and "other Protestant" groups. There is also evidence from Eastern and Central Europe that institutions became entrenched social policy under Communist regimes and remain so as these countries deal with poverty and HIV/AIDS.

In many countries, the idea of institutional care was imported from the industrialized world in the belief that it was modern and therefore better. Paradoxically, most Western countries have now largely abandoned congregate care in favor of family-based alternatives. Even those institutions still open – in the United States and the United Kingdom, for example – typically do not house orphans; rather, they provide time-limited social treatment mainly for adolescents with serious emotional or behavioral problems and function as "family" units with many community ties.

In countries severely affected by HIV/AIDS, the development of residential care is sometimes justified on the grounds either that families and communities are so overwhelmed by the problems of children orphaned by AIDS that there is no alternative, or that other forms of substitute family care (such as fostering or adoption by unrelated families) are nontraditional and expose children to an unacceptable risk of abuse and exploitation. Donors sometimes favor residential care because it provides tangible and visible manifestation of their investment, and residential institutions provide philanthropic organizations with an opportunity to actively exercise surrogate parenting. Institutions also have high media appeal, are perceived to be easier to monitor than family care, and can be favored by social service professionals because they are organizationally convenient (Defence for Children International 1985; Tolfree 1995).

The research literature, however, provides extensive data on the principal disadvantages and negative impacts of residential care (Tolfree 1995). At its worst, there may be serious violations of children's rights, whether in the form of systematic sexual abuse or exploitation, malnutrition, inadequate hygiene and health care, educational deprivation, strict regimentation, and harsh discipline. Even where physical conditions are good and the standard of education excellent, a number of problems are almost inevitably associated with residential forms of care. These include lack of stimulation and personal care and affection, institutional dependence, and difficulties in adjusting to the outside world on leaving. Postinstitutional problems are greater when there are risk factors in the new environment (MacLean 2003). Significantly, there is virtually no empirical evidence to contradict these findings.

Table 1.1 outlines some of the key features of institutional care. These points are illustrated, with one exception, by the voices of children who through participatory research have shared their experiences in a wide variety of residential care situations. Age is a key variable in the psychological impact of institutional care: Evidence strongly suggests that the experience of institutional care is most damaging to children under the age of five or six. Personality and temperament are also important variables, but few significant gender differences have been found. None of the features of institutions in the table is invariably present; however, research suggests that it is extremely rare to find any residential institution that fully respects children's rights and that offers adequate conditions for comprehensive child development.

Moreover, it is clear that institutional care, once established, tends to act as a magnet, drawing in children who do have parents or other potential family caregivers and undermining traditional family and community responsibility for parentless children (Foster et al. 1995; Tolfree 1995; USAID et al. 2002). In some African countries a significant percentage of children in orphanages had traceable relatives and were there primarily because of poverty (Phiri and Webb 2002).

Institutional care is inappropriate not just because it contravenes children's rights and undermines their development. From a policy standpoint, it also produces poor results for small numbers at high cost per child. Cost is an important consideration because of the vast scope of the epidemic. Institutional care costs are estimated to be between five and ten times more than foster care by unrelated caregivers (see, for example, Barth 2002; Government of Eritrea 1998; Tobis 2000). Where the institutional providers are government agencies, the diversion of a disproportionate percentage of state funding into the care of relatively small numbers of children distracts attention and much-needed resources away from the greater priority of supporting family- and community-based care. Unfortunately,

TABLE 1.1. *A Critique of Institutionalization*

Institutional Characteristic	Perspective Based on UN Declaration on Rights of the Child	Child Development Perspective	Illustration in Children's Words
1. Institutions tend to segregate children, leading to a powerful sense of discrimination and stigma.	The principle of nondiscrimination (Art. 2)	Stigma and discrimination have a strong negative effect on the growing child's identity and self-esteem.	"We always felt humiliated because of living in the home." "They would always treat us like orphans."
2. The placement of the child in an institution is frequently driven by the wishes of the family, not the best interests of the child.	The principle of the child's best interests (Art. 3)	Placement in an institution may be perceived by the child as a form of rejection by the family, resulting in feelings of abandonment and loss of self-esteem.	From a researcher: "Admission was sought partly because their children were assured of a good diet and access to a quality of education unavailable in refugee camps."
3. Even if a child in an institution has one or both parents, the evidence suggests that contact with parents and the wider family decays over time.	The right to maintain regular contact with both parents (Art. 9.3); the right to preserve his or her identity (Art. 8) and the right to family reunification (Art. 10)	Placement may result in loss of personal and family identity; loss of a sense of belonging to a community and consequent loss of support networks for the future.	"I felt I needed my family, even though I always had other people around me." "We didn't have any relatives visit."
4. Institutions lack individual and personal care, attention, and affection, and institutional needs take precedence over those of individual children.	The right to grow up in an atmosphere of happiness, love, and understanding (Preamble); the right to express an opinion (Art. 12)	Opportunities for attachment and for reasonably continuous relationships with parental figures are fundamental to child development, especially in the early years.	"We never had any affection; we had all the material things – a bed, food, clothing – but we never had love."
5. Many institutions do not provide adequate stimulation and purposeful activity for children.	The right to leisure, play, and recreational activities appropriate to the age of the child (Art. 31)	Stimulation is vital for the development of motor skills, intellectual capacity, and social skills. Deprivation can have profound and long-term effects.	"It was like a prison." "The babies . . . were left in their cots most of the day."

The child should be fully prepared to live an individual life in society (Preamble)	Childhood experiences are partly aimed at equipping the child with the knowledge and skills required of adulthood.	6. Children who grow up in institutions may be denied opportunities to learn about the roles of adults within the particular culture.	"I have no idea what it is like to live in a family." "We called the director 'Daddy' ... but he really had little time for us."
The right to freedom of association (Art. 15)	A variety of peer-group relationships and exposure to "normal" family life are important for children's development.	7. Institutions frequently provide little or no opportunity for mixing with children outside of the institution.	"A large children's village ... has the appearance of a homely fortress surrounded by a high barbed-wire fence."
The right to protection from all forms of abuse and neglect (Art. 19) and from sexual exploitation (Art. 34)	Child abuse has been demonstrated to have a devastating impact on children's development and well-being, often with long-term implications.	8. Child abuse of various kinds is common in institutions – even in well-resourced institutions in the industrialized nations – and often persists for years without being revealed to the outside world.	"They would beat us even with the iron, with no clothes on." "The priest ... started to touch my stomach and private parts...." [Several others said he had sexually abused them.]
The right to rehabilitative care (Art. 39)	Experiences such as caring for a dying parent followed by bereavement can have a seriously negative impact on children's development.	9. Residential institutions often fail to respond adequately to the psychological needs of children.	"They told me I should try to forget everything. And I told them 'How can I forget this? Could you forget your own child's death?'"
The right to assistance to enable the child to fully assume his or her responsibilities within the community (Preamble and Art. 18)	Institutions tend to encourage dependence and discourage children from thinking and solving problems themselves, leaving them ill-equipped to live independently.	10. Many children in institutions experience considerable problems in adjusting to life outside the institution; many end up in prisons or psychiatric institutions.	"They don't give proper tools to survive in society." "They throw you out into society with no kind of structure to survive."

Source: Adapted from Tolfree 2003.

disinvesting in institutional care always seems to be more difficult than investing in it. By contrast, community-owned initiatives that aim to promote local solutions based on family and community resources (supplemented by modest external resources where necessary) achieve good results for large numbers at low cost per child.

THE NEED FOR STRATEGIES TO SUPPORT
FAMILIES AND COMMUNITIES

The foundation of an effective response to the problems of orphan care must be the families and communities that are on the front lines of response. One often hears claims in public forums that families and communities have disintegrated and are no longer able to support orphans. Even in the most affected countries, however, the vast majority of orphans live in families and communities. Only a tiny minority – perhaps 2 to 3 percent – live on the streets or in orphanages and children's homes (Foster 2002). According to unofficial reports, even that small number may be an overestimate.

In Africa, the community is a kind of "extended-extended family." The close links of families, clans, and communities in sub-Saharan Africa make for an enduring resource. Compared with children raised in communities, those brought up in institutions are likely to have tenuous cultural, spiritual, and kinship ties with their families, clans, and communities. Kinship ties are especially important in Africa because they form the foundation for people's sense of connectedness and continuity. They are the basis upon which are built the social, cultural, "all round life" skills for navigating the complexity of life on the continent. By asserting that they should be raised in communities, we are promoting children's ability to realize many of their fundamental rights.

Even living with close relatives, however, often has its own problems for children. Living with family members other than the birth parents is extremely common in many parts of the world, often for reasons other than orphanhood. But the very ubiquity of such a phenomenon must not blind us to the potential for discrimination. Gillian Mann's (2003) research in Malawi, documenting the views of children affected by HIV/AIDS, revealed a startling picture of what many children regarded as discrimination and abuse within the extended family. Moreover, these children reported that they had little opportunity to express their concerns. They also expressed clear and informed preferences about the most appropriate caregivers, opinions that often were at variance with those of the adults who made the decisions.

While these findings are important, they do not override the central importance of care within the extended family and community. Rather, they highlight the reality that some orphaned children have particular problems that require monitoring and support if their needs and rights are to be met adequately. Families increasingly are feeling the strain of shouldering a disproportionate burden of taking in more children when, strangled by pervasive poverty, they already live in extremely difficult circumstances. The impact of this inordinately heavy strain is manifesting itself in various ways. These families and communities need help. To understand and appreciate the range and potential that families and communities might have, it is useful to suggest a framework that comprises three mutually dependent elements that have a direct bearing on the quality of family and community response (Phiri 2001; Phiri, Foster, and Nzima 2001):

- The front line, made up of families and communities
- The influence arena, made up of catalysts and capacity builders, including nongovernmental organizations (NGOs), grassroots support organizations, and similar groups
- The enabling arena, made up of national and regional as well as international participants, including governments and international organizations.

The Front Line: Building on Existing Coping Strategies

To provide effective assistance, it is important to understand how families and communities are responding to the HIV/AIDS crisis in the midst of poverty. Often community groups (mostly charitable, faith-based, and concerned women's groups) respond to the situation of their brethren, kin, or neighbors. In some countries, Christian women's "guilds" or Moslem sisters organize assistance. (*Dawa* sisters are missionaries for Islam but, like their Christian counterparts, help all children.) Often the response emanates from a sense of religious or traditional obligation to care for persons in need (see also Chapter 6). The Bible and Quran enjoin the faithful to do good by caring for widows, orphans, and the poor.

In addition, a traditional religious and spiritual dimension emanates from a sense of continuous connection to the past, the present, and the future. In African traditions, respect for ancestors connects the extended family and community to the past, and concern for children connects them to the future. Motivation to care may also be driven by a sense of expected reciprocal altruism: If I care for orphans today, someone will care for my children when I die. The expectation of something in return is especially important in the case of families fostering an unrelated child.

Members of the extended family usually assume responsibility for orphaned children when both parents have died or when the surviving parent is unable to look after the children without assistance. The immediate extended family comprises the uncles, aunts, cousins, or grandparents on both sides of the marriage. Beyond this close circle of kin, there are other relatives – twice or even thrice removed – who are also part of this extended family or the clan. If the close circle fails, these other relatives may be called upon to take in or assist with the care of orphaned children. In the rural setting, another circle may assist, including distant relatives, neighbors, and members of the same community.

Even in cultures where the care of children by members of the extended family is common, children may experience discrimination or abuse (Mann 2003). Guardians in this study, however, frequently asserted that orphaned children were not disadvantaged. They felt that the children were ungrateful, considering the difficulties of adding their care to the family's other responsibilities, and they often expressed frustration at the orphaned child's disobedience and lack of respect, which, in their view, reflected a previous lack of parental guidance.

These contrasting perceptions are typically rooted in the unexpressed distress experienced by children at the loss of their parents and at the extremely difficult circumstances that attended the illness. The difficulties experienced by guardians in responding appropriately to children's emotional needs are reflected in their frustrations at the children's attitudes and behavior, resulting in an increasing tension and lack of communication within the family. These findings suggest that families who take in orphaned children, whether related or not, may benefit from additional psychosocial support to enable the reconstituted family to cope with the challenges posed by the inclusion of children traumatized by their experiences of caring for and losing their parents. (See Chapter 4.)

It is clear that caring for someone else's children, especially children who have had psychologically damaging experiences, is not the same as caring for one's own children. This conclusion is mirrored in research on children separated from their families in armed conflict and forced migration: The past experiences of children are likely to intrude into the substitute families and become manifest as emotional or behavioral difficulties. Caregivers are often at a loss to understand such behaviors, and consequently their responses may be inadequate or inappropriate. Research has shown the value of mobilizing networks of support around such children and their caregivers. For example, in a refugee camp setting in Sinje, Liberia, caregivers formed the Association of Concerned Carers in order to provide support for themselves and the children in their care (Abdullai, Dorbor, and Tolfree 2002). This association had a number of components, including offering mutual support, holding informal meetings with children, responding to allegations of abuse or exploitation, advocating for the needs of separated children, and providing them with skills training. Clubs for boys and for girls were also created, and these evolved into more self-directing associations of mobilized young people. Youths played an active role in child protection in the community. They provided a well-informed network of support and formed a system of young advocates who accepted responsibility for providing peer-support to the children within their particular block in the camp. Underpinning the whole approach was a community mobilization strategy, which strongly emphasized the importance of diffusing knowledge of children's needs and rights in all sections of the refugee community. This approach holds great promise for AIDS-affected communities.

At the community level, responses are characterized by collective decision making, coalition- and consensus-building elements, local visionary leadership, internal material and financial resource mobilization, and local issue-based advocacy. Specific activities have included:

- Facilitation of care by extended and, where necessary, unrelated family members within the community
- Community vegetable or nutrition gardens
- Material support
- Spiritual and emotional support
- Assistance with household chores such as sweeping, cooking, bathing, fetching water and firewood, and providing child care
- Income-generating activities
- Assistance with school fees or costs
- Issue-based advocacy, such as enrolling children in schools and keeping them from dropping out, and reducing or eliminating school fees
- Monitoring the situation of children
- Referral services
- Community schools
- Community-managed child care centers
- Recreational and cultural activities

The Influence Arena

The front-line response of families and communities must be sustained through strategic support with resources, skills, and capacity building. NGOs and other actors in the influence arena are well-placed to mobilize, catalyze, and strengthen the front line.

Several factors contribute to the ability of external agencies to provide effective support to the front line. A thorough understanding of how communities and families are coping is indispensable and can be provided through situation analyses that are comprehensive, local, collaborative, and participatory. This provides a basis for a common assessment of concerns, a recognition of existing responses, and an analysis of strengths and assets as well as gaps and weaknesses. The process of developing a situation analysis can act as a vehicle for consensus and constituency building and as a means of developing a vision for the future. In addition, external agents should avoid imposing their own definitions, structures, and monitoring systems on communities. Many community groups have located their own index of vulnerability, so that an external definition of orphans or children needing care is neither needed nor appropriate.

Actors in this arena should work to assist communities to identify and prioritize their concerns and to reinforce their existing responses to the needs and rights of children and families affected by HIV/AIDS. External agents might provide training and technical assistance in developing and strengthening skills, in organizational and institutional development, in financial and material resource provision, and in technical exchange and networking.

The basis of any viable mobilization effort is community ownership and responsibility. Before they access external resources, mobilized communities should muster internal resources and embark on activities that are intended to identify the children most in need.

Agents of community mobilization should utilize existing structures that have been shown to be effective, such as congregation-level faith-based groups, women's support groups, youth groups, credit and savings groups, farmers' clubs, funeral committees, development committees, water and sanitation and health committees, income-generating activities, home-based care groups, groups for people living with AIDS, and other support and solidarity groups. These types of groups are already implementing activities that assist orphans and other vulnerable children. Apart from being owned by the communities, these structures have high social capital and legitimacy, factors that are critical for sustainability.

Building on these foundations, actors in the influence arena may also catalyze the formation of community coalitions that involve different players concerned with children's welfare. Community coalitions will typically include existing organizations or groups, plus government departments, business leaders, and traditional, civic, and religious leaders. A number of lessons have been learned from practical experience.

Key Factors in Improving Response. Several factors contribute to improving communities' responses to vulnerable children. In Eastern and Southern Africa, programs such as Families, Orphans, and Children Under Stress (FOCUS) in Zimbabwe, Scaling Up HIV/AIDS Interventions through Expanded Partnerships (STEP) in Malawi, Thandanani ("Love One Another") Children's Foundation in South Africa, SCOPE-OVC (Strengthening Community Partnerships for the Empowerment of Orphans and Vulnerable Children) in Zambia, and UWESO (Uganda Women's Effort to Save Orphans) in Uganda have contributed to a better understanding of these factors.

A number of programs mobilize community support, most often through women volunteers recommended by the community (Lee et al. 2002). These women are often well-known, respected congregation members, and they may be caring for orphans themselves. The main emphasis of many programs is to identify and monitor vulnerable children through regular household visits and follow-up activities. Part of the objective is to ensure that children are kept in school and that there is enough income to support needy families. Volunteers identify unmet basic needs of the households and provide essential material support, including maize seed, fertilizer, food, clothing, blankets, and school fees. They also offer to bathe children, sweep the house, repair leaky roofs and faulty bathrooms, and fetch firewood or cook.

These visits also enable volunteers to observe and monitor the children's well-being. Children who are not in school, who are in psychological and emotional distress, or are in abusive situations are identified. The volunteers, community groups, or leaders then take appropriate follow-up action. Experience indicates that the likelihood of abuse, exploitation, and maltreatment of orphans lessens in communities with frequent visiting. In addition, visits are important because they provide the space and opportunity to provide spiritual, emotional, and cultural support. Spiritual activities such as prayer, scripture reading, and "praise songs" often provide a powerful support process. Psychosocial support is provided through weekly craft, cultural, and sporting activities. Volunteers are also involved in advocacy and in raising awareness about orphan issues (Phiri et al. 2001).

Volunteers typically visit the guardians, however, rather than the children themselves. There is a need for a more direct focus on young people and the promotion of children's participation as a key program theme. STEP in Malawi works at the district and village level and makes use of existing structures or organizations, including community-based religious organizations or local NGOs. One of these is a multisectoral, multistakeholder structure at the district level that is mirrored at the subdistrict level by the Community AIDS Committees (CACs) – usually defined by a health catchment area or traditional authority comprising as many as one hundred villages – and at the village level by the Village AIDS Committees (VACs). At every level, four technical subcommittees are responsible for different areas of response: orphans, youth, home-based care, and prevention. STEP strengthens the District AIDS Coordinating Committees, which in turn work to establish or strengthen existing CACs. The CACs are then responsible for catalyzing the communities.

As part of the mobilization strategy, these community-managed care coalitions are strengthened through various capacity-development strategies and activities. These include:

- leadership development and training,
- partnership development,
- organizational development,
- agricultural skills development (drought-resistant crop propagation, animal husbandry, vegetable farming),

- development of business, credit, and savings-related skills,
- promotion of income-generating activities,
- training in writing grant proposals,
- training in basic accounting; and
- training and skills development in home-based care.

These activities strengthen the coalitions to undertake projects for responding to the diverse needs of affected children and families. At the CAC and VAC level, coalitions typically include traditional leaders, religious leaders, teachers, and community-based government workers in social services, community development, agricultural extension services, and health. They also include business leaders, widows, and youth. STEP and similar programs have used coalitions of individuals from a cross section of the community. The diversity of the skills and the authority of the constituent members are significant factors in the strength and effectiveness of the coalition.

Several lessons have been learned. First, home-based care activities should be developed as an entry point for working with children before they become orphans. This allows issues such as succession planning and ensuring the inheritance and property rights of orphans to be raised with parents.

Second, coalitions engaged in community-managed child-care centers provide community care, stimulation, and psychosocial activities for children under six – both orphans and non-orphans. These centers offer caregivers respite and an opportunity to pursue other economic or social activities. For adolescents, vocational skills, apprenticeships, and unstructured life-skills training provide an opportunity to relate to consistent adult role models who offer mentoring and the connection needed by children who have lost a parent.

The STEP program, along with others such as the National Association of Women Living with AIDS (NACWOLA) in Uganda, have learned that keeping alive the memories or milestones in the lives of children and families helps create a sense of connection. NACWOLA adapted the approach of creating a "memory book" – a journal of favorite memories of the mother and father, family traditions, weddings, births, and special events, along with a record of health and education and a family tree. The parents can complete it and then take the child through the steps, or the child can be part of the process of completing it (Alidri 2001; Phiri and Webb 2002).

Succession planning is also integrated into the memory book activities. With the participation of the child, parents or guardians discuss who will be the caregiver after the parent's death, most often an uncle or aunt of the child (Gilborn et al. 2001). Mothers also identify others who might play significant roles in the child's life. This mirrors reality, where the child is parented not just by the biological mother and father but also by relatives, neighbors, and other significant adults (Phiri and Webb 2002). Connecting the past, present, and future helps the child maintain a sense of continuity and belonging.

Most of the programs specifically focus on orphans, with components that include enumeration, prioritization, visiting, assistance, and monitoring. Other non-orphaned but vulnerable children comprise a significant minority of those who also receive assistance, with communities defining their own indices of vulnerability. Typically, double orphans (whose father and mother have both died) and children living on their own are at the top of the list. Others given priority include children who have lost one parent and have no assistance from the extended family, and children living in a grandmother-headed household. Some of the children deemed to be the most vulnerable might not necessarily be orphans: children with a parent who is terminally ill, for example, or whose mother is ill and whose father is rarely at home or has remarried. Sometimes children whose parents are alive are referred to as orphans in the local language because of their dire situation. These children may be termed "social" as opposed to "biological" orphans.

Children's Participation. Among the challenges in the influence arena is encouraging children's participation. Young people have considerable insight into their problems, needs, resources, and priorities, and should participate in the decisions that affect them. They have clear and well-informed opinions on the most appropriate caregiver, and may be resentful if adults fail to ask their views on important choices. Programs should have more direct focus on children themselves and their relationship with their caregivers (Mann 2003).

Gender. Another challenge relates to gender. Most programs depend on women. More than 95 percent of the members of FOCUS committees, for example, are women. In STEP, more than 60 percent of the members of the DACC-CAC-VAC structures are women. Men, in contrast, have more leadership positions on committees. This limited and unbalanced involvement of men is a weakness that programs should address in a nonthreatening way, but still recognizing that cultural standards are fluid and can adapt to new dynamics, threats, and opportunities.

Volunteers. A fundamental challenge is the extent to which volunteers feel they are responding to a personal commitment rather than to a directive from external agents. Volunteers should not be motivated only by economic incentives or material gain – otherwise they may begin "helping" children for selfish reasons, which creates an inherent risk of abuse, neglect, and exploitation. It can be argued that people should not be made to feel or say they are volunteering, but rather that they are doing what is their duty – familial, filial, traditional, communal, religious, or otherwise – because volunteering in the African context engenders other expectations. This is a critical challenge that most programs have to face.

The Enabling Arena

To ensure effectiveness, continuity, and sustainability of initiatives and responses at the front line, governments and national and international organizations provide a supportive and facilitating program environment. In the context in which children are cared for, many conditions can negatively affect them. Some practices are an outcome of existing policies, laws, traditions, and attitudes, including abuse, violence, and discrimination against women, property dispossession, and unaffordable health and school costs. Action is needed in areas of concern, to amend specific laws and policies, for example:

• Policies and laws upholding the property and inheritance rights of orphans and widows
• Free primary school education, including the waiver of school fees for orphans and other vulnerable children, and the subsidizing of other school costs
• Recognition of community schools, and the related provision of financial and technical support for their establishment and development
• Gender-sensitive school policies, including the waiver of uniforms for girls (who are already at greater risk than boys of leaving school), and reversing policies that expel pregnant girls from school
• Support and endorsement of community-based care for orphans
• Decentralization that involves devolution to local governments and engagement in good governance, community participation, consensus building, and stewardship
• Development of female economic empowerment programs (credit and other microfinance programs)
• Efficient stoves to reduce time women spend collecting firewood
• A strong emphasis on children's rights and the empowerment of young people to express their concerns and to have a voice in program planning
• Female literacy programs
• Food security programs
• Well-targeted health insurance; prepayment schemes for health services; letting people pay in-kind after they harvest
• Preventive health care to reduce morbidity and mortality (Foster 2002; Mutangadura, Mukurazita, and Jackson 1999; Phiri 2001; USAID et al. 2002)

Political leadership, will, and commitment are crucial to create an enabling environment. Unfortunately there has been a lack of leadership in the response to orphaned children; most leaders have paid only lip service to the problem. With strong and sustained leadership commitment and responsiveness, it is easier to inspire and galvanize the rest of the government bureaucracy. In the front line arena, leadership directly or indirectly affects the capacity of groups to undertake specified action in a sustained, accepted, coordinated, effective manner. While government leadership is clearly pivotal, traditional and religious leaders are also critical in mobilizing communities and reducing stigma (Phiri et al. 2001; Phiri and Webb 2002).

FOSTERING, ADOPTION, AND OTHER FAMILY-BASED CARE ARRANGEMENTS

Even with an optimistic forecast of the spread and impact of HIV/AIDS, it seems likely that, in some contexts, the needs of children lacking protection and care will exceed the capacity of the extended family and the community to provide for them. If alternative forms of care need to be developed, placement within a family setting is almost always preferable to institutional care.

In some situations, fostering occurs spontaneously by families who take on the care of an unrelated parentless child, possibly because of preexisting friendships between the families, or because of religious or humanitarian motivation. However, in situations where large numbers of children need families, and especially in cultural contexts in which it is not common to care for an unrelated child, an organization may need to promote the development of fostering or adoption. Evidence from a number of African countries demonstrates that when the need for substitute families is well publicized through appropriate media, large numbers of people come forward to offer to foster or adopt a child, even when care outside of the extended family and community is a relatively unfamiliar concept.

In Western societies, adoption and fostering have different meanings. In adoption, a court transfers the legal rights and responsibilities of one set of parents permanently to another caregiver or couple. Fostering, by contrast, is a less permanent form of substitute care, usually implemented by a government agency, that does not involve the final transfer of parental rights and responsibilities. This distinction can become quite blurred, however, in countries in which legal adoption is either not available or not readily accessible. This section refers mainly to fostering, but the intention may be a permanent form of care, even involving changing the child's name – a form of de facto adoption (Tolfree 1995). In any case, most of the issues raised will also relate to more formal, legal adoption.

Fostering

Anthropological studies demonstrate that in some cultures, the care of children by strangers is an unfamiliar practice; in others, it may be culturally acceptable but not based on the best interests of the child (Bledsoe 1990). In West Africa, many children are cared for by unrelated families, but the arrangement is often based on a notion of *exchange*. For example, the child benefits from the caregiver's teaching or training, and the caregiver benefits from the child's labor. Young children receive care and nurturing, especially from older women, releasing the child's mother for productive work. In exchange, it is expected that when the child grows up, he or she will support the foster mother in her older years. Some cultures sanction the less favorable treatment of fostered children and may even positively value it, as illustrated by the proverb in Mende, the language of Sierra Leone: "No success without hardship." In terms of children's rights, however, less favorable treatment may involve discrimination or even exploitation.

Nevertheless, fostering – whether occurring spontaneously in the community or arranged by an agency – must be approached with care, and steps must be taken to ensure the child's protection and well-being. Children being cared for by relatives may also receive an inferior quality of care compared with the family's own children. Any alternative care arrangement for orphaned children may need to be monitored and supported, either by members of the local community through established care coalitions or by staff employed by an agency, or in some cases both.

The Save the Children Alliance's global study into the care and protection of separated children in emergency situations examined the concept of fostering (Tolfree 2004). The main focus has been on situations of armed conflict and forced migration, but many of the findings are equally relevant to the situation of children orphaned by HIV/AIDS. In both contexts there is an urgent need to promote family-based care for potentially large numbers of children who have lost or become separated from their own families. The research suggests that fostering is a very heterogeneous concept and is highly context-related; the degree of risk involved will vary from one situation to another. In some contexts, widespread assumptions that children cared for by strangers will be abused or neglected are not always borne out in practice. However, fostered children often feel that they are treated less well than other children in the family, especially with regard to the burden of household work and access to education. A crucial variable is the extent to which fostered children are monitored and supported by individuals outside the family.

In order to protect children's rights, fostering programs must be based on thorough cultural understandings, with an acknowledgment of the potential risks as well as benefits to children. Fostering has been successfully promoted in the emergency contexts of armed conflict and forced migration despite the considerable difficulties involved, including the lack of information about the whereabouts of the child's own family, large numbers of separated children, and the urgency to provide for their care and protection. In the context of HIV/AIDS, the situation is possibly somewhat easier because it will be known that the child's natural parents have died, leaving substitute caregivers the potentially more manageable task of providing permanent care rather than facing the uncertainties of indeterminate care. One tentative finding of the global study is that where fostering is perceived to be permanent, the quality of care of the child is likely to be higher. In such situations, fostering is more akin to a form of de facto adoption. Mann's (2003) study in Malawi has indicated, however, that children orphaned by HIV/AIDS tend to have particular emotional and behavioral problems. Even when these children are placed within the extended family, their problems can place great strain on a family already struggling to survive.

Given the potential for abuse or exploitation, or the less favorable treatment of fostered children, what steps need to be taken to ensure that adequate care and protection are provided? Save the Children's research suggests four key safeguards. First, programs designed to support and protect children who are in a potentially vulnerable situation should be based on a detailed knowledge of cultural norms concerning the care of parentless children, together with a solid knowledge of both child rights and child development. This is important not only in establishing effective frameworks for managing the fostering process, but also in educating the wider community about the needs and rights of children so as to facilitate substitute family care.

Second, the program should be firmly embedded within the local community, with a strong sense of community ownership of responsibility for the care and protection of children. In her book on global child abuse and neglect, Jill Korbin (1981: 208–9) concludes:

A network of concerned individuals beyond the biological parents is a powerful deterrent to child abuse and neglect. The shared responsibility for child rearing acts in many ways to reduce the likelihood of child maltreatment. If a wide network of individuals is concerned with the well-being of the group's children, general standards of child care are more likely to be ensured. An extended network further helps to guarantee that someone will intervene when standards of child care are violated. A network of individuals provides alternative caretakers, thus relieving... parents of the entire burden of child care.

The involvement of respected members of the community in both selecting foster caregivers and monitoring and supporting them and the children, is a key component in facilitating protection and adequate care. The importance of mobilizing networks of support around substitute families and orphaned children has already been discussed.

Third, preparing foster caregivers for their responsibilities will lead to more favorable outcomes. Such preparation raises their awareness of the needs and rights of children who have lost their parents. In the context of

AIDS, it is likely that this will also involve promoting an understanding of the emotional issues faced by children who may have watched their parents die, and who may need emotional support to grieve and come to terms with their changed situation. It is also helpful if preparation includes a consideration of the behavioral reactions of children to death, loss, and change, and addresses the skills and techniques required to manage these behaviors. It also needs to involve discussion of the longer-term issues of initiation, marriage (including the provision of a dowry where this is traditional), and inheritance.

Gender issues will be significant, as will the acceptance of the foster child by the family's own children and extended family. In addition, it is also important that there be a planned process for transition. Children often have very clear preferences for their care, and a remarkable capacity for weighing the options. Their active participation in the process of planning for their care is a vital and often neglected aspect of good practice.

While no universal template can be applied to all fostering programs, the following are the typical components of such a program:

- Effective community mobilization to identify separated children, advocate for family-based care and protection, identify families willing to foster children, and mobilize networks of support for both children and families
- A system of approving prospective foster caregivers – normally involving both individual assessment and the approval of the wider community – and preparation for fostering that often includes an education in some of the expected difficulties, with an emphasis on the caregivers' role as "duty-bearers" in respecting the children's rights
- The identification and preparation of children for fostering, including the active participation of the children using methods appropriate to their age and stage of development
- The actual placement of the child. The involvement of the wider community – through some kind of ceremony involving community leaders and neighbors, for example – may be important. A formal fostering agreement is sometimes helpful in setting out the rights and responsibilities of the various parties
- Continuing monitoring and support of the child and the foster family

This last is possibly the most important and usually the most difficult. Continuing responsibility for fostering may be located within the community, the agency, or the government, according to the particular context. The issue of material support to foster families is a difficult one. Experience in post-genocide Rwanda (Doná 2001) suggests that when the need for foster caregivers is well publicized, with strong government backing, people come forward despite very limited means, and commit themselves to foster care without material support.

In some situations, community-based organizations have taken on responsibility for implementing fostering programs, with the support of an agency that is firmly rooted in child rights and knowledgeable in child development (Abdullai et al. 2002; Tolfree 2004). In others it has been necessary for an NGO or a government ministry (or sometimes both, working in partnership) to assume long-term responsibility for the fostering program, depending on the existence of a framework of legislation to regulate fostering and the capacity of government staff to implement state policies. In the longer term, it may be necessary for governments to enact legislation to define the status of fostered children and provide a statutory framework for their protection; this may include, for example, the provision for some form of legal adoption or guardianship.

Legal Adoption

Many less economically developed countries do have adoption legislation, but in many cases these laws stem from the colonial era in which Western legal provisions and procedures were incorporated into local legislation but in practice were rarely used by the indigenous population. South Africa is a case in point. Other countries have no adoption framework, including many Islamic states in which the concept of adoption, and in particular the change of the child's name, is prohibited by the Quran. In some African cultures, a legal change in parental rights and responsibilities is an alien concept. If the idea of legal adoption is to be accepted, cultural values would have to change.

South Africa, however, provides a good example of a country in which legal adoption – originally introduced primarily for the benefit of white people wanting to adopt white children – has been promoted successfully among the black population by agencies concerned about offering this option for children, especially those orphaned or abandoned in the context of the HIV/AIDS epidemic (Harber 1999). By creating an adoption service that is more appropriate and accessible to the black population, some agencies have found that legal adoption becomes a highly acceptable option, not least because of the lack of permanence and security that fostering may imply. This option is particularly important to more urbanized childless couples wanting to use adoption as a means of creating their own family.

An important aspect of the development of legal adoption has been the need to use appropriate means to raise awareness of adoption within the community, and to shed some of the assumptions upon which adoption in Western societies traditionally was based. Single people, unmarried couples, and families living in poor quality or overcrowded accommodation were not automatically excluded from adopting, for example. Similar easing of restrictions has also occurred in the United States as a result of the epidemics of HIV/AIDS and drug use: Nontraditional families have been encouraged to adopt, especially "hard-to-place" older, disabled, or troubled children.

In some contexts, people willing to care for an additional child may be reluctant to take on the long-term financial costs (such as the costs of marriage arrangements and providing inheritance on the same basis as the biological children of the family) associated with the permanent, legal responsibility for the child. This may lead to a situation in which long-term fostering may be more acceptable than adoption. Although this may provide an inferior sense of security and permanence from the child's point of view, it is vastly preferable to long-term residential care.

In situations where legal adoption is either not available or is difficult and expensive to access, the notion of long-term fostering can be similar to a form of de facto adoption. It may, for example, involve a change in the child's name (in practice rather than through any legal means) and an arrangement similar in all respects to legal adoption except that it is not formalized in law. From the point of view of agencies involved in facilitating the placement of children in long-term fostering, the key issues are probably less the child's legal status and more the nature of the commitment. The ideal situation would provide the child with optimal opportunities and offer a quality of life equal to that of the family's biological children. Safeguards must be built into the system, especially the careful assessment and preparation of caretakers and the establishment of adequate procedures for monitoring and support.

Finally, the issue of intercountry adoption deserves a brief mention. In some extreme situations, it is possible that this may provide the only route to enable a child to enjoy a normal family life. In practice, however, intercountry adoption is, at best, an expensive way of responding to the needs of relatively small numbers of children. At worst, intercountry adoption can be abusive and exploitative, based more on the needs and interests of adopters and their lawyers than on the best interests of children. It is most likely to be unsatisfactory where the countries involved have not ratified the Hague Convention on Protection of Children and Co-operation in Respect of Intercountry Adoption (Hague Conference on Private International Law 1993), which seeks to eliminate the worst malpractices in this field. Perhaps the greatest danger in supporting intercountry adoption is that it tends to distract much-needed resources and attention away from the more urgent need to promote local, family- and community-based options for children needing care.

Other Community-Based Approaches for Children Lacking Protection and Care

Some agencies have experimented with other approaches, sometimes producing a model of care that is a hybrid between a foster home and a small family-group residential home. In some instances this is a specifically short-term arrangement, pending the establishment of a permanent form of care; in others it is seen as a long-term arrangement. Save the Children Norway has developed the model of a community-based foster home that has been promoted in various countries in Africa (Tolfree 1995).

The model consists of establishing a small group of children under the care of foster caregivers (usually a widow or married couple) who are respected members of their own community. It is used as a means of keeping sibling groups together and maintaining children's member-ship in their own community. The group normally comprises between two and seven children who live together in as normal a family envi-ronment as possible. Emphasis is placed on integration with the local community, including attendance at local schools, and it is anticipated that a considerable degree of support from the local community will be given. The "family" follows the same life cycle as a normal family, with children remaining until they can achieve independence. The character-istics of, recruitment procedures for, and methods of supporting foster caregivers vary. The preferred means of support is through the provision of a house and the materials necessary to enable the family to achieve self-sufficiency – land, agricultural implements, animals, household equip-ment, or a grant to set up a small business, along with the material neces-sities to get the family established. Achieving family self-sufficiency is important if the agency is to avoid the necessity of ongoing funding and support.

In a similar model in South Africa, up to six children are placed with a foster mother in a home purchased and furnished by an external agency. The foster mother is paid an allowance and receives foster grants for the children, with periodic assistance from a "relief mother." There is a con-scious effort to keep siblings together where possible. Community leader-ship structures are involved in the process of monitoring. Another variation is cluster foster homes typically run by volunteer women or couples who keep up to six children each and receive foster care grants, health services, income-generating activities, and material and child care support. Less common is collective foster care, where religious groups of women or cou-ples collectively agree to act as surrogate mothers for children who remain in their own deceased parents' houses (Loening-Voysey and Wilson 2001; McKerrow 1996).

Other broadly similar models have been promoted by various agen-cies. In some countries, lay Catholic sisters have taken on the care of groups of children. In other contexts, the foster caregiver has been pro-vided with a small salary and a house. However, the sustainability of such arrangements may be problematic if they require long-term rev-enue support, and this in turn may detract from a sense of community ownership.

Family Placements for Older Children. Many adoption agencies only consider the placement of very young children, while some fostering programs have assumed that older children cannot be successfully fostered. In any case, most prospective foster caregivers or adopters express a strong preference for very young children. One exception to this is the Family Attachment Program (Derib 2002) for separated refugee children from South Sudan. Here the approach was to encourage children to select their own foster family from their existing social networks. Subject to approval by the Foster Care Supervisors, children were then placed, often in small friendship groups. In accordance with Sudanese custom, older children normally lived in separate huts close to those of the parents, and this tradition was followed in fostering. What is particularly interesting is that the system allowed for the gradual evolution of the relationship between the fostered children and the foster caregivers. Sometimes this led to a gradual integration into the life of the family, while for other (often older) young people, the system also allowed for a degree of separateness and independence, which some adolescents found more acceptable.

Another form of care for older children that builds on traditional practice was found in Sierra Leone. Here it was common for skilled artisans to provide both training and accommodation for their apprentices. Some organizations developed this idea by placing groups of young people who had been separated from their families with an artisan. They worked in exchange for training, accommodations, and pocket money. The organization provided tools so that when the youths had finished their training they could establish themselves in small business; it also helped them find accommodations.

Self-Care Arrangements. Save the Children's research into the care and protection of separated children in emergencies has revealed that some children and adolescents express a strong preference for various forms of self-care, including the care of children by older siblings. As Gillian Mann (2001: 51) suggests: "In communities where shared management child care is the norm, child rearing tasks are distributed among a large sibling and family group, and exclusive parental care is extremely rare. In these circumstances, children may rely as much, or more, on their siblings for nurture and support than they do on their parents." Sibling caretaking preserves important attachment relationships, ensures that siblings remain together, preserves the continuing occupancy of the family home and land and, hopefully, continued involvement in community life. Such an arrangement may be more appropriate for some children than the replacement of sibling caretakers with unfamiliar adult caretakers.

Clearly, however, there are many problems, including the need to ensure an adequate livelihood, vulnerability to abuse and exploitation, and the difficulties in sustaining school attendance that often result from an inadequate economic base and the need for practical and emotional support. If these difficulties can be satisfactorily resolved by providing community support, these self-care arrangements may be preferable to the alternatives for some children.

CONCLUSIONS

The community-based care options for orphaned children outlined in this chapter – especially fostering – are neither risk-free nor easy to implement. The evidence, however, points toward the successful introduction of fostering and adoption, even in societies where care by strangers is either relatively unfamiliar or not necessarily based on the child's best interests. The existence of traditional, spontaneous forms of fostering should be seen to imply neither that fostering is always protective of children nor that discrimination and abuse are inevitable consequences. A key role for agencies is to take every possible step to ensure that risks are minimized and that protection and care are of an acceptable standard.

A community-based strategy to support and protect vulnerable children must be based on an understanding of the cultural norms regarding the care of children who cannot be cared for by their own families. It requires public awareness campaigns to educate the community in children's rights and the needs of parentless children. It demands a consistent attempt to involve the community in the care and protection of children in a vulnerable situation. The strategy should be integrated with other community-based approaches to address the range of problems posed by HIV/AIDS.

Research suggests that children themselves have a considerable capacity for identifying their own preferred care option. Their resilience in the face of enormous adversity and their ability to help to shape their own destiny is sometimes hidden – especially when agencies lump orphans together as a group of "vulnerable" children. It is not children who are intrinsically vulnerable, but rather the situation they are in, which is rarely of their own making. Labeling them may add to the stigma associated with orphanhood and HIV/AIDS and further undermine their own coping capacities.

Some writers continue to argue for residential forms of care, while others state that in a small number of cases of children who fall through the cracks, institutions are inevitable. There is a clear and urgent need to ensure that governments and resourcing organizations create a policy and implementation environment in which the need, or argument, for any such response is eliminated. It is vital that governments develop and implement clear policies to support, strengthen, and sustain community-managed and community-based care. Governments need to aggressively support and promote the location of responsibility for orphaned children within the wider family and community, while at the same time facilitating the provision of appropriate community support.

Even short-term institutional care, as advocated by some (for example, Grainger, Webb, and Elliott 2001: 89), makes little sense considering that institutional experiences almost always result in children finding it incrementally more difficult to adjust to normal family life in the community (Barth 2002; Tolfree 1995). Institutional responses encourage families and communities to disown children who have lost their parents. All our efforts must be directed to supporting and strengthening community ownership of and sense of responsibility for their children.

References

Abdullai, M., E. Dorbor, and D. Tolfree. 2002. *Case study of the care and protection of separated children in the Sinje Refugee Camp, Liberia*. Stockholm: Save the Children Sweden.

Ali, S. 1998. Community perceptions of orphan care in Malawi: Children in Distress Project of the Family Health Trust (CINDI). http://www.cindi.org.za/papers/cindi_paper_index.htm

Alidri, P. 2001. Community and home-based care practices for HIV/AIDS infected and affected children in Uganda: Lessons learned from Kasese and Arua Districts. Paper presented at the First African Great Lakes Conference on Access to HIV/AIDS Care and Support, Entebbe, September.

Barth, R. P. 2002. *Institutions vs foster homes: The empirical base for the second century of debate*. Chapel Hill: University of North Carolina, School of Social Work, Jordan Institute for Families. http://www.jimcaseyyouth.org/docs/GroupCareLong.pdf

Bledsoe, C. H. 1990. No success without struggle: Social mobility and hardship for foster children in Sierra Leone. *Man* 25:70–88.

Defence for Children International (DCI). 1985. *Children in institutions*. Geneva: DCI.

Derib, A. 2002. *Group care and fostering of Sudanese children in Pignudo and Kakuma refugee camps: A CPSC case study*. Stockholm: Save the Children Sweden.

Doná, G. 2001. *The Rwandan experience of fostering separated children: A CPSC case study*. Stockholm: Save the Children Sweden.

Foster, G. 2002. Supporting community efforts to assist orphans in Africa. *New England Journal of Medicine* 346; 24:1907–9.

——. 2004a. Understanding community responses to the situation of children affected by AIDS: Lessons for external agencies. In *One step further: Responses to HIV/AIDS*, ed. A. Sisask, 91–115. SIDA studies no. 7. Geneva: United Nations Research Institute in Social Development. Available at http://www.unrisd.org

——. 2004b. *Study of the response by faith-based organizations to orphans and vulnerable children*. New York: World Conference of Religions for Peace and UNICEF. http://www.unicef.org/aids/FBO_OVC_study_summary.pdf

Foster, G., C. Makufa, R. Drew, S. Kambeu, and K. Saurombe. 1996. Supporting children in need through a community-based orphan visiting program. *AIDS Care* 8:389–403.

Foster, G. , R. Shakespeare, F. Chinemana, H. Jackson, S. Gregson, C. Marange, and S. Mashumba. 1995. Orphan prevalence and extended family care in a peri-urban community in Zimbabwe. *AIDS Care* 7:3–17.

Gilborn, L., Z. R. Nyonyintono, R. Kabumbuli, and G. Jagwe–Wadda. 2001. Making a difference for children affected by AIDS: Baseline findings from operations research in Uganda. Washington, DC: Population Council.

Government of Eritrea. 1998. *Evaluation of the Orphans Re-Unification Programme in Eritrea*. Asmara: Government of Eritrea, Ministry of Labour and Human Welfare.

Grainger, C., D. Webb, and L. Elliott. 2001. *Children affected by HIV/AIDS: Rights and responsibilities in the developing world*. London: Save the Children UK.

Hague Conference on Private International Law. 1993. *Convention on protection of children and co-operation in respect of intercountry adoption*. The Hague: Hague Conference on Private International Law, May 29. http://www.hcch.net/e/conventions/menu33e.html

Harber, M. 1998. *Who will care for the children? Social policy implications for the care and welfare of children affected by HIV/AIDS in KwaZulu Natal*. Research report no. 17. Durban: University of Natal.

———. 1999. Transforming adoption in the "new" South Africa in response to the HIV/AIDS epidemic. *Adoption and Fostering* 23 (1): 6–15.

Korbin, J. 1981. *Child abuse and neglect: Cross-cultural perspectives*. Berkeley and Los Angeles: University of California Press.

Lee, T. , G. Foster, C. Makufa, and S. Hinton. 2002. Care and support of children and women: Families, orphans, and children under stress in Zimbabwe. *Evaluation and Program Planning* 25:459–70.

Loening-Voysey, H., and T. Wilson. 2001. *Approaches to caring for children orphaned by AIDS and other vulnerable children: Essential elements for a quality service*. Johannesburg: UNICEF and Institute of Urban Primary Health Care South Africa.

MacLean, K. 2003. The impact of institutionalization on child development. *Developmental Psychopathology* 15 (4): 853–84.

Mann, G. 2001. *Networks of support: A literature review of care issues for separated children; A CPSC case study*. Stockholm: Save the Children Sweden.

———. 2003. *Family matters: The care and protection of children affected by HIV/AIDS in Malawi: A CPSC case study*. Stockholm: Save the Children Sweden.

McKerrow, N. 1996. *Implementation strategies for the development of models of care for orphaned children*. New York: UNICEF.

Mutangadura, G. B., D. Mukurazita, and H. Jackson. 1999. *A review of household and community responses to the HIV/AIDS epidemic in the rural areas of sub-Saharan Africa*. UNAIDS Best Practice Collection. Geneva: UNAIDS, June. http://www.iaen.org/files.cgi/241_una99e39.pdf

Phiri, S. N. 2001. The case for an expanded response: Scaling up community mobilization interventions to mitigate the impact of HIV/AIDS in the Southern Africa Development Community (SADC) countries. Master's thesis, Duke University.

Phiri, S. N., G. Foster, and M. Nzima. 2001. *Expanding and strengthening community action: A study of ways to scale up community mobilization interventions to mitigate the effect of HIV/AIDS on children and families*. Washington, DC: Displaced Children

and Orphans Fund, USAID. http://www.usaid.gov/our_work/humanitarian_
assistance/the_funds/pubs/ovc.html

Phiri, S. N., and D. Webb. 2002. The impacts of HIV/AIDS on children: Program and
policy response. Chapter 15 in *AIDS, public policy, and child wellbeing*. Florence:
UNICEF/Innocenti Research Centre.

Tobis, D. 2000. *Moving from residential institutions to community-based social services
in Central and Eastern Europe and the former Soviet Union*. Washington, DC: World
Bank. Available at http://www.worldbank.org

Tolfree, D. 1995. *Roofs and roots: The care of separated children in the developing world*.
Aldershot: Ashgate.

———. 2003. *Community-based care for separated children*. Stockholm: Save the Children Sweden.

———. 2004. *Whose children? Separated children's protection and participation in emergencies*. Stockholm: Save the Children Sweden.

USAID (United States Agency for International Development), UNICEF, and
UNAIDS (Joint United Nations Programme on HIV/AIDS). 2002. *Children
on the brink: A joint report on orphan estimates and program strategies*. Washington, DC: TvT Associates/Synergy Project. www.unicef.org/publications/
pub_children_on_the_brink_en.pdf

2

Strengthening Households and Communities

The Key to Reducing the Economic Impacts of HIV/AIDS on Children and Families

Jill Donahue

There is widespread and well-founded concern about the impacts of HIV/AIDS on children and families. Most major studies that discuss the effects of the pandemic share many of the same conclusions:

- The HIV/AIDS pandemic is an evolving and broad-scale disaster.
- AIDS is not only a health issue but also a development crisis.
- The pandemic is unraveling years of hard-won gains in economic and social development.
- The economic toll of AIDS starts with eroding the resources of the person living with the disease, then depletes the resources of the immediate and extended family, and eventually threatens to overwhelm the capacity of communities to act as a "safety net."
- Agencies and donors pay too little attention to the massive scale of the impact, and their efforts reach only a small fraction of individuals, families, and communities affected by HIV/AIDS.
- The fundamental challenge is to develop coordinated, multisectoral interventions that make a difference over the long haul at a scale that approaches the magnitude of the HIV/AIDS pandemic.

There is deep concern in both the most affected regions and the industrialized world about young people affected by AIDS. It is clear that these children and adolescents face daunting challenges. Many analysts fear that the unprecedented strain on extended families and communities will cause societal breakdown, and that the wider world is not doing much to help.

While these concerns are well-founded, they reflect only part of the reality. Despite seemingly overwhelming challenges, families and communities are responding creatively in devising ways to sustain their initiatives. The safety net role played by individual households and communities is crucial to the well-being and quality of care afforded to orphans and other vulnerable children.

If we perceive AIDS-affected children and families as helpless victims, we risk creating programs that treat them as passive recipients of our goodwill, rather than as active participants in addressing their needs, problems, and challenges. We must recognize, celebrate, and actively support the hundreds of small, humble, yet collectively powerful local initiatives through which ordinary people are responding in extraordinary ways. Overlooking these efforts would be a grave disservice to their integrity, courage, and care for young people.

Consider the following examples of grassroots action:

- Throughout Zimbabwe, communities are rediscovering a traditional community safety net mechanism called Zunde RaMambo, "the chief's field." In this tradition, the harvest from a communal garden provides food for those who cannot afford their own.
- Many communities in Zambia have established their own schools for children unable to go to more expensive or more distant government schools.
- In the Kibera slums in Nairobi, a group of women widowed by AIDS raises money and pools its resources and time to run a day-care center. They also have a savings club and take out loans from a microfinance institution to finance their individual livelihoods.
- Young Voices, a local youth organization in Dedza, Malawi, provides positive role models for younger orphans and other vulnerable children in the community. These teenagers organize recreational activities such as writing songs and poems or playing games with younger children.
- In another Malawi village, a teenage girl, an orphan herself, teaches younger children (some are orphans, others have parents who are seriously ill) how to jump rope, sing traditional songs, and play hopscotch. The Village AIDS Committee supports, encourages, and honors this young woman.
- The selflessness of "hero moms" is extolled in a South African newspaper in Guateng Province. The local government honored three women with the title "Foster Mother of the Year." Each has taken in numerous children whose parents have died of AIDS, and they manage to provide for the children's needs through their own earnings, government grants, and support from their communities (*Johannesburg Sunday Times*, March 10, 2002).

These examples are admirable, but they are not exceptional: Throughout Africa many thousands of people are helping those in greater need than themselves. As Choice Makufa, a colleague from Zimbabwe, observed, "The poor are helping the destitute." Such stories of hope and courage should be the inspiration that we keep in our minds and spirits when we think of children affected by HIV/AIDS. It is also true, however, that children, families, and communities are experiencing extreme hardships and difficulty because of AIDS, and they need active support. Our efforts to help will be more appropriate and effective if they recognize and build upon people's capacities, instead of being motivated by images of helpless, hopeless victims.

In addition to exploring the economic impact of HIV/AIDS, this chapter also describes coping mechanisms that households use in response to economic stress. Of particular interest are the ways that some households move from coping over the short term to successfully adapting or permanently changing their mix of strategies to fulfill their basic needs. The chapter also discusses the role of community safety nets in this mix of strategies employed by households in crisis. Finally, it describes project approaches that can bolster household and community safety nets.

THE ECONOMIC IMPACT ON CHILDREN OF HIV/AIDS-RELATED ILLNESS AND DEATH

When HIV/AIDS strikes a household, the stress of illness, death, and uncertainty about the future can be overwhelming. HIV/AIDS puts enormous economic stress on households as they care for sick family members, experience the loss of productive adults, or take in orphans. The slide from relative comfort to destitution can be frighteningly quick. Illness usually does not cause poverty, but it worsens its legacy.

HIV/AIDS is not only an increasing cause of death among adults, infants, and young children, it is also slowly impoverishing and dismembering families. At every stage of the HIV/AIDS epidemic, most of the social and economic consequences fall on families. In fact, the greatest economic impact of HIV/AIDS comes from the high costs of treatment and the need to assist surviving family members. Families and communities coping with AIDS-related illness and death shoulder a heavy burden, and the epidemic takes its greatest toll at the household and community level (Over 1998).

As other chapters in this book make clear, there are many dimensions to the impacts of HIV/AIDS on children and families. Loss of educational opportunities for many AIDS-affected children is of particular concern. Families who decide to keep children out of school do so for a variety of reasons. Children may be needed at home to help care for sick family members or to work in the fields. Children also drop out of school if, because of reduced household income, their families can no longer afford school expenses (Mutangadura 1999). Some children may opt out of school because they are too worried about a parent's condition or because they feel stigmatized by the nature of a parent's illness.

Regarding children's attendance in school, a study in Uganda found that women placed a very high priority on accumulating money for their children's school fees and that they planned other expenditures with whatever was left over. Some families negotiated with school authorities to pay in installments so their children were able to continue in school despite the household's financial hardships. Some women interviewed during the study went so far as to say that they were not working for themselves, but for the future of their children. They see very clearly that education is the main determinant of social status and future opportunities in Uganda (Wright et al. 1999).

Parents in other countries echo similar sentiments. The following excerpt from a World Bank study on poverty conducted throughout the world (Narayan 2000: 43) describes it well: "In Swaziland, parents make considerable sacrifices, including rationing food to reduce household expenses so that their children can go to school. In Guinea–Bissau a man said about his children's schooling, 'I think that, God willing, they'll do well so they'll be able to get good jobs. I do all in my power to make sure they don't miss class. I hope God will point the way to success for them. Without an education, life is difficult because you can't get a good job.'" In Vietnam, investment in education is seen as the most important way out of poverty; lack of money for education and not having a stable job are identified as the number one problems.

The economic impacts of HIV/AIDS on children also manifest themselves through the reduced capacity of their mothers to care for them. Ordinarily, it is a woman's duty to care for children and for sick family members or relatives. This obligation forces many women to neglect subsistence crop production and activities that generate income for the household, as well as the direct care of their own children. Diverting labor from economic activities can lead to food insecurity. After a husband's death, his widow and children may lose household assets and even their home itself, due to "property grabbing" by his relatives. Claiming property may have some justification under traditional law, but it can disenfranchise women and children and push them quickly into poverty. In addition, in many countries, widowed grandmothers take on the burden of caring for their grandchildren and experience severe economic stress as a result (Donahue 1998).

A study by Mutangadura (2000) in Zimbabwe examined the impact of a woman's death on the welfare of her household. She points out that a mother's capacity to spend time with her children, the energy she can devote to them, the conditions of home life, and her knowledge and skills strongly influence children's passage from childhood to maturity. Other studies have shown how important the mother's role is to the welfare of the household:

- Women are typically responsible for health care (de Bruyn 1992).
- Women (in Africa) produce 70 percent of food consumed (Neema 1998).
- Women are more likely to use their income to meet children's needs, including schooling (UNAIDS, 1999).
- Children are likely, in the short run, to replace the labor of a woman who dies (Ainsworth and Filmer 2002).

Consequently, a mother's early death from HIV/AIDS will have a profound effect on her children.

Household surveys in Côte d'Ivoire, Tanzania, and Thailand have shown that HIV/AIDS can reduce income by 40 to 60 percent (Mutangadura, Mukurazita, and Jackson 1999). This finding is further supported by focus group participants interviewed during a study that I led in Uganda and Kenya for MicroSave (Donahue, Kabuccho, and Osinde 2001). The participants identified several HIV/AIDS-related crises, including prolonged illnesses of an extended family member or spouse, multiple deaths in close succession, death and burial, and orphan care and education costs.

My colleagues and I explored the economic impact of AIDS on microfinance clients. We focused specifically on the impacts experienced by clients who were caregivers of a person living with AIDS or who had taken several orphaned children into their household. Figure 2.1 presents an overview of the responses of clients regarding crises that cause the greatest financial pressure. AIDS-related crises were the most frequently mentioned. Participants also pointed out that although crises not related to HIV/AIDS (such

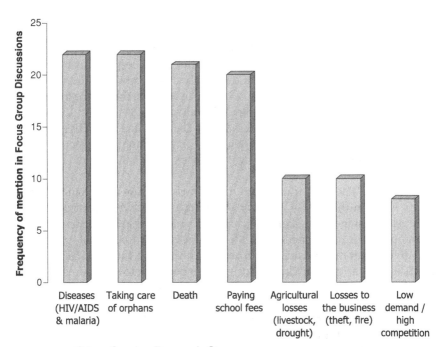

FIGURE 2.1. Crises Causing Economic Stress

as business or agricultural losses) happen more frequently, they come in isolation. HIV/AIDS, on the other hand, triggers a series of crises that requires an entire arsenal of coping mechanisms.

Findings from this study further suggest that as the effects of the disease and the demands of caregiving evolve within a household, there are distinct peaks of financial pressure. Focus group participants generally identified five phases in this evolution: (1) *early stages*, when a person living with AIDS first calls on the family or the caregiver for assistance; (2) *frequent opportunistic illnesses*, when the person living with AIDS is in and out of hospital; (3) *bedridden*, either at home or in the hospital; (4) *death and burial*; and (5) *care for orphaned children* and their education. The most severe economic stresses occur:

- before the person infected with HIV is diagnosed, and the caregivers spare no expense in looking for a cure,
- when the family member with AIDS is bedridden and the caregivers must assume financial responsibility for health and child care, at the expense of spending time in economic activities, and
- when a caregiver assumes responsibility for the children whose parent(s) have died.

Early stages. During the early stages of progression of HIV to AIDS, caregivers may not be aware of the crisis looming on their horizon because the HIV-infected person is still economically active and may or may not know (or wish to find out) her or his HIV status. However, the first signs of declining health and the first calls for financial assistance begin in this stage.

Frequent hospital visits. This phase of the illness can be particularly expensive when family members are in denial about the cause of illness. There is pressure on the family to spare no expense because they want to believe that there will be a recovery. They will liquidate not only all the assets of the person who is ill, but also many of their own. As the disease progresses, the individual is more frequently ill and caregivers increasingly spend their time providing care, leaving less time for their own economic activities.

Bedridden. The most financially strenuous time for caregiving households is when the family member suffering from AIDS becomes bedridden. At this stage, it is likely the caregivers have exhausted most of their economic resources, especially if the patient is in hospital. Not only must caregivers shut their businesses to be with the patient, they must also cover medical bills and other daily household expenses. Households liquidate remaining assets to pay these expenses. In cases where the person living with AIDS is a sibling or an extended family member, the caregiver often takes responsibility for the individual's children. All of this occurs during an income lapse for the caregiver.

Death and burial. This can also be an expensive time for survivors because food must be provided for all the relatives and friends who participate

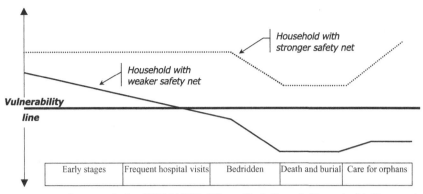

FIGURE 2.2. Stages of the HIV/AIDS "Care Cycle" and Household Economic Decline

in the funeral. However, in some countries with mature epidemics, people generally have developed ways of handling the financial pressures imposed by death. Community, extended family members, and other well-wishers may share the financial burden of burial. Everyone sees this practice as a reciprocal arrangement: Contributors to someone else's burial expenses can count on support if death comes to their household. Many people belong to some type of informal burial association where they make regular savings deposits toward funeral and burial expenses. Nonetheless, households affected by HIV/AIDS tend to be at their most economically vulnerable when the family member they have been caring for dies.

Care for orphaned children. The obligation to arrange care for orphans follows the death of a surviving or single parent. The financial pressure on caregiving households at this stage grows more intense as they struggle to incorporate new dependants. School fees are the most common financial pressure. Figure 2.2 suggests the pattern of economic decline in a household with a weaker economic safety net compared with a stronger household during the stages of caring for someone living with HIV/AIDS.

Ultimately, the economic decline experienced by caregivers is not much different from that experienced by the person with AIDS. In fact, the economic caregiving burden continues after the person with AIDS dies in the form of their orphaned children and unpaid debts or outstanding hospital bills. How extensive the financial impacts become appears to depend on:

- the presence or absence of physical assets, income, and credit or savings opportunities,
- the economic resources (including business strength and stability) a caregiver has when the crisis begins to take its toll,
- the duration of a given crisis – how many crises occur and the amount of time between them,
- the quality and number of available coping mechanisms,

- the informal networks to which a caregiver belongs, and
- knowledge of available resources.

Here are some typical comments from the focus groups of microfinance clients (Donahue et al. 2001) describing the impact of HIV/AIDS:

You may have followed family planning, but if your brother didn't and he dies – you still get his children.

You don't know about the burden that someone had to carry until they die and their burden becomes yours.

You don't inherit the skills or the business of the person who died, just their responsibilities.

Your business is the same size, but you now have more people to support. Where you used to buy one kilo of sugar, now you must buy three.

Your own child will accept going to bed hungry, but an orphan will cry and complain, "If my parents were alive, they wouldn't allow me to go hungry." This creates a lot of pressure on you. It makes for a very complex family.

HOW POOR HOUSEHOLDS COPE ECONOMICALLY IN RESPONSE TO CRISES

In their paper examining the dynamics of household economic portfolios, Chen and Dunn (1996) explain household economic coping behavior in terms of reducing risk and managing loss.

Risk reduction strategies include:

- choosing low-risk income-generating activities that earn modest, but steady, returns,
- diversifying household, crop, or income-earning activities,
- building up savings and in-kind assets (such as livestock, jewelry, and household goods), and
- preserving extended family and community ties.

Loss management techniques fall into three stages. Stage one is made up of reversible steps that involve the liquidation of "protective assets" (expendable resources). Stage two involves the sale of "productive assets" that produce income for the household. The sale of such resources is difficult to reverse and undermines future household capacity to generate income and produce food. Stage three occurs when a household has become destitute, with few if any coping mechanisms available. Avoiding stages two and three depends on the effectiveness and resiliency of stage one strategies, and stage one depends on successful risk reduction activities. Therefore, strengthening risk reduction activities of affected households and helping them to avoid stages two and three will reduce their vulnerability to poverty – and, by extension, the impacts of AIDS.

The extent to which a household will be able to cope economically with the effects of HIV/AIDS infection depends on the range and type

TABLE 2.1. *Sequence of Asset Liquidation*

Protective assets	Most quickly liquidated	• Cash savings • In-kind savings that are quickly liquidated (chickens, goats, sheep, stored harvests)
	Less easily transformed into cash	• TV, radio, kitchen utensils, furniture • Jewelry • Social capital (goodwill from relatives, friends, and neighbors)
Productive assets	Selling has negative impact on income flows to household	• Business capital • Draft/dairy animals • Rental property • Land
	Will sell only after having exhausted all other avenues	

Source: Donahue et al. 2001.

of economic coping options available to it before, during, and after the crisis. It is vitally important to identify mechanisms that appear to reduce economic pressures caused by HIV/AIDS. Such an examination can provide insight into the ways people are moving from coping (getting through a crisis in the short term) to adapting (permanently changing the mix of strategies used to fulfil the household's basic needs). Recognizing the types of asset that households accumulate and how these are used is extremely important in this regard. In our MicroSave study (Donahue et al. 2001), focus group participants frequently said that liquidating assets provides a household with options in the face of a crisis.

Generally speaking, studies on household strategies to minimize the impact of crises or fulfil needs for lump sums of cash categorize assets as protective or productive. Protective assets are those that households can easily liquidate and thus are the most immediately available. The more a household can accumulate protective assets, the more easily it is able to avoid liquidating productive assets. Households protect the assets that they use to produce income. Productive assets are important because they represent future income-generating potential. Focus group participants in the MicroSave study said that they liquidate savings and protective assets first; they sell productive assets only when they have run out of other options (see also Chen and Dunn 1996; Sebstad and Cohen 2000). The sequence of asset liquidation that our focus group described (shown in Table 2.1) clearly progressed from protective to productive assets.

TABLE 2.2. *Economic Coping Strategies*

Strategy	Examples of Specific Actions
Reducing household consumption	• Cut down on nonfood items to reduce expenditure (e.g., hosting or attending social events) • Drop more expensive foods from diet • Switch to less expensive staple foods • Set limit on daily expenditures • Reduce the number of meals • Find cheaper accommodations • Remove children from school
Mobilize assets for income	• Capitalize on household and family relationships • Call in "favors" from those assisted in the past • Divide responsibilities between husband and wife for meeting different expenditures • Match different savings mechanisms to predictable life-cycle events (e.g., weddings, baptisms, graduation) and for protection against unforeseen costs. • Subdivide house into rental units • Use house for different purposes at different times of day (e.g., hair salon during the day, bar in the evening, and a place to sleep at night)
Increase income	• Seek new sources of income for each expense as it arises • Match specific income-generating activities or sources to specific expenditures, (e.g., income from rental property goes to pay school fees, money gained from a rotating saving and credit scheme goes to pay hospital bills, major business activity pays for day-to-day expenses or for medicine) • Increase the number of working hours • Take out an informal loan • Take on "piece work" (cash paid on the spot in exchange for labor, e.g., working in other people's fields)

Source: Wright et al. 1999.

Another study, by Wright et al. (1999), provides insights into the rich array of economic coping strategies Ugandan women use when faced with crises. This qualitative study mirrored much of what economic impact research has described. Table 2.2 summarizes and provides examples of the major strategies employed.

In essence, what the studies by Wright et al. (1999), Chen and Dunn (1996), and Donahue et al. (2001) illustrate is that there is no single strategy that poor households employ to counter increasing vulnerability and economic crises successfully over the long term. Rather, it is the piecing together of various kinds of social and financial capital that enables households to plan and adapt, as opposed to merely coping. Adapting emerges from the combined strength of many strategies, woven together so that if one falters, another sustains.

BUILDING THE RESILIENCE OF HOUSEHOLD ECONOMIC
SAFETY NETS

Poor households have always engaged in a multitude of economic activities to manage income flows and to meet crisis needs for cash. Over years of involvement with poor communities, development organizations have learned that the most successful initiatives are those that incorporate or build upon existing economic capacities and behavior that enable poor households to adapt to risk and crises. Generating income and building up savings are long-standing coping mechanisms that poor households employ to respond to times of economic stress, whatever the cause.

Microenterprise development is the technical field of assistance that seeks to strengthen poor entrepreneurs who rely on a range of economic activities. There are two major categories – microfinance and business development services – which are compared in Table 2.3.

The following section describes some of the aspects of microfinance and business development services that potentially can help mitigate the impacts of AIDS at household and community levels. The services described are initiatives that:

- have proven consistently useful in facilitating income generation and asset accumulation for poor households,
- are capable of reaching large numbers of poor households, and
- seek to deliver services in a cost-effective manner in order to reach operational and financial sustainability.

Microfinance Services

Loans offered by microfinance institutions can strengthen clients' income-earning activities, and are one of the few interventions with the potential to reach massive numbers of poor clients in a sustainable and cost-effective manner. The loans are deliberately kept small to attract the poorest households, who typically already engage in short-term, rapid-turnover trading activities that are the very endeavors most likely to benefit from infusions of small amounts of working capital. Having a greater financial cushion to

TABLE 2.3. *Microfinance and Business Development Services Compared*

Microfinance is the delivery of financial services to poor clients.	Business Development Services are considered to be everything that isn't a financial service.
Services include: • Small loans • Savings • Insurance Financial services can be: – Credit-led, where entrepreneurs gain immediate access to loans through a microfinance institution. External grants from donors capitalize the loan portfolio. – Savings-led, where the accent is on mobilizing client savings first, which later forms the capital for loans. Methodologies for delivering credit services include: • Lending to individuals • Peer lending through solidarity groups Entrepreneurs can be clients of a microfinance institution, which takes on the responsibility of managing the delivery and collection of credit repayments. An alternative approach is for entrepreneurs to form self-managed savings and credit groups using members' savings as capital for loans.	Services include: • Training • Market development and linkages • Brokering or subcontracting commercial arrangements between large and small businesses • Improved technology that brings added value to entrepreneurs' products Business development is a very young field. Practitioners in this field have not yet developed a "package" for widespread replication, as they have with microfinance services. However, the aim is to work toward initiatives that are demand-driven and that reach large numbers of entrepreneurs in a cost-effective manner.

hedge against loss can enable loan recipients to initiate higher-risk, higher-return businesses that can result in the building up of household resources (MkNelly and Dunford 1996).

Microfinance services can help mitigate the economic impacts of HIV/AIDS because access to small loans can enable clients to:

• maintain or increase income,
• accumulate savings that are secure, easy to liquidate quickly, and that retain value,
• liquidate savings and assets when necessary, which reduces vulnerability by providing alternatives to irreversible coping strategies that eliminate future income-earning and productive capacity,

- obtain lump sums of cash that can help them avoid eating into their business capital, and
- restore business activities that help clients bounce back once a crisis is over.

Impact evaluations of microfinance services show that access to credit enables businesses to survive crises and helps households smooth income ebb and flow and accumulate assets (Sebstad and Chen 1996; Wright et al. 1999). In addition, a literature review and analysis conducted by Freedom from Hunger (MkNelly and Dunford 1996: 5) concludes: "Poverty lending [microfinance] is unlikely to produce major economic gains for poor households. However, in relative terms, these modest gains seem likely to make very important contributions to household survival, such as income smoothing and insurance against emergencies. And these are precisely the types of livelihood strategies that, if strengthened, are most closely associated with increased household food security and nutritional status."

An impact evaluation of a microfinance program in Burkina Faso (Adelski et al. 2001: 9) compared "clients" (women who had previously obtained three or more loans), and "trainees" (women who had received training so they could join the program but who had not yet received a loan). The evaluators found that "both the quantitative and the qualitative evaluation-data show that the microfinance activity definitely has had a positive impact on women's lives.... Clients reported spending 2.5 times more on their children's education than trainees, having 6.5 times more savings than trainees, and spending 2.5 times more on health care than trainees. The clients stated that most of their profits are spent on their children and other household expenses. These are proxy indicators for increased income, which is linked to improved food security."

Microfinance services are most appropriate for those who support orphans, are widowed, are single heads of household, or are supporting someone in their family suffering from AIDS and related illnesses. Microfinance services can also enable households not seriously affected by HIV/AIDS (but that, at any given time might well become so) to shore up their resources ahead of time.

These are potentially very important elements in lessening the epidemic's impacts on families and communities. Microfinance can play a valuable role in helping households build up resources before the worst consequences arrive. This is especially crucial for households that are already poor or are still at risk of falling back into poverty, but there are definite limits to what microfinance can be expected to do: It is widely seen as improving livelihoods, reducing vulnerability, and fostering social as well as economic empowerment, but it is not for everyone.

Microfinance is not a panacea for mitigating the economic impacts of AIDS or for alleviating poverty. The client, not the financial service, creates economic opportunity. Access to savings and credit services is not appropriate for households so debilitated that their immediate survival is at stake. To make use of credit and savings opportunities, a household must be able to carry out some kind of financially productive activity, usually one with a fairly quick turnover of capital. It is not for households whose members have no productive capacity. Such clients may need to leave the microfinance institution until they are back on their feet financially (Parker, Singh, and Hattel 2000).

The survival of a microfinance institution depends on clients paying back loans in full and on time. Microfinance is not a type of social service program, and donors must avoid pressuring microfinance institutions to make changes in their methodology without an adequate assessment of the implications for institutional sustainability.

While microfinance does work in communities seriously affected by AIDS, it does not work when an organization tries to target loans to individuals or groups that it selects based on members' serostatus. With good reason, best-practice standards in microfinance advise against deliberately targeting loans to specific types of clients. To do so would compromise the integrity and sustainability of their services. Furthermore, attempts to engineer the composition of solidarity groups would undermine the delicate mix of peer pressure and group accountability on which successful lending programs are built. Targeting specific types of clients with preferential loan terms or products also tends to create a negative dynamic of the general population resenting the perceived preferential treatment of the targeted group. Targeting also can increase stigma when others feel that their economic circumstances, too, should warrant special consideration.

Savings Mobilization

Savings schemes or savings-led credit initiatives can help households for which credit is inappropriate. These include households that do not want or are not able to repay debt, and those in rural and remote areas whose income may be seasonal or unpredictable. Such households generally rely on in-kind savings, such as livestock or stored crops that they can sell later to stabilize income throughout the year and provide lump sums of cash.

Building savings reduces economic risk and enhances ability to cope with loss, because in a crisis, households are able to liquidate these reserves rather than the productive assets on which their future income-earning ability may rely. Stockpiling savings is an important risk reduction and loss management strategy.

People living at lower socioeconomic levels create informal means to plan for times in their lives when they will need a significant amount of cash, for example for weddings, funerals, baptisms, sending children to school, starting a business, and retirement. Emergencies – medical, natural disaster, or man-made – also create urgent needs for cash. Many societies have informal savings mechanisms that enable participants to access lump sums of cash. Two of these are described next.

Rotating Savings and Credit Associations (ROSCAs). A ROSCA is a voluntary, self-selected group in which all members put in equal amounts of money that is pooled and rotated equally in turn to each person in the group. These traditional savings mechanisms exist in one form or another all over the world. In Africa, there are *tontines* in Francophone countries, *susus* in Ghana, merry-go-rounds in Kenya, *chilembas* in Zambia, and *stockveldt* in South Africa (Rutherford 2000).

Accumulating Savings and Credit Associations (ASCAs). ASCAs are similar to ROSCAs except that members in the group must treat their turn at receiving the pooled money as they would a loan and pay it back with interest. The interest charged allows the pooled funds to accumulate. In time, members divide the interest payments and pay themselves dividends.

For both savings mechanisms, the group must simply agree on the following items and abide by the agreement:

- the amount of money each member will save,
- the regularity with which the money will be saved, and
- either the schedule for rotating the cumulative savings to each member of the group or the rules for taking a loan from the savings of the members.

There are many other ways that poor households manage their savings to access informal credit. Rutherford (2000) presents a very thorough and readable look at the rich diversity of these methods. Formal savings mobilization schemes base their methodologies on ROSCAs and ASCAs. Some of the better known institutional models are credit unions, savings and credit cooperatives, financial service associations, and self-managed savings and credit groups.

Like microfinance programs, savings mobilization programs must be appraised cautiously, because while it may appear that they would be a more appropriate mechanism for assisting households unable or unwilling to risk using credit, the managing of formal savings institutions can be more complicated than managing microcredit only (Christen et al. 1995). In addition many countries have strict legal limitations on the types of institutions allowed to take, hold, and lend members' savings. Some microfinance institutions appear to offer savings and loans, but more often than not the savings are in reality a buffer against defaults and are not available on demand, which limits their effectiveness as risk-reduction and loss-management strategies. Further, the provision of externally generated capital (through soft loans or donor grants) to savings-led institutions for the purposes of bolstering loan portfolios has had mixed results. The more unsophisticated and low-tech version of savings-led models – self-managed savings and credit groups – tend to perform poorly when a donor adds external capital to members' savings to stretch groups' capacity to provide loans.

Table 2.4 presents a generalized summary of microfinance models and methodologies.

Business Development Services

Business Development Services (BDS) include training, introducing improved technology that adds value to business activities, and facilitating better linkages of microenterprises to growing markets or to more economical sources of raw materials in order to increase their profits. Recent innovation within BDS involves developing links between agricultural producer groups and markets to which traditionally they have not had access.

Another type of linkage program involves art or craft products. With some approaches, producers simply obtain more or better access to market information; with others, they receive assistance to organize and pool their production in order to do business with a more commercially oriented client. To date, among BDS programs that create market-driven linkages, agricultural opportunities show the best potential to reach significant scale, in part because there are more households in developing countries that depend on agriculture for their livelihood.

Closely related to market linkages are initiatives that broker arrangements for small businesses to provide services to larger businesses. For example, a larger business might engage a smaller food preparation business to provide lunch for its workers.

Another innovative BDS involves providing business management training through voucher schemes. With this approach, an organization provides vouchers to entrepreneurs for a preselected range of institutions or private companies that offer business management training. Entrepreneurs turn in their vouchers in exchange for courses, which the training provider redeems with the organization that issued them.

Although business training has been a long-standing element of BDS, provision of such services has yet to achieve desired results in terms of increased revenue, particularly for those entrepreneurs operating microbusinesses in the survival economy. In an effort to improve on BDS performance, microenterprise practitioners have introduced such elements as brokering, facilitating commercial linkages, and introducing improved technology. These are relatively new areas, however, and very few organizations specialize in them, which limits the possibility of providing such services on a large scale. Another consideration is that the reach of BDS providers to the so-called poorest of the poor is very limited. Most BDS

TABLE 2.4. *Comparison of Microfinance Models and Methodologies*

	Methodologies	
Individual Lending	**Peer Lending**	
	• Borrowers mutually guarantee each other's loans in lieu of collateral. Group formation is the loan guarantee mechanism • Potential clients are screened by their peers • Little or no analysis is made of the business by program staff • Loan size and terms closely follow a predetermined gradual growth curve • Staff workload and cost of lending small amounts of money are reduced by lending to groups of peers.	
	Models Using Peer Lending Methodologies	
	Solidarity Groups	**Self-Managed Organizations**
• Loans are guaranteed by collateral and/or cosigners • Potential clients are screened by program staff • Loan amount is based on thorough business viability analysis • Loan size and term can be tailored to needs of business • Loan size tends to be larger than those offered through peer lending • Clients tend to operate small and medium (as opposed to micro) enterprises • Each client requires a significant investment of staff time and energy	• Program does not develop the self-management capability of the group • Participants are considered long-term clients of the program and must take loans to retain membership • Loan capital starts with an external grant	• Program develops the members' capability for self-management • Program works toward the goal of operational and financial independence of the organization • Loan capital comes from member savings

Source: Adapted from C. Waterfield and A. Derval, 1996, *CARE Savings and Credit Sourcebook.* Washington and Atlanta: CARE and PACT Publications.

programs reach small to medium-sized businesses, not microentre-
preneurs – and certainly not those self-employed for their very survival.

COMMUNITY MECHANISMS THAT SUPPORT HOUSEHOLDS
UNDER STRESS

The grim reality of HIV/AIDS is that its economic impact can become so
severe that adult members of a household can no longer continue income-
earning activities. This is equally the case for household members who
experience AIDS-related illnesses and for those taking caring of them.
When the adult members of a household reduce or stop productive activities, children's welfare is at its most tenuous. In fact, a recurring theme
among communities seriously affected by HIV/AIDS is their concern about
the circumstances in which a growing number of vulnerable children live
(Donahue and Williamson 1999).

A community safety net emerges when neighbors, friends, traditional
leaders, and church groups rally around extremely vulnerable children
and their guardians. Often, a sense of urgency and the need to join forces
to assist households in crisis motivates people to form informal or formal
coalitions, committees, or community associations. The members of these
spontaneous community coalitions may take turns visiting households
that are most in jeopardy, at times providing food and soap or school
supplies and fees for children, at other times running errands, taking care
of household chores, or watching the children. Community groups also
typically engage in activities to create a source of funds for the material
needs (food, clothes, soap, school fees) of households in crisis. Having
access to this type of relief assistance can make the difference between a
household disintegrating or being able to bounce back.

In forming these coalitions, communities build social capital, which is
defined as relationships that serve as assets and resources, which in turn
enable residents to undertake collective action for mutual benefit.[1] Simply forming groups does not create social capital. Instead, social capital
emerges through the practice of taking action – of acquiring and using
skills that enable community members to coordinate activities to achieve
their mutually defined goals. Social capital can play a subtle but critical
role in cushioning shocks.

A concrete illustration of the importance of social capital emerges from
the discussions among focus group participants in the MicroSave study
on the economic impact of AIDS on microfinance clients (Donahue et al.
2001). It was evident that women count on a variety of groups from which
they draw social capital, including religious groups, informal savings

[1] Information on social capital comes from the "Let's Talk Social Capital" discussion list at the
World Bank and the World Bank Web site, http://www.worldbank.org/poverty/scapital

clubs, Munno Mukabi,[2] burial groups, informal insurance groups, local government councils, government programs, savings and credit cooperatives, and nongovernmental organization (NGO) programs, among others. When asked why they joined groups, the women gave varied answers that included convenient access to credit, mutual encouragement, emotional support, feelings of importance, access to vital information, and learning household management skills. These associations are particularly useful in responding to periodic but unpredictable risks related to death, sickness, and celebrations that can impose significant financial pressure on a household (Wright et al. 1999).

BUILDING THE RESILIENCE OF COMMUNITY SAFETY NETS

Community groups typically engage in activities to create a source of funds for the material needs of households in crisis. To create a source of funds that are sustainable over the long term, communities need to embark on an ongoing resource-mobilization campaign to identify and tap into first internal resources, and then external resources. This *community resource mobilization* could include fund-raising activities, community asset mapping, and community participation.

Fund-Raising Activities

Operating a group-run, income-generating activity successfully requires full-time and year-round attention. Identifying and holding a variety of one-time fund-raising events, however, will probably take less financial resources and time, which increases the chances for success. The most successful fund-raising is based on skills and resources that already exist within the community.

Activities can range from simple cash or in-kind donations scraped together within the community to sophisticated formal events like raffles or (even further) creating foundations. Community gardens or fields are a very common form of generating in-kind or cash assistance. Engaging casual labor is also a very common form of generating cash.

Fund-raising strategies should evolve continually to avoid depending on one sort of activity or one group of donors. For example, in an effort to gain donations and generate cash from a variety of sources, village AIDS committees in Malawi have:

- organized "big-walks," where walkers are sponsored by businesses or individuals and proceeds go toward the community fund,

---

[2] Munno Mukabi is a Ugandan term that means "friend in need." It is used in some parts of Uganda when referring to informal groups of mutual self-help. Munno Mukabi is a very old practice that, according to some focus group participants in the MicroSave study, saw a renewed popularity in Uganda when AIDS became a feature of everyday life.

- approached the Muslim and Christian communities to donate offerings collected during their respective religious services,
- created links with an agricultural research project to get free, improved-variety cassava and sweet potato cuttings for their community garden, and
- collected membership fees from people joining their AIDS committee (Donahue and Williamson 1999).

Community Asset Mapping

Assistance to community groups should help develop strategies to tap into local and external resources. A community may first need to appreciate the resources available to it before it can effectively mobilize those resources. Community asset mapping is a tool that uncovers hidden or undervalued resources. The mapping exercise includes an inventory of community skills and talents, a map of physical resources controlled by community members, and identification of resources controlled by external parties. After conducting one such exercise, a community living next to Lake Malawi realized they had not even thought of the lake as a resource. Upon reflection, the resource-mobilization committee decided to build fish-drying tables next to the lake and rent them out to fishermen. The proceeds went into their community fund.

Community Participation

Although not an explicitly economic strategy, building strong community cohesion, participation, ownership, and management of all activities are important aspects of sound practice for orphans and vulnerable children programs. Moreover, successful community resource mobilization cannot occur in communities where ownership and participation do not exist.

Community groups that act as a catalyst around which the rest of the community rallies tend to be the most successful. Any community group, no matter how dedicated or energetic, needs the participation of the wider community; it will not be able to create a truly resilient safety net alone. Simply possessing the good intention of catalyzing community ownership, however, is not enough, nor is it an intuitive ability. Eliciting community participation requires specific skills that can be learned.

Several sound participatory development tools already exist, including (among others) Training for Transformation, an outgrowth of the Development Education Leadership Teams in Action (DELTA), started in Kenya in 1974 (Hope and Timmel 1995); UNICEF's Triple "A" approach of "assessment, analysis, and action" (UNICEF 1998); the Participatory Rural Appraisal (PRA) approach (World Bank n.d.), and Participatory Learning and Action (IAPAD n.d.).

Community groups are often encouraged or assisted to initiate community-run microenterprises (often referred to as income-generating projects or activities, also known as IGPs or IGAs) to finance their activities. Such an approach, although often tried, rarely seems to succeed. Group businesses are notoriously risky endeavors that have enormous difficulties generating significant profit, and that frequently require more management skills than a community can offer. Similarly, the time and effort necessary to achieve the desired profits consumes members' time, which is then not available for the initial goal of helping vulnerable children. Finally, most of these initiatives reach very small numbers of families caring for children affected by HIV/AIDS and are expensive to scale up.

Fund-raising activities can be a less taxing way to raise funds for social purposes, and offers a promising alternative. A community needs to think creatively, however, and vary the ways in which they raise funds so as to avoid "charity fatigue" within their community.

INTERRELATIONSHIP BETWEEN HOUSEHOLD AND COMMUNITY SAFETY NETS

Interventions by project designers, policymakers and others will have significant, sustainable impacts on children's vulnerability and well-being largely to the extent that they strengthen ongoing capacities of affected families and communities to protect and care for vulnerable children (USAID, UNICEF, and UNAIDS 2002). The capacity of households to provide for children depends, in turn, on maintaining or stabilizing livelihoods. Wages from formal or self-employment, physical assets, and savings provide a *household safety net*, but, these resources erode quickly as parents become caregivers for sick family members, become sick themselves, or take in additional dependents.

When the safety net fails them, households look to relatives, neighbors, or the community for relief: Individuals concerned for their friends, neighbors, and families often organize to provide moral support and material relief to households affected by HIV/AIDS. This is the foundation of a *community safety net*.

Household and community safety nets are inherently interrelated. The extent to which each can provide an economic buffer to the impact of HIV/AIDS depends on how successfully they interact to support one another. It also depends on how well people are able to piece together social and financial coping mechanisms so that households can deal with HIV/AIDS crises over an extended period.

Strong household safety nets help families maintain their assets and remain economically productive, which in turn allows them to be part of a community safety net for both extended family and others in crisis. If too many households are unable to support themselves, however, their

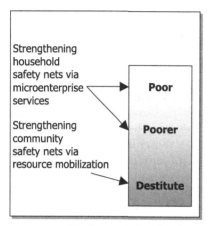

FIGURE 2.3. The interrelationship between household and community safety nets

needs rapidly overwhelm community safety nets. Minimizing the number of families in need of relief increases the chances that the community can maintain a safety net for its most vulnerable members (Donahue 1998, 2002). (See Figure 2.3.)

Social capital is an important asset for poor households. Reciprocal social relationships form the backbone of community safety nets: They are a key component of the social capital of an individual or household. Reciprocity means that in assisting someone else, the giver can expect assistance when she or he needs help. These relationships provide wells of financial, social, and political support that can be drawn on in times of need. Most frequently, poor people cope in times of dire need by turning to their extended family (Narayan 2000).

Another important aspect of community safety nets, social capital, and reciprocity is the relationship between the "better-off" and the "less well off" in a given community. For instance, according to a study conducted in Makueni, Kenya, households at the top end of a community's wealth range are essential to the food security of those at the bottom end. The study found that for every better-off household affected by illness, access to food will diminish for at least five poor households. As someone in a richer household experiences chronic bouts of HIV/AIDS-related illnesses, more of that household's resources go toward medical care and less toward hiring people to help in various agricultural activities (Marsland 2002).

COMBINING FORCES: "WHERE THERE IS A WILL,
THERE IS A WAY"

Given the interrelationship between them, finding new ways of strengthening both household and community safety nets simultaneously is a challenge development agencies must face. The task is daunting because experience shows that the design approaches and technical assistance needs are quite different for activities aimed at the household level than they are for the community level. Similarly, the skill set required for rigorous analysis and design of income-generating schemes is not at all the same as that required for designing effective child welfare or community-mobilization programs.

Nevertheless, because of strong demand for such services, child-focused organizations feel compelled to respond. In part, the demand for services is exacerbated by the fact that, in most developing countries, microfinance service coverage has not yet reached its potential, and services do not reach all potential clients. In the absence of a specialized institution that knows how to deliver microfinance services, many social welfare organizations take on the task without the benefit of experienced staff or sound technical assistance – and their programs suffer the consequences.

The study for MicroSave in Uganda (Donahue et al. 2001) provides a concrete illustration of the tension between technical proficiency and demand for economic support services for poor households. The study team spoke to programs that mixed credit with targeted social welfare services for people living with HIV/AIDS. In each case, the organizations started out by providing social and health services to persons living with HIV/AIDS, widows whose husbands had died of AIDS, or caretakers of children whose parents had died of AIDS. The common evolution toward credit programs generally involved:

- initial access to free goods and services,
- an inability to sustain services because of donor need to spread resources more widely, as well as increasing pressure from target clientele to address the economic effects of HIV/AIDS,
- the decision to "help people to help themselves" through encouraging or supporting their income-generating capacity using training, grants, or credit, and
- the eventual expansion of service from those infected to their caretakers.

The common trends as the organizations interviewed implemented the mixed programs included poor repayment rates, eroding loan capital or a devolving loan fund, very limited outreach capacity, and mission drift.

Poor repayment rates. The repayment rate among the organizations interviewed ranged between 65 and 86 percent (95 percent is considered the minimum acceptable for a sustainable program). Staff observed that when late payers suffered no consequences from nonrepayment, those previously paying on time began falling behind on their payments.

Eroding loan capital or a devolving loan fund. Most program staff referred to their loan capital as a revolving fund. However, in most cases the loan fund decreased by as much as 50 percent in two years. Staff recognized that eventually capital would have to be replenished, but plans to do so were sketchy at best. Programs had simply delayed addressing the sustainability issue and still were faced with the need to replenish funds.

Very limited outreach capacity. Because organizations had other services to provide to their clients, staff were typically dividing their time among the various services (including credit), which limited the number of clients they could reach. Organizations interviewed for this study served between fifty and twelve hundred clients. Microfinance institutions in East Africa typically reach between three thousand and twenty-eight thousand clients.

Mission drift. Organizations were asking themselves such questions as, "Are we an NGO providing social services or are we in the business of giving out and recovering credit?" All program staff reported that their clients identified the financial services with the social aspect of the organization, and consequently expected it to have "soft" policies on repayment. Some organizations were able to drop from the program people who were merely taking advantage of the policies, but that took up an inordinate amount of staff time. In one case, the organization tapped into community knowledge of potential borrowers and avoided lending to opportunists. Another organization observed that their target clientele no longer seemed interested in the original purpose of serving the best interests of children; they simply wanted access to credit.

Most organizations trying to play both social service and microfinance roles concluded that if they were going to offer financial services to their target clients, they needed to establish a separate mechanism for that purpose. They also learned that such a mechanism must adhere to sound lending and savings practices. They discovered that serving the poor does not justify relaxed policies on repayment or loan terms, and that peer pressure and group solidarity are essential aspects of maintaining the necessary financial discipline. Where policies were relaxed, operators of the loan scheme could no longer determine clearly why people were not repaying. In the microfinance industry, examples abound where slow or nonpayers affect the repayment behavior of other clients. When one person does not pay and suffers no consequences, other clients wonder why they should repay. This attitude can then spread to other microfinance service providers in the country. Our study in Uganda found that most social welfare service organizations eventually conclude that they are not well-suited to deliver microfinance services, and either abandon the effort or seek out a specialized institution who can serve clients more effectively.

APPLYING THE "RULE OF THE TOOL"

How can concerned development practitioners rise to the challenge of building community and household safety nets? The "rule of the tool" (an old adage) informs us, "For every job, there is a correct tool. And for every tool there is an artisan who knows how to use it." To determine how to combine technical strategies to form the best match to strengthen household and community safety nets, project designers should follow three steps:

- *Define the job.* Is the goal to provide relief assistance or to increase household capacity for generating income? Is it aiming to strengthen household or community safety nets? Who is the project trying to reach – the most destitute who are no longer able to engage in productive activity, or those who are very poor but still economically productive? Is the geographic target urban and periurban or rural and remote?
- *Match the tool to the job.* What does the development world already know about strengthening household and community-level safety nets? Which tools have performed best at each level?
- *Pick the artisan most proficient in the use of the tool.* Once practitioners identify the tools that work best, it is extremely important to identify what type of organization or practitioner knows best how to use the preferred tools and has the capacity to do so.

Strengthening safety nets at the household and community levels does not have to be an either/or proposition. Two organizations can initiate a strategic alliance to target the same geographic area with activities that are operationally separate but coordinated. This allows each to do what it does best, yet still benefit from the other's activities. While one organization carries out activities to mobilize and strengthen community support for children and households whose own economic safety nets have failed, the other delivers financial and business development services to strengthen household economic safety nets. While it is possible for one organization to do both, there must be two clearly distinct program elements involved that are seen by the community as separate.

Donors and organizations concerned with orphans and other vulnerable children should actively explore such experiments. The following figures, supplied by the managing director of a microfinance institution (MFI) in Faulu, Nairobi (personal communication, May 1999), suggest the potential for such collaboration:

- The MFI reaches 9,140 registered members in 333 groups.
- The MFI has given out over 10,641 loans.
- The average cost per loan is 22 cents.
- For every 10 loans, 3 jobs are created.
- At least 9,800 jobs, along with income for that many households, have been stabilized.
- Those indirectly benefiting from income stabilization multiplies by a factor of five (49,000) and three out of those five are children (16,333).

TABLE 2.5. *Guide for Microenterprise Options*

Type of Intervention	Target Population* (In Terms of Productive Capacity and Vulnerability to Poverty)
Microfinance institutions	• Everyone in the community who meets the MFI's eligibility criteria • Household has adults capable of productive activity • Is vulnerable or somewhat vulnerable to poverty (poor or not-so-poor)
ROSCAs	• Open to everyone in community who is interested and has some productive capacity, but is unable or unwilling to absorb debt. • Is vulnerable or very vulnerable to poverty (poor and poorer)
Market linkages	• Open to everyone in community who is interested • Has some productive capacity, but is unable or unwilling to absorb debt. • Is vulnerable or very vulnerable to poverty (poor and poorer)
Advice/guidance and training on economic opportunities (perhaps coupled with provision of small grants)	• Could be productive but has sold off all assets and liquidated all savings (covering, for example, medical or funeral expenses, paying for care of orphans). • Is destitute but has not always been so. Needs temporary boost to get back on feet. Needs to switch to economic opportunity that is less demanding or time-consuming
Relief assistance (permanent or temporary)	• Needs temporary assistance to avoid break up of household or is permanently disabled and needs assistance indefinitely (household or individual is coping with advanced stages of AIDS). • Is destitute and has no productive capacity

Note: ROSCAs = rotating savings and credit associations; MFI = microfinance institution.
*HIV/AIDS-affected categories such as widows, orphans, orphan caregivers, and people living with HIV/AIDS cut across all the targets.

Table 2.5 presents an illustrative guide for a range of microenterprise options for households affected by HIV/AIDS. The table could form the basis of a conceptual framework to guide collaboration between microenterprise practitioners and programs for children and communities affected by HIV/AIDS.

Besides the operational challenges inherent in combining projects from different technical sectors, devising effective economic strengthening strategies is complicated further by two other factors: (1) The financial and social needs of households and communities change as HIV/AIDS-related crises evolve; and (2) HIV/AIDS does not affect each household in the same way. Therefore, it is not possible to propose a "one-size-fits-all" solution, no neat package of responses to the financial stress brought on by HIV/AIDS. However, a judicious blending of appropriately targeted interventions can make a critical difference.

Families and communities are not only on the front line of the impacts of HIV/AIDS, they *are* the front line of response to the impact that children encounter. Communities are not only concerned about the impacts of HIV/AIDS on children, they also are prepared to take leadership, demonstrate ownership, and devise ways of sustaining the activities they initiate. Communities are the key stakeholders.

The burden is on development professionals to find ever more innovative ways to demonstrate solidarity with the households and communities we support. Another old adage says, "Where there is a will, there is a way." There are ways, albeit not easy ones, to collaborate with one another and to forge multisectoral alliances. What is required is the will to make them happen.

References

Adelski, E., P. Bourdeau, J. B. Doamba, T. Lairez, and J. P. Ouedraogo. 2001. Final impact evaluation report on development activity proposal. Catholic Relief Services, Burkina Faso, May.

Ainsworth, M, and D. Filmer. 2002. Poverty, AIDS, and children's schooling: A targeting dilemma. World Bank Policy Research Working Paper 2885. Operations Evaluation Department and Development Research Group, World Bank, September. Available at http://www.worldbank.org

Chen, M. A., and E. Dunn. 1996. Household economic portfolios. AIMS paper. Harvard University and University of Missouri-Columbia, June.

Christen, R. P., E. Rhyne, R. Vogel, and C. McKean. 1995. *Maximizing the outreach of microenterprise finance: The emerging lessons of successful programs.* Arlington, VA: Interactive Multimedia and Collaborative Communications Alliance for USAID/Center for the Development of Information and Evaluation, July.

de Bruyn, M. 1992. Women and AIDS in developing countries. *Social Science & Medicine* 34 (3): 249–62.

Donahue, J. 1998. Community-based economic support for households affected by HIV/AIDS. Discussion Paper on HIV/AIDS Care and Support no. 6. Arlington, VA: Health Technical Services Project for USAID, June.

————. 2002. Children, HIV/AIDS and poverty in Southern Africa. Paper presented at the Southern Africa Regional Poverty Network, Pretoria, April 9–10.

Donahue, J., K. Kabuccho, and S. Osinde. 2001. *HIV/AIDS: Responding to a silent crisis among microfinance clients in Kenya and Uganda.* Nairobi, Kenya: MicroSave and at www.microsave.com. September. Available at http://www.alternative-finance.org.uk/

Donahue, J., and J. Williamson. 1999. *Community mobilization to mitigate the impacts of HIV/AIDS.* Washington, DC: Displaced Children and Orphans Fund, USAID, September 1.

Hope, A., and S. Timmel. 1995. *Training for transformation: A handbook for community workers.* London: ITDG Publishing.

IAPAD (Integrated Approaches to Participatory Development). n.d. Participatory Learning and Action. Available at http://www.iapad.org

Marsland, N. 2002. Household food economy analysis and the effect of HIV/AIDS on food security at the household level. Paper presented to the Southern Africa Regional Poverty Network, Pretoria, April. [Based on study conducted by Save the Children UK Food Security Unit in conjunction with the Famine Early Warning Systems Network in Kenya and Zambia.]

MkNelly, B., and C. Dunford. 1996. Are credit and savings services effective against hunger and malnutrition? A literature review and analysis. Freedom from Hunger Research Paper no. 1, February. http://www.ffhtechnical.org/publications/pdf.Cw_E_R1_Review.pdf

Mutangadura, G. B. 1999. The economic impact of AIDS. Paper prepared by the POLICY Project of The Futures Group International for the Agency for International Development, March 16.

————. 2000. Household welfare impacts of mortality of adult females in Zimbabwe: Implications for policy and program development. Draft report prepared for UNAIDS, May.

Mutangadura, G. B., D. Mukurazita, and H. Jackson. 1999. *A review of household and community responses to the HIV/AIDS epidemic in the rural areas of sub-Saharan Africa.* UNAIDS Best Practice Collection. Geneva: UNAIDS, June.

Narayan, D., ed. 2000. *Voices of the poor: Can anyone hear us?* New York: Oxford University Press, published for the World Bank.

Neema, S. 1998. Afflicted and affected: Consequences of HIV/AIDS on women in a farming community in Uganda. Paper presented at the East and Southern Africa Regional Conference on Responding to HIV/AIDS: Development Needs of African Smallholder Agriculture, Harare, June.

Over, M. 1998. Coping with the impact of AIDS. *Finance and Development*, March, 22–4.

Parker, J., I. Singh, and K. Hattel. 2000. *The role of microfinance in the fight against HIV/AIDS.* UNAIDS Background Paper. A report to The Joint United Nations Programme on HIV/AIDS (UNAIDS). Bethesda, MD: Development Alternatives, Inc., September. Available at http://www.dai.com/pdfs/UNAIDS_policy_Paper_on_Microfinance.pdf

Rutherford, S. 2000. The poor and their money. Paper distributed by the Institute for Development Policy and Management, University of Manchester, January.

Sebstad, J., and M. A. Chen. 1996. Overview of studies on the impact of microenterprise credit. AIMS paper. Management Systems International, Washington, DC, June.

Sebstad, J., and M. Cohen. 2000. Microfinance, risk management, and poverty. *AIMS Synthesis Study Commissioned for World Development Report* 2000/2001, World Bank, Washington, DC, March. http://www.usaidmicro.org/pdfs/asims/wdr_report.pdr.

UNAIDS. 1999. A review of household and community responses to the HIV/AIDS epidemic in the rural areas of sub-Saharan Africa. Best Practices Collection. Geneva, Switzerland.

UNICEF. 1998. *The state of the world's children 1998.* New York: UNICEF. http://www.unicef.org.sowc98/approach6.htm

USAID, UNICEF, and UNAIDS. 2002. *Children on the brink 2002: A joint report on orphan estimates and program strategies.* Washington, DC: TvT Associates/The Synergy Project, USAID. http://www.unicef.org/publications/pub_children_on_the_brink_en.pdf

Williamson, J., and J. Donahue. 2001. *A review of the COPE program and its strengthening of AIDS committee structures.* UNAIDS Displaced Children and Orphans Fund. Arlington, VA. May.

World Bank. n.d. Participatory Rural Appraisal (PRA). http://www.worldbank/poverty/impact/methods/pra.htm

Wright, G. A. N., D. Kasente, G. Ssemogerere, and L. Mutesasira. 1999. Vulnerability, risks, assets, and empowerment: The impact of microfinance on poverty alleviation. Commissioned in preparation for the *World Development Report 2001,* MicroSave-Africa and Uganda Women's Finance Trust, March. http://www.undp.org/sum/MicroSave/ftp_downloads/UWFTstudyFinal.pdf

3

The Response of the Educational System to the Needs of Orphans and Children Affected by HIV/AIDS

Michael J. Kelly

> Everyone has the right to education. Education shall be free, at least in the elementary and fundamental stages. Elementary education shall be compulsory.
> – *United Nations Universal Declaration of Human Rights*,
> Art. 26, December 1948

> States Parties recognize the right of the child to education, and with a view to achieving this right progressively and on the basis of equal opportunity, they shall, in particular . . . make primary education compulsory and available free to all.
> – *United Nations Convention on the Rights of the Child*,
> Art. 28, November 1989

Despite international declarations asserting that children have a basic right to free elementary and fundamental education, this essential foundation for life is denied to millions of children around the world. As the international aid organization Oxfam has observed, "No human right is more systematically or extensively violated by governments than the right of their citizens to a basic education" (Watkins 2000: 1). Currently, more than 113 million children of primary school age are not in school, while as many as 150 million may not complete their primary schooling, dropping out before they have achieved sustainable mastery of basic literacy, numeracy, and social competencies (World Bank 2002). Moreover, in a disastrous feminization of illiteracy, two-thirds of those not attending school or dropping out early are girls.

Vacillating political commitment, inadequate vision, and lack of financial resources have helped create this situation, but over the past two decades the HIV/AIDS pandemic has played a major role in sustaining it. Moreover, HIV/AIDS continues to hit hard at children's access to school, their educational performance, and their ability to complete school. Of the thirty-two developing countries unlikely to reach the international development target of having all children in primary school by

2015, twenty are among those most affected by HIV/AIDS (World Bank 2002).

In the absence of significant and comprehensive interventions, HIV/AIDS will continue to undermine the educational prospects of children and the potential of schools to assist young people to achieve a fulfilling adult life. This chapter advocates changing this situation through interventions within and outside the current educational framework.

There are four imperatives for existing educational structures:

- Eliminating all primary school cash costs.
- Easing the cash and labor losses sustained by poor families when children attend school.
- Establishing school conditions and an environment in which every child can experience real and relevant learning.
- Involving a wide variety of partners in a collaborative education process.

More radically, however, we need an expanded vision that sees the answer to the needs of all children, including those affected by HIV/AIDS, as lying within communities. This expanded vision would place the school at the heart of the community and the community at the heart of the school.

HIV/AIDS AND SCHOOLING

HIV/AIDS makes it difficult for many children to enroll in or complete school, attend school on a regular basis, or perform as they should in school. Three different groups of children are affected by these difficulties: HIV-infected children, orphans and other children affected by HIV/AIDS, and children who become heads of household when their parents or guardians die. The situations faced by each of these groups are considered in the next three sections.

HIV-Infected Children

Some HIV-positive school-age children may have already been infected before they began school. A small percentage infected perinatally may survive to school age and into adolescence and adulthood. Others are infected later as a result of sexual abuse or exploitation, a pattern found in many countries. The plight of abused and exploited children is often made worse because they are afraid to report what has been done to them. They fear the perpetrator, fear they will not be believed, or fear that disclosure will cause discrimination and ostracism. Sexual abuse increases children's risk of HIV infection. When sexual abuse occurs within the family, solidarity and shame can pressure children and parents into silence (UNICEF 2002). Silence makes the crime less visible to the community at large, thus both limiting any effort to prevent it and compounding the victims' emotional pain. In South Africa, which reportedly has one of the highest rates of violence against women in the world, both rape and sexual abuse of children are increasing rapidly, causing grave concern. From 1996 to 1998, girls aged seventeen and under constituted approximately 40 percent of reported rape and attempted rape victims nationally. Girls aged twelve to seventeen experienced the highest rape ratio (471 cases per 100,000 females in the population), while the ratio for girls aged eleven and below was alarming (130 rapes for every 100,000) (Human Rights Watch 2001: IV-6).

One girl who did speak out said:

I am seventeen years old. I believe that teachers can have a huge impact on the lives of learners who are affected and infected by AIDS. I lost my mother and sister in 1999 and in 2000 I was raped by my father. A year later I discovered that I was HIV positive. The first person who knew about this was a teacher and the attitude that she had is the cause of my positive thinking in life.

(Children's Testimony 2002)

Some children become infected during their school years. The well-documented HIV prevalence among fifteen-to-nineteen-year-olds, especially the higher rates for girls in many countries, provides stark evidence of adolescent infection. Because there is a latency period of several years between initial HIV infection and progression to AIDS, the occurrence of AIDS in fifteen-to-nineteen-year-olds means that many girls and some boys became HIV-infected in early adolescence or as children. The higher rates of HIV prevalence among those in their early twenties show that teenage infection with HIV is extensive, among both boys and girls, though more so among girls. The reality for young people of school age, "the AIDS generation" (Kiragu 2001), is that appreciable numbers of them in Africa are HIV-infected. Families, communities, and schools must face the reality that HIV infection occurs at young ages, and must give these children and teenagers the support that they need.

Moreover, school-related circumstances aggravate the risk to students of becoming HIV-infected. Numerous factors are at play here, singly and in combination:

- the early sexual activity of a substantial proportion of those attending school,
- schools serving children of widely divergent ages,
- sexual harassment on the way to or from school,
- sexual harassment and pressure by fellow students and teachers,
- unsupervised boarding or other school accommodation arrangements,
- pressure to conform to the perceived expectations and practices of peers and colleagues,
- failure of adult society to set appropriate standards and expectations,
- double societal standards for the sexual behavior of males and females,

- transactional sex, whereby sex is traded for material, financial, or academic favors from "sugar-daddies," "sugar-mummies," and individuals who control valued resources,
- school or college as the locus for rape or coerced sex (Jewkes et al. 2002), and
- reluctance of adults to acknowledge these factors and provide guidance and support to children.

The majority of infected children may not be aware of their HIV status, but as the symptoms of AIDS start appearing, they begin to experience extensive school-related problems. In addition to suffering and trauma, their condition will often occasion fear, anxiety, and uneasiness in their schoolmates and teachers. Academic and administrative leaders are seldom prepared to respond to the special needs of young people living with HIV/AIDS. Students may find that uninformed school authorities place unnecessary restraints on their participation in school activities. They may experience stigma, discrimination, and social ostracism. Recurring bouts of illness interrupt their attendance and diminish their learning opportunities. Eventually they may stop attending school. The evidence from institutions of higher learning is that many students who learn that they have AIDS simply fail to return after a vacation. It may well be the same in primary and secondary schools.

What action should schools take concerning their HIV-positive students? The first step is to establish an accepting and welcoming atmosphere in which there is no suspicion, no anxiety, and certainly no stigma or discrimination. It may take considerable skill to educate all members of a school community, as well as parents and other stakeholders, but the human dignity of infected students cannot be maintained by anything less.

Establishing an understanding and open-minded atmosphere requires, in turn, resolute efforts by school authorities and teachers to learn more about HIV/AIDS, the modes of HIV transmission, the ethic of confidentiality, and the need for the complete rejection of any form of stigma or discrimination. School staff members also need information on standard infection control precautions, as well as training to build confidence in their ability to manage issues relating to HIV-positive children. All of this occurs more easily in a school that has incorporated HIV/AIDS into its curriculum.

Equipped with these understandings, school staff have the challenge of ensuring the full integration of HIV-positive learners into the institution's life and activities. The principle of inclusiveness requires that they do so with every learner, regardless of the individual's special needs, and it is no different for the child who is HIV-positive. The full institutional assimilation of such a child brings the added advantage of affirming powerfully and naturally the inherent dignity and value of every person living with HIV/AIDS, which is a crucial component in the global struggle against the disease.

The school will also need to make special provisions to enable those whose learning is interrupted by illness to make up for lost time and catch up on delayed opportunities. Responding to this need can be a very practical expression of acceptance. Because such provisions require extra effort by teachers and accommodation by other students, they become a measure by which the humanity of an institution can be gauged.

Schools can also manifest support for those with HIV by emphasizing in appropriate parts of the curriculum the importance of a healthy lifestyle. Healthy living is one way of slowing down the progression from HIV to AIDS. All other things being equal, people with HIV who maintain a healthy lifestyle – eat balanced, nourishing meals, do not smoke, drink alcohol, or use harmful drugs, and get adequate exercise and rest – are likely to enjoy more years of life than those who do not follow this regimen.

A person living with HIV/AIDS testified:

> I was diagnosed HIV positive 10 years ago, and I have not yet developed AIDS. Like tuberculosis, a person can have the virus for years without developing symptoms. I do not get any medical treatment. The medication I get is by eating the right food. I strictly get the right diet to make me live long. I use food as my treatment if I get sick on a day. There is a purpose of knowing that you're HIV positive if you don't yet have AIDS. It helps you a lot to know, in order to change your behaviour, so you can live long. HIV destroys your immunity, so knowing you have it early helps you change your lifestyle, like what you eat.
>
> (Hall 2002: 10)

Information about the significance of living in a healthy way is an important message that educators can always communicate because it is valuable to all learners, irrespective of their HIV status. For those infected, it can be a life-prolonging message. The message by itself, though, will not be meaningful to impoverished students unless they have sufficient resources to put it into practice. Schools can cooperate with programs that support home care or with social support services; they may even make food available directly to students. Living in a healthy way can help keep a learner alive until the time an effective treatment or a vaccine for HIV-infected persons becomes available.

Finally, schools should enable social welfare and medical providers to play their proper roles when their services are needed. They could also involve the wider community of parents, local groups, faith-based organizations, and others in providing direct assistance or supporting vulnerable children's access to formal services.

Orphans and Other Children Affected by HIV/AIDS

Prior to the HIV/AIDS pandemic, traditional social mechanisms generally were sufficient to provide some level of care for orphans and other children affected by outbreaks of disease. However, HIV/AIDS is creating orphans in numbers that exceed anything that communities hitherto have had to manage. The highest numbers of orphans are in countries where public welfare systems are inadequate, where the traditional extended family coping system has been weakened through poverty and urbanization, and where the sheer weight of numbers is threatening to overwhelm communities. Moreover, in the absence of courageous visionary measures to stem the growth in the number of orphans,[1] the problem and challenge will grow incomparably greater over the coming two to three decades. Children not yet orphaned but whose parents are ill can be as vulnerable as orphans – perhaps even more so. If they are caring for sick parents they are likely to be facing extreme economic pressure as their family tries to cope with increased health expenses and reduced income. (See Chapter 2.)

HIV/AIDS interferes with what schools can do for orphans and HIV-affected children in at least four ways: The children may be prevented from attending or remaining in school. If they do attend, their ability to learn may be compromised. The school's ability to respond to their real learning needs may be impeded. And finally, HIV/AIDS generates special psychological and emotional needs.

The Importance of Schooling to Orphans. Orphaned children in particular need schooling. With the loss of a parent or significant adult, their lives may be on the verge of disintegration, leaving them frozen in a state of uncertainty, bewilderment, confusion, and anxiety. A Zambian survey found a high proportion of orphans who feel unhappy, have trouble sleeping, and experience nightmares (FHI and SCOPE-OVC 2002). Even uncomprehending, they try to cope with a life governed by a new set of parameters, but they are not sure of the extent to which they can trust this life that has cheated and deprived them so painfully.

School attendance is one of the greatest antidotes to this sense of insecurity and worry. Schooling is characterized by normality and routines, factors that help an orphaned child cope with disturbing and bewildering events. It provides a social milieu where a child can relate to peers and adults in an atmosphere of ordinariness and predictability. Thus schooling helps the child develop a renewed sense of efficacy in relation to life and its circumstances, restores some lost confidence, and offers hope that life can move forward. "School restores structure to young lives; it provides a

---

[1] One such measure would be to take steps to keep mothers alive. In the circumstances of HIV/AIDS, keeping mothers alive means being prepared to provide antiretroviral treatment not only to HIV-positive pregnant mothers but also to all HIV-positive mothers with young children who still need their mother's care. Keeping a mother alive prevents the disintegration of the family and the growing number of orphans. Providing antiretroviral therapy for these mothers throughout life would be at significant economic cost, but it is a cost that would preempt even more costly social consequences and economic outlays if families fall apart and orphan numbers continue to swell.

measure of stability in the midst of chaos; it trains the mind, rehabilitates the spirit, and offers critical, life-sustaining hope to a child in the face of an otherwise uncertain future" (Donovan 2000: 3).

In addition to the stability that it can bring into the life of an orphan, a school environment can enable a child to develop socially and emotionally and gain knowledge and skills to progress through adolescence to adult life. World leaders (World Summit for Children 1990: 1) added a further dimension in the *World Declaration on the Survival, Protection, and Development of Children* when they affirmed that the time of childhood "should be one of joy and peace, of playing, learning and growing." Zambia, the country where I have done most of my work, has reformulated this statement by affirming that "the school environment should be such that it ensures each young person's right to a joyful, safe and formative childhood and early adolescence" (Ministry of Education 1996: 29). One hopes that school might also be a place where an orphan would be free to play, experience joy, and know happiness.

Barriers to School Participation. Because of HIV/AIDS, many children never enroll in school; those who do frequently arrive late or miss class altogether, and may eventually drop out. Chief among the many factors leading to this situation are costs, family responsibilities, and doubts about the value of schooling. Costs include: school fees; levies imposed by parent-teacher associations for school operations, maintenance, and development; the costs of educational materials (books, writing paper, pencils); material items that learners are asked to provide (brooms, printing paper, garden tools, and so forth); school uniforms; and (sometimes) supplementation for teachers' salaries. Typically, the cash costs associated with primary school attendance in many developing countries range from fifteen to sixty dollars a year – seemingly a small amount, but unavailable to large numbers of households that eke out their existence on less than a dollar a day. For Western observers, it is astonishing to find out how pathetically small an amount prevents orphans and vulnerable children from attending school.

Poor families in rural areas and in urban shantytowns have always found it difficult to meet the cash costs associated with schooling, a difficulty aggravated by HIV/AIDS. Evidence from various parts of Africa shows significant declines in both family income and food consumption when a family member has AIDS. Very frequently these declines occur because adults must reduce their working time to take care of the person who is sick. A Tanzanian survey found that in households where one person was sick with AIDS, 29 percent of labor was spent on AIDS-related matters. The average household loss from agricultural activities was 43 percent if two household members were devoted to nursing duties (UNAIDS-UNECA 2000). In Côte d'Ivoire, following an AIDS death, average household consumption fell 44 percent from the previous year. Households with a member living with AIDS spent twice as much on medical expenses as other households (Béchu 1998). The United Nations Food and Agriculture Organization (FAO 2001: 6) has observed: "Classically, a downward spiral of the family/household's welfare begins when the first adult in a household falls ill. There is increased spending for health care, decreased productivity and higher demands for care. Food production and income drop dramatically as more adults are affected. Once savings are gone, the family seeks support from relatives, borrows money or sells its productive assets."

In such difficult circumstances, school expenses fall low in a family's order of priorities. Often, children drop out because the family cannot afford the costs. From a household perspective, school costs also include opportunity costs – the value of the domestic, farm, or trading activities that the child must forgo when attending school. A significant proportion of poor households affected by AIDS find it difficult to do without the contribution to their domestic economy that their children, particularly girls, can make. Consequently, many children must break off their schooling to shoulder the tasks of caring for the sick, caring for younger siblings, doing household chores, carrying water, collecting firewood, tending animals, weeding crops, and engaging in petty trading. Girls who have reached the age of puberty may also leave schooling for an early marriage, which may bring bride price resources to the household or provide the girl a more secure livelihood.

Children from poor families have always been vulnerable to the inroads of these demands on their potential school time, especially in rural areas where the age at which children attend school is less well established than in urban areas. AIDS has increased and intensified household reliance on children's labor.

In addition to forcing some children to drop out, HIV/AIDS increases absences among those who stay in school. Children may miss school because of:

- Periodic home demands for the child's help arising from the sickness of a household member. A study of sixty-five primary schools in Malawi found that one-third of all the children stated that they sometimes missed school to care for someone who was sick (Harris and Schubert 2001).
- Children's illnesses for which treatment cannot be obtained because of AIDS-compounded poverty.
- A death in the family or local community, followed by funeral attendance and periods of mourning.

Family doubts about the value of schooling also contribute to low participation rates, particularly in rural areas. The poor quality of education available in many schools is a significant factor. Poor families often say that they would be prepared to pay for their children to go to school if they felt that worthwhile learning was taking place, but what they perceive to be poor educational quality deters them from paying school costs and from sacrificing their children's time to school attendance. HIV/AIDS undermines quality and escalates this problem because it erodes teaching time, as we will discuss. A second influence, more directly AIDS-related, is a fatalistic disillusion with education. Older people ask: Why bother sending children to school when they will die young from AIDS and not reap the benefits of their education?

The School Participation of Orphans. In the precarious educational circumstances of children affected by HIV/AIDS, orphans are at least as vulnerable as other children, and many are even more so. However, evidence about their access to school is mixed. While studies at the community level frequently have found that orphans are disadvantaged in terms of school attendance, some large surveys are less conclusive. A study in the Copperbelt (Rossi and Reijer 1995) – one of the regions in Zambia most affected by HIV/AIDS – found that of the 44 percent of school-age children who were not attending school, proportionately more orphans (53.6 percent) than non-orphans (42.4 percent) were not attending. A 1998 national survey in Zambia (Living Conditions Monitoring Survey 1998), however, found that paternal orphans actually had slightly higher enrollment rates than those with both parents living, while the enrollment rates for double orphans were much the same as those for children whose parents were alive. The reason may be that targeting educational assistance to orphans has given them an advantage in a poor society. Or it may be that children in the most difficult circumstances, such as those on the street or in child-headed households, can easily be overlooked by a national-level household survey.

Research by the World Bank (Ainsworth and Filmer 2002) comparing the school enrollment of orphans to other children in twenty-eight countries (in Africa, Asia, the Caribbean, Central America, and South America) found considerable variation. Orphans were enrolled at lower rates in twenty-two of the countries, at the same rate in four, and at higher rates in two (see Table 3.1). Among the countries where orphans were disadvantaged, significant differences were found between countries where all orphans were enrolled at lower rates and those where lower rates were found only among children who had lost their mother, father, or both parents.

The Ainsworth and Filmer (2002) study found that enrollment was strongly influenced by income level, and the authors question whether orphan status by itself should be used to target educational assistance. They recommend that, because of the variations identified in the situation of orphans, interventions to improve orphan participation in education should be country-specific. To increase school participation, as in other

TABLE 3.1. *Comparison of Orphan School Enrollment in 28 Countries*

Enrollment Differential	Number of Countries
All orphans have lower enrollment rates than non-orphans	10
Only maternal orphans have lower enrollment rates than non-orphans	2
Only paternal orphans have lower enrollment rates than non-orphans	1
Only two-parent orphans have lower enrollment rates than non-orphans	2
Maternal and two-parent orphans have lower enrollment rates than non-orphans	4
Paternal and two-parent orphans have lower enrollment rates than non-orphans	3
Orphans and other children are equally likely to be enrolled	4
Orphans have higher enrollment	2
TOTAL	28

Source: Adapted from Ainsworth and Filmer 2002, Table 2.

areas of orphan care and support, "there appears to be no single 'best practice' option applicable to all countries in all circumstances" (Subbarao, Mattimore, and Plangemann 2001: viii). The variations found in the situations of orphans underscore the programming principle that, rather than targeting orphans exclusively, programs for AIDS-affected children should be directed to the communities most seriously affected by HIV/AIDS, and that the most vulnerable children within them should be identified by community members (USAID, UNICEF, and UNAIDS 2002: 35).

The Learning Capacity of Children Affected by HIV/AIDS. In poor households further impoverished by AIDS, children's capacity to learn is imperiled by a combination of poor nutrition, hunger, trauma, and emotional distress. On its own, each of these factors has a negative effect on learning capacity. Taken together, they impair thinking, ability to attend to environmental stimuli, and performance on school tests.

The learning capacity of all children from poor families is endangered by poor nutritional status and hunger, but the situation of orphans in poor households is likely to be even worse. Data from Zambia, for example, show that 56 percent of orphaned children and 49 percent of non-orphaned children were short for their age (Government of Zambia 1999). Research led by K. Subbarao (Subbarao et al. 2001: 10) in Tanzania also shows that "the loss of either parent and the deaths of other adults in the household will worsen height for age and [increase] stunting of children."

Some qualitative studies show that orphans may be the last to receive their share of food, forcing them to make do with leftovers. Their already compromised nutritional status may decline further, and with it their capacity to learn. For orphans, the inhibiting effects of malnutrition and hunger on learning are aggravated by trauma and emotional distress.

The pain of losing a parent remains for a long time. Many children have had the experience of seeing a parent or other loved adult enduring the devastating effects of AIDS, culminating in remorseless suffering and a dehumanizing death. The child's distress is often compounded by denial and silence within the household, as well as by community talk and gossip. After a parent's death, children's emotional pain may be increased by separation from siblings and familiar surroundings and worsened by family dissension over claims to the dead parent's property. Coming to terms with loss is inhibited in some cultures where boys are discouraged from expressing their grief. In some cases, survival demands prevent bereaved children from having sufficient time to grieve or adjust to their loss. (See also Chapter 4.)

This emotional turmoil affects children's ability to learn. Often, teachers report that orphaned children are apathetic, listless, excessively reserved or inappropriately serious in the classroom, and do not play and laugh as much as other children. They are often unable to mix freely with their schoolmates.

The distress and barriers to learning faced by some children affected by AIDS are increased by their schoolmates' teasing and a lack of response by the school community to their emotional needs. Orphans have reported such barbed comments as, "So your father died of that disease," or "Why do you want me to lend you a pencil? Ask your mother to buy one for you – oh, I forgot, you have no mother." Teachers sometimes aggravate the situation by insensitive remarks or by unwillingness to make allowances for children's late arrival, absenteeism, or shabby clothing. Such prejudice can push AIDS-affected children further into the isolation of their own melancholy world.

Children Who Become Heads of Households

In addition to orphans, infected children, and others affected by the disease, HIV/AIDS has led to the emergence of a relatively new sociological phenomenon – the child-headed household: All the adult members of the household have died, leaving the children to fend for themselves. Generally the oldest child assumes economic and quasiparental responsibility for the others, most of whom are siblings or at least have close blood ties. Similar groups are also formed by street children whose bond is their common need to survive. In 1998, there were an estimated forty-five thousand child-headed households in Rwanda, while in communities in Swaziland severely affected by AIDS, about 10 percent of homesteads were headed by children (Brody 2002; Subbarao et al. 2001).

Access to school is very uncertain for such children. They often have no way of meeting school-related costs, and the demands of sheer survival may take precedence over going to school. As difficult as the situation is for child-headed households, there have been numerous accounts of older children making superb, generous efforts to ensure that at least some of their younger siblings attend school.

THE ABILITY OF SCHOOLS TO RESPOND TO THE NEEDS OF LEARNERS

AIDS is also undermining the capacity of educational systems to serve all students, and particularly to meet the special needs of students affected by the epidemic. An adequate response is currently beyond the capacity of many schools and educational systems because they have been devastated by sickness, absenteeism, declining morale, and an increasing number of deaths among teachers and other education personnel.

Permanent Teacher Losses

There is some debate about whether teachers are at higher risk than others of HIV infection (World Bank 2002, Bennell 2005, Kinghorn and Kelly 2005). But at a minimum, HIV/AIDS affects at least the same proportion of educators (teachers, administrators, finance and planning personnel, inspectors, etc.) as adults in the general population. Thus, in the most severely affected countries, a quarter or more of the educators are HIV-positive and likely to die in the decade ahead.

The illness or death of educators who hold nonteaching positions can seriously weaken an educational system, but the death of a teacher brings immediate consequences to classrooms. Unless there is a prompt replacement (something that seldom happens in the most severely affected countries) a whole class is left without a teacher for a considerable period. UNICEF (2000) has estimated that 860,000 children in sub-Saharan Africa lost teachers to AIDS in 1999. In the Central African Republic alone, 107 primary schools had to close in the 1998–99 school year (Tassa 2000). The loss of personnel due to AIDS in the private sector and other branches of government service has further contributed to the loss of educators, as better-paying jobs lure them out of the school system to replace those who have died.

Teacher Absenteeism

Teacher absenteeism due to illness associated with HIV/AIDS is also responsible for an extensive loss of teaching time. For many months prior to AIDS-related deaths, the progressive nature of the disease results in periodic bouts of illness that keep teachers from school. The World Bank (2000: 21) has estimated that the professional service of each infected educator is reduced by an average of six months before HIV progresses to AIDS; another twelve months are lost thereafter.

Recurrent teacher absences could well be more detrimental to learning than the permanent absence that follows death, when schools may be able to amalgamate classes so that the affected children get some form of teaching. Such measures may not be undertaken when an ill teacher is expected to return soon to the classroom.

Teacher absenteeism also occurs when healthy teachers must help care for ill family members or attend funerals. But no matter the reason, AIDS-related teacher absenteeism has at least two negative consequences for educational systems: It reduces student learning opportunities, and it gives administrators the false impression that teaching and learning are continuing satisfactorily because the absences are not permanent.

Teacher Morale

The frequent experience of serious sickness and death in teachers' families, communities, and schools undermines teacher morale. The decline is aggravated when teachers see their incomes consumed by medical and funeral expenses within their families and sometimes by local fund-raising ventures to support orphans and other vulnerable children. There is also an underlying sense of uneasiness and fear arising from what they observe around them, from concern that they too may have the virus, and from a fatalistic sense of hopelessness about the value of HIV testing when there is little prospect that effective treatment will be available. Many yearn to know their HIV status but are also afraid to find out.

Sickness, absenteeism, death, and falling morale among teachers combine to undermine both the quality of teaching provided and the quality of learning possible. This is detrimental for all learners, but for orphans and children affected by HIV/AIDS it can be calamitous.

The Impact of HIV/AIDS on Resources for Education

While the HIV/AIDS epidemic is increasing the demands on educational systems, it is at the same time reducing the financial and other resources these systems need for their operations. HIV/AIDS reduces the public funds available for education by reducing national resources overall and influencing their allocation. Models of the impact of HIV/AIDS on national economies generally show the annual gross domestic product (GDP) growth rate as lower than it would have been in the absence of AIDS but do not show any actual decline in GDP (Barnett and Whiteside 2002: 283–94).

A lower growth rate means fewer resources for public spending. A country's HIV/AIDS epidemic affects the allocation of resources among and within sectors. It may result in an increased proportion of public resources going to health services and a smaller proportion to education and other services. Within the education sector, HIV/AIDS tends to increase the need for resources at secondary and tertiary levels. While teacher losses at these levels are not necessarily higher, training and replacement costs are.

THE APPROPRIATENESS OF THE SCHOOL CURRICULUM

Mainstreaming HIV/AIDS Issues

HIV/AIDS has particular implications for school curricula. The first and basically correct response of education ministries to the HIV/AIDS crisis has been to strive to incorporate aspects of HIV/AIDS, sexual and reproductive health, and life skills education into school curricula. A review of studies from seventeen countries found that education ministries were seeking to integrate these areas into school instruction with a view to preventing HIV infection (Akoulouze, Rugalema, and Khanye 2001). Regrettably, these efforts have not yet been very effective (Bennell, Hyde, and Swainson 2002; UNECA 2000). However, with a deeper understanding of how to mainstream HIV/AIDS instruction into school curricula, education ministries continue to implement initiatives they hope will empower learners to live sexually responsible, healthy lives (Kelly 2002).

Sexuality and healthy living are the two principal areas around which HIV/AIDS-related programs must be developed. These involve (1) learning behaviors to protect against contracting or passing on HIV, and (2) knowing how to maintain a healthy lifestyle both to prevent HIV and to slow the progression from HIV infection to AIDS. From these must flow the values and attitudes that can change the trajectory of an HIV/AIDS epidemic.

Every young person has a right to this kind of knowledge. According to the United Nations *Convention on the Rights of the Child*, "The child shall have the right to freedom of expression; this right shall include freedom to seek, receive and impart information and ideas of all kinds" (1989, Art. 13). Schools are bound by this statement to equip learners with information about HIV/AIDS, about protecting oneself against infection, and about practical ways of coping in the event of infection.

Learning in this area is especially important for orphans and children otherwise affected by HIV/AIDS. The harm that the disease has already caused these children, and their own risk of HIV infection, demand that they gain the knowledge and have access to the resources they need to protect themselves against further harm (UNICEF 1999). They need to grasp in practical ways that maintaining a healthy way of living is in itself a substantial step in the direction of preventing HIV infection, and coping with the disease should it occur.

The Need for a More Practically Oriented Curriculum

Schools must also equip children more purposefully for the life they face. Essential competencies needed by children at the end of primary school should include:

*   literacy, comprising adequate reading, writing, and expository skills in their own and one international language,
*   numeracy, comprising basic computational skills and the ability to interpret simple numerical data and charts,
*   some knowledge about the approach, methods, and procedures of science and technology,
*   how to learn (how to find, extract, and use information),
*   how to live with others, accepting diversity, interdependence, and a common basic humanity, and
*   how to live healthy and sexually responsible lives.

But where the level of HIV infection is high, there is additional need for practical skills more immediately oriented toward the work and household environments. Depending on the economic environment, these may include horticultural, agricultural, household economy, mechanical, entrepreneurial, electronic, or other skills. One reason schools must teach such skills is that AIDS is forcing children prematurely to find ways to support themselves and younger siblings. It is also reducing the number of adults who normally would transmit such skills to young people. Recognizing that AIDS disrupts intergenerational mechanisms for transferring knowledge, values, and beliefs, the United Nations Food and Agriculture Organization (FAO 2001: 14) has raised the concern that "agricultural skills may be lost since children are unable to observe their parents working. Due to gender divisions, a surviving parent is not always able to teach the skills and knowledge of the deceased partner."

In response to the needs of individual HIV/AIDS-affected learners, as well as in response to the needs of a society in danger of losing certain crucial skills, school systems should be asking what they can do. Regrettably, few seem to be doing much, and most continue to see their mandate as providing an education with a heavy academic bias that is strongly oriented toward further progression within the education system. In the climate of HIV/AIDS, such an education does not meet the needs of children generally, and it particularly fails children affected by AIDS.

Some educators, pointing to past failures and the vastness of the challenge, balk at the notion of a more practically oriented primary school curriculum. While their misgivings might have been valid in a world without

HIV/AIDS, the onset of the epidemic calls for a radical change. In education, as in virtually every other sphere of life, the imperatives of HIV/AIDS necessitate the reappraisal of earlier understandings and practices. Kofi Annan, Secretary General of the United Nations, has called for an unprecedented response to the unprecedented HIV/AIDS crisis (United Nations 1999). Education systems and curriculum contents have yet to respond with meaningful efforts to equip the generation of young people – the HIV/AIDS generation – with economic survival skills in a world that the epidemic has changed irrevocably.

Addressing Psychological Needs of Children Affected by AIDS

It has already been noted that the trauma and psychological distress that HIV/AIDS causes orphans and other affected children can impair their capacity to learn. Dealing with this reality calls for considerable ability on the part of teachers and school administrators to provide emotional support to learners in distress. The stigmatization from which infected or affected learners can suffer causes deep wounds, leading them to question their efficacy and worth as persons. Affected children may suffer from depression, unresolved anger, resentment, fears, worries, and anxieties, which can generate behavioral problems such as excessive attention seeking, class disruption, fighting, ignoring school work, and risky sexual activity.

The epidemic has made emotional and psychological trauma part of the educational environment. HIV/AIDS brings to school "increasing numbers of intellectually, socially, and psychologically dysfunctional learners" (Coombe 2002: 20). Reports from some schools describe administrators and teachers as being almost overwhelmed by the seemingly endless experience of behavioral, emotional, and psychological problems brought into the classroom by infected and affected learners. The outcome is unsatisfactory all round. Children in need of understanding, guidance, and counseling are not having their needs met, while teachers feel frustrated, guilty, or demoralized by their inability to do more for learners who are in obvious need. Moreover, many teachers are themselves in need of counseling and support as they experience AIDS-related psychological turmoil.

Some initiatives to respond to the psychological needs of HIV/AIDS-traumatized children are within the immediate reach of school authorities and teachers. Others require more purposeful programs. Even without additional material resources, a committed and understanding school administrator can:

- help school staff recognize that in addition to providing for the cognitive needs of children they must also be prepared to respond to their emotional and psychological needs,

- develop a caring environment at both school and classroom levels that will stimulate children's sense of worth and self-esteem,
- ensure that the school genuinely offers security and safety for all learners and educators, with zero tolerance for every form of discrimination, violence, or abuse (Coombe 2002), and
- make rebuilding children's ability to trust life a task for everyone in the school, through establishing good relationships with children and giving them appropriate feedback and by playing, listening, supporting, keeping promises, and involving children in real tasks (International Save the Children Alliance 1996: 14).

Beyond these fundamental actions, the realities of HIV/AIDS require more purposeful preparation of all teachers in elements of counseling and care. In high prevalence countries, basic training in counseling skills should be integrated into preservice and inservice teacher training programs. In addition, there is a need for individuals with more specialized skills to help orphans and other HIV/AIDS-affected children. This points to the need for a cadre of guidance and counseling personnel, qualified to provide the support children need, and with the space and time to do so effectively (Bennell et al. 2002: 46). Counselors in educational settings should be able to provide services not only to learners in distress but also to educators who are themselves in need of support.

Expanding the cadre of counseling personnel will require enlarged, revamped programs in universities and training institutions. Hard decisions will have to be made to give priority to this area ahead of more traditional concerns. But HIV/AIDS is demanding a reexamination of priorities in every area. The needs of society and of learners will never be satisfied by addressing only situations that existed before the advent of the epidemic. A meaningful response requires adjustments in curricula and teacher preparation programs to respond to the new burdens. Such changes increase demands for already limited resources, but nothing less can provide for the emotional and psychological health of future generations.

Integrating AIDS-Affected Children into School Systems

Clearly, HIV/AIDS is making it increasingly difficult to ensure children's access to formal education. In response, various innovative efforts are being made or have been proposed to meet the basic educational needs of orphans and other vulnerable children. In some countries, communities have established their own free schools for children who for a variety of reasons do not attend public or government schools. The pressure to establish free schools can be gauged from their mushroom-like growth in Zambia, from 38 schools enrolling 6,600 children in 1996, to 1,149 schools with over 140,000 children in 2001 (Ministry of Education 2002). During the same period, enrollments in schools that charged fees increased only marginally, suggesting a major reason for the popularity of community schools. Being community owned and managed, they are often more adapted to the needs of local children and the economic realities in their daily schedule, management, and other arrangements. Community members with some minimum level of education serve as teachers, but typically they have had no formal training in education, a factor that may have adverse effects on the quality of education that such schools can provide.

Distance learning is another approach that has been used in some developing countries as a way to extend opportunities for education to remote or underserved areas. Interactive radio and other media programs are being used in mentored group settings to provide some of the basics of primary education to out-of-school children (World Bank 2002). The beneficiaries of these programs include orphans and some of the most disadvantaged children in a community.

Innovations such as community schools and distance education are appropriate responses to help meet the basic educational needs of orphans and other vulnerable children. However, caution must be taken to avoid establishing a different and possibly less complete form of education for children at risk. Targeting special education toward orphans and vulnerable children can have several disadvantages:

- the isolation of these children from their age-mates,
- their possible marginalization or stigmatization, and
- the danger that the special provision being made on their behalf might fall below the standards prevailing in more conventional settings.

Furthermore, governments hard-pressed for resources might see such alternative forms of education as community initiatives that need not attract the same level of public support provided to the formal school system. Moreover, the stability and normality that school should bring into the disoriented life of an orphan or HIV/AIDS-affected child are more likely to be experienced in a conventional educational setting than in one that consists largely of fellow orphans and other disadvantaged children.

These concerns highlight the need to ensure, where possible, that orphans can attend the same type of school as children with living parents. Programming principles for children affected by HIV/AIDS advise strongly against singling out children as "AIDS orphans" (USAID et al. 2002: 35). Education programs should not be singled out as intended for orphans or vulnerable children. Instead, as much as possible, the principle of inclusivity should rule. Unless there are very compelling reasons not to do so, these children should attend the same type of school and participate in the same programs as their community age-mates. Differential provision and specialized programmes could intensify their sense of social alienation and, if the alternative programmes are not adequately resourced, reduce the children's educational and life prospects.

This is not, however, to argue against community schools as an appropriate response by communities that lack other options. Indeed, there is much to be learned from community schools and the profound commitment to which their very existence testifies.

PAST, PRESENT, AND FUTURE

The response that school systems have made to the educational needs of children affected by HIV/AIDS can be conveniently summarized in answers to two questions: What have education systems done for orphans and HIV/AIDS-affected children in the past, and what are they doing for them now? The answers to a third question – what should school systems do for these children in the future? – help chart the way forward.

What Have Education Systems Done for Orphans and HIV/AIDS-Affected Children in the Past?

When the nature and impacts of HIV/AIDS first began to emerge, and for a long time thereafter, the formal education sector did not know how to respond. Education systems simply did not comprehend the extent of the epidemic, and the way it permeated and threatened to undermine the entire sector and its operations. The need to mobilize all available resources to protect students, educators, and the system itself was not yet understood. This lack of response was no different from that of most other public sectors and, indeed, no different from that of the majority of individuals.

The education sector was only dimly aware that orphans and children affected by HIV/AIDS were going to confront schools with a new challenge of immense proportions. Two global education conferences bear witness to this state of denial. The World Conference on Education for All (1990) in Jomtien, Thailand, does not even mention HIV/AIDS in its key reports, *World Declaration on Education for All* and *Framework for Action*. Article Three of *The World Declaration*, on universal access and equity, lists a number of groups that are underserved educationally, but orphans are not among them. Ten years later, with stunning obliviousness, the Dakar World Education Forum (2000) reaffirmed the Jomtien World Declaration and committed the world to the achievement of the Education for All goals and targets – but was all but silent on the rapidly growing number of orphans. Not mentioned in the *Dakar Framework for Action*, orphans are referred to only once in the more than forty pages of the final conference report (in the section reporting on a subplenary session titled "Overcoming the Effects of HIV/AIDS on Basic Education").

By late in the 1990s, some within the education sector had recognized that AIDS was causing lack of access to education for many orphans and other affected children. Most educators, though, seemed content to leave response measures to communities and nongovernmental organizations (NGOs). Essentially the only action by the education sector was to recognize that orphans and other children affected by AIDS were among various categories of vulnerable children (such as the poor, rural children, those in urban squatter areas, and girls), while giving little explicit consideration to their special access and learning needs. Recommendations for action now must take into account that for most of the first two decades of the epidemic, the education sector ignored the magnitude and complexity of the problems and the imperatives for action.

What Are Education Systems Doing for Orphans and HIV/AIDS-Affected Children Now?

Education systems are only gradually emerging from a state of denial regarding HIV/AIDS and orphans. Despite warnings on the need for action (Schaeffer 1994), the education sector has allowed the dimensions of the situations of orphans in the AIDS epidemic to grow to almost unmanageable proportions where schooling is concerned. There is some halting recognition of the magnitude of the challenge posed by orphans and HIV/AIDS-affected children, but as yet there is little indication that this challenge is seen as qualitatively and quantitatively different from anything that education ministries have previously experienced. Indeed, some still cling to willful ignorance. In general, education authorities have accepted the importance of including instruction on HIV/AIDS in school programs, but they are only slowly coming to grips with the possibility that the epidemic undermines and might jeopardize system survival. Few have accepted that radically new management structures are essential.

Among the emerging responses within the education sector is increasing attention to the barriers that cash costs create for vulnerable children. There is less attention, however, to the lost opportunities faced by AIDS-affected children who do not attend school, or to the relevance of curricula, and almost none to the emotional and psychological needs of AIDS-affected children.

Although education authorities generally welcome the participation of NGOs in responding to the educational needs of children made vulnerable by HIV/AIDS, they are more grudging in sharing access to public resources. Partnership between the education sector and civil society is lauded in principle, but the modalities for implementation are still being developed.

Nor has there been much collaboration within the public sector. Education ministries continue to guard closely their role in meeting the needs for primary and secondary education and so far have done little to collaborate with health, social welfare, community development, and other governmental sectors, even though the involvement of the government is crucial to supporting AIDS-affected children. One exception has been in South Africa, where a multisectoral education coalition against HIV/AIDS was established in June 2002. Hopefully, this will lead to real progress in that country and provide an example to others.

There are, however, some positive current developments regarding the education for children affected by HIV/AIDS. These include:

- more widespread action to provide free primary education through the abolition of fees and other school costs (as has been done in Kenya, Malawi, Uganda, and Zambia),
- more determined action to ensure that schools provide safe and secure learning environments for young people, especially those who are affected by HIV/AIDS,
- new partnerships between grassroots organizations and international agencies in evaluating and responding to orphans' needs,
- growing recognition of how serious and difficult the orphan issue appears to be, and
- a groundswell of opinion that ways must be found to stop further increase in the number of orphans.

These developments are welcome, but they do not obscure the reality that, as summarized in a World Bank report (Subbarao et al. 2001: 32), "Current efforts to address the orphan crisis are inadequate and piecemeal. The enormity of the problem demands a coordinated response." Participants must include all those concerned with the well-being of children and with the educational, social, psychological, and economic character of the next generation of adults. This coordinated response is not yet in place.

What Should Education Systems Do for Orphans and HIV/AIDS-Affected Children in the Future?

The education sector can take some steps within its current framework to improve its response to the educational needs of children affected by HIV/AIDS.

Eliminate Learner Costs. The first imperative is to ensure that every child can attend a conventional school and complete the relevant education cycle. The school participation of AIDS-affected children will remain problematic until educational costs and the need for child labor to support the household are addressed. Key interventions would include:

- the abolition of all primary school fees,
- the elimination of all other compulsory cash costs associated with school attendance, and

- the provision of support to enable poor families and child-headed households to cope without the labor of students (or, less desirably, significant adjustment of school hours and functioning to allow working children to attend).

School fees and cash costs should be abolished for all children, not just orphans or children affected by AIDS; otherwise, significant "stigma through privilege" would be generated. As required by the *Convention on the Rights of the Child*, primary education must be "compulsory and available free for all" (United Nations 1989: Art. 28). As another safeguard against stigma, orphans should attend conventional schools where possible and not special institutions. Implementation of these measures will require extensive resource mobilization at national and international levels.

Enable Real and Relevant Learning. The second imperative for the education sector is to establish conditions in schools that enable every child to experience real and relevant learning. In the strictly educational domain, this means ensuring that every class is taught by an appropriately qualified and motivated teacher, that there is minimum disruption in the continuity of teaching, that there are adequate educational materials and supplies, and that what is taught is relevant to the immediate and future needs of learners. The relevance of what is taught must also include effective HIV/AIDS education, reproductive health, and life-skills, as well as vocationally relevant knowledge and skills.

The establishment of an enabling school environment requires the adequate provision of school buildings and furnishings, a source of clean water, and suitable gender-segregated toilet facilities. At all levels, a minimum requirement is the establishment of a school environment shaped by human rights, including positive attitudes toward those infected or affected by HIV/AIDS. Such attitudes would manifest themselves in the nondiscriminatory integration of infected or affected learners and educators into every aspect of school life. Schools must also show zero tolerance for all forms of stigma and discrimination and ensure a safe and secure learning environment (and living environment in boarding schools), with no place for sexual exploitation, abuse, or any other form of violence.

Strengthen Partnerships. Responding to the challenges of HIV/AIDS is not something that the education sector can accomplish on its own. Responses require the collaborative involvement of central and local government institutions, NGOs, faith-based organizations, and communities themselves. The need for partnerships is particularly true with regard to issues relating to physical health, psychological and emotional well-being, and family difficulties that affect students. For response to these needs, a school needs viable, working partnerships with health, social welfare, community development, and other government departments. A school also needs arrangements with communities, NGOs, and faith-based organizations to make and support responses to the particular needs of orphans and vulnerable children, during and outside school hours. Such community bodies can work powerfully with schools to develop a safe and secure environment, as well as in helping schools respond to the emotional and psychological needs of distressed children. Also, rural schools need to work with agricultural extension services to foster improved and more stable nutrition and relevant instruction.

AN EXPANDED VISION: THE SCHOOL AT THE HEART
OF THE COMMUNITY

The overwhelming majority of orphans and children affected by HIV/ AIDS live with a surviving parent or with extended family members; it is within their communities that real and lasting solutions to the challenges faced by these children must be found. This applies to educational challenges as much as to others. The implication is that if they are to respond to the needs of orphans and vulnerable children, schools must be well integrated into the communities they serve.

The current reality, however, is that in many societies, especially in rural areas, a large gap exists between school and community. Apart from involvement in the development and maintenance of the school infrastructure, communities often play little part in the life of the school. The role of parents in the actual education of their children is typically confined to making the necessary payments, ensuring that the children attend and do their homework, and reviewing end-of-term reports. Moreover, in areas where literacy levels are low, the school may be culturally quite remote from the community, with parents not understanding much of what goes on in classrooms.

One immediate negative outcome of the continuing gap between school and community is that many school children learn in two very distinct environments: the school, where an analytic, Western, urban, middle-class approach often dominates, and the home and community, where a holistic approach rooted in traditional values and beliefs may hold sway. The failure to harmonize the learning that occurs in these two environments may be part of the reason why school-based HIV/AIDS education has often failed to generate responsible, life-protecting sexual behavior.

The danger of HIV/AIDS, the burgeoning number of orphans, and the pressing needs of children affected by the epidemic all call for the gap between school and community to be bridged. The crucial responses must occur at the community level, but they must be buttressed by the type of institutional support that schools, and only schools, can give. Most communities of any size have a school, a ready-made institutional and physical framework that makes an ideal center for responding in a holistic manner to community needs.

A new vision is needed with the school at the heart of the community, and concrete action is required to bring this about. In this new vision, the school would be transformed into a multipurpose development and welfare institution that would serve as a center where, in cooperation with its staff, communities would develop their own initiatives for responding to their education, health, food production, and other welfare needs. In this new role, the school would become the place where families, community members, educators, health workers, agricultural extension workers, social workers, other specialist staff, local religious bodies, and NGOs come together to develop an integrated response to the threats of HIV/AIDS to children and its impacts on them. By working together, they could develop holistic solutions that would respond to the full range of children's needs, including their education.

The potential of such a development has been eloquently expressed by Paula Donovan (2000: 4), the UNICEF regional HIV/AIDS advisor for Eastern and Southern Africa: "It is exciting to imagine such expanded schools of the near future: no longer isolated and dangerous, no longer dependent on just the few adults employed to teach, but active social and social service centres, bases of operations for the full spectrum of local organizations and caregivers working within communities. Such schools will evolve into places where everyone in the community – including those who have been excluded or marginalized, and children without support systems – can turn." In short, what we want to see is every child in a school, a school in every community, and every school a multipurpose development and welfare institution.

One implication of this solution is that *every school would become a community school*. Instead of being outliers, responding precariously to the needs of specially identified groups, community schools would become the norm. Indeed, the opportunity is there for existing community schools to transform themselves into expanded institutions responding to the full spectrum of needs within a community, including those of orphans and HIV/AIDS-affected children.

In Zambia, some of these schools have already reached into their communities to provide Training for Transformation programs that build the capacity of local communities to manage their schools efficiently and effectively. As a result, some have established revolving credit funds, trained mobilizers to promote the involvement of the wider community in school affairs, increased awareness of HIV/AIDS and health issues, and organised community action on human rights (ZOCS 2001). Apart from bridging the gap between schools and communities, this approach has generated tangible benefits, with the interest from loans being directed to school needs.

Transforming such an expanded vision of the school into reality can take place only within the community, with the specific components and linkages being established at the local level. To be sure, national and international understanding, encouragement, and material support would be needed to scale up this new vision, but communities would have to make it a reality. Enabling the school to become the heart of the community by transforming it into a multipurpose development and welfare institution attuned to every community need offers hope of effective, enduring solutions to the needs of children and families affected by HIV/AIDS.

References

Ainsworth, M., and D. Filmer. 2002. Poverty, AIDS, and children's schooling: A targeting dilemma. World Bank Policy Research Working Paper 2885. Operations Evaluation Department and Development Research Group, World Bank, September. Available at http://www.worldbank.org

Akoulouze, R., G. Rugalema, and V. Khanye. 2001. Taking stock of promising approaches in HIV/AIDS and education in sub-Saharan Africa: What works, why, and how; A synthesis of country case studies. Paper presented at the Association for the Development of Education in Africa Biennial Meeting, Arusha, Tanzania, October 7–11.

Barnett, T., and A. Whiteside. 2002. *AIDS in the twenty-first century.* Basingstoke: Palgrave Macmillan.

Béchu, N. 1998. The impact of AIDS on the economy of families in Côte d'Ivoire: Changes in consumption among AIDS-affected households. In *Confronting AIDS: Evidence from the developing world*, ed. M. Ainsworth, L. Fransen, and M. Over. 341–8. Washington, DC: World Bank; Brussels: European Commission.

Bennell, P. 2005. The impact of the AIDS epidemic on teachers in sub-Saharan Africa. *Journal of Development Studies* 41(3): 440–66.

Bennell, P., K. Hyde, and N. Swainson. 2002. *The impact of the HIV/AIDS epidemic on the education sector in sub-Saharan Africa: A synthesis of the findings and recommendations of three country studies.* Brighton: Centre for International Education, University of Sussex Institute of Education.

Brody, A. B. 2002. Combating HIV/AIDS: Intervention strategies, impact mitigation, and policy issues. Paper presented at the International Conference on Commitment to Combat HIV/AIDS, University of Swaziland, Kwaluseni Campus, July 2–4.

Children's Testimony. 2002. National HIV/AIDS and Education Conference, Midrand, South Africa, May 31.

Coombe, C. 2002. Mitigating the impact of HIV/AIDS on education supply, demand, and quality. Chapter 12 of *AIDS, policy, and child well-being*, ed. Giovanni Andrew Cornia. Florence: UNICEF-Innocenti Research Center, June. 52 pages. Available at http://www.unicef-icdc.org/siteguide/indexsearch.html

Donovan, P. 2000. The impact of HIV and AIDS on the rights of the child to education: Discrimination and HIV/AIDS-related stigma and access to education; The response. Paper presented at South African Development Community–European Union Seminar on the Rights of the Child in a World with HIV and AIDS, Harare, Zimbabwe, October 23.

FAO (United Nations Food and Agriculture Organization). 2001. The impact of HIV/AIDS on food security. Report of the Committee on Food Security, 27th session, Rome, May 28–June 1.

Fassa, M. 2000. HIV/AIDS and education: Sharing experiences, views, and ideas from the Côte d'Ivoire and Central African Republic HIV/AIDS impact assessment, measure, and response. Presentation to Impact of HIV/AIDS on Education workshop, International Institute for Educational Planning, Paris, September 27–29.

FHI (Family Health International) and SCOPE-OVC (Strengthening Community Partnerships for the Empowerment of Orphans and Vulnerable Children). 2002. Psycho-social baseline survey (data highlights). FHI, Lusaka, March.

Government of Zambia. 1999. *Zambia: A situation analysis of orphans.* Joint USAID/UNICEF/USIDA study fund project. Lusaka: UNICEF.

Hall, J. 2002. *Life stories: Testimonies of hope from people with HIV and AIDS.* Manzini, Swaziland: UNICEF.

Harris, A. M., and J. G. Schubert. 2001. Defining "quality" in the midst of HIV/AIDS: Ripple effects in the classroom. Report prepared for Improving Educational Quality Project, American Institutes of Research in collaboration with the Academy for International Development, Education Development Center, Juarez and Associates, and University of Pittsburgh. Washington, DC: USAID. http://www.ieq.org/pdf/Defining?Quality_HIV/AIDS.pdf

Human Rights Watch. 2001. *Scared at school: Sexual violence against girls in South African Schools.* New York: Human Rights Watch.

International Save the Children Alliance. 1996. Promoting psychosocial well-being among children affected by armed conflict and displacement: principles and approaches. Working Paper no. 1. Working Group on Children Affected by Armed Conflict and Displacement, Save the Children Fund, London.

Jewkes, R. , J. Levin, N. Mbananga, and D. Bradshaw. 2002. Rape of girls in South Africa. *The Lancet* 359:319–32.

Kelly, M. J. 2002. Preventing HIV transmission through education. *Perspectives in Education* (University of Pretoria), June.

Kinghorn, A. and M. J. Kelly. 2005. 'The impact of the AIDS epidemic' articles by Paul Bennell: Some comments. *Journal of Development Studies* 41(3): 489–99.

Kiragu, K. 2001. *Youth and HIV/AIDS: Can we avoid catastrophe?* Population Reports, Series L, no. 12. Population Information Program, Bloomberg School of Public Health. Baltimore: The Johns Hopkins University.

Living Conditions Monitoring Survey. 1998. *Living conditions in Zambia (1998). Preliminary Report.* Lusaka: Central Statistical Office.

Ministry of Education, Zambia. 1996. *Educating our future: National policy on education.* Lusaka: Ministry of Education.

———. 2002. *Strategic plan, 2003–2007.* Lusaka: Ministry of Education.

Rossi, M. M., and P. Reijer. 1995. Prevalence of orphans and their geographical status. Research report for the AIDS Department, Catholic Diocese of Ndola, Zambia.

Schaeffer, S. 1994. The impact of HIV/AIDS on education: A review of the literature and experience. Background paper presented to International Institute for Educational Planning seminar, Paris, December 8–10, 1993.

Subbarao, K., A. Mattimore, and K. Plangemann. 2001. *Social protection of Africa's orphans and other vulnerable children: Issues and good practices; Program options.*

Africa Region Human Development Working Paper Series, Africa Region, World Bank. Washington, DC: World Bank.

UNAIDS-UNECA (Joint United Nations Programme on HIV/AIDS – United Nations Economic Commission for Africa). 2000. *AIDS in Africa, country by country.* Report prepared for delegates to African Development Forum 2000, Addis Ababa, December 2000. Geneva: UNAIDS.

UNECA (United Nations Economic Commission for Africa). 2000. *HIV/AIDS and education in eastern and southern Africa: The leadership challenge and the way forward.* Synthesis Report for African Development Forum 2000. Addis Ababa: UNECA, October.

UNICEF. 1999. *Children orphaned by AIDS: Front-line responses from eastern and southern Africa.* New York: UNICEF.

———. 2000. *The progress of nations, 2000.* New York: UNICEF.

———. 2002. *Rapid assessment of the incidence of child abuse in Lusaka.* Report to UNICEF, Zambia, by Children in Need Network (CHIN). Lusaka: UNICEF.

United Nations. 1989. *Convention on the rights of the child.* UN General Assembly Res. 44/25, UN GAOR, 44th sess., 41st plen. mtg., annex, UN Doc. A/RES/44/25 (December 12). Geneva: United Nations. http://www.unchr.ch/html/menu3/b/k2crc.htm

———. 1999. Opening Address by the United Nations Secretary General, Kofi Annan, to the International Partnership Against AIDS in Africa, New York, December 6.

USAID (United States Agency for International Development), UNICEF, and UNAIDS (Joint United Nations Programme on AIDS) 2002. *Children on the brink 2002: A joint report on orphan estimates and program strategies.* Washington, DC: TvT Associates/Synergy Project, USAID. http://www.unicef.org/publications/pub_children_on_the_brink_en.pdf

Watkins, K. 2000. *The Oxfam education report.* Oxford: Oxfam Publishing.

World Bank. 2000. *Exploring the implications of the HIV/AIDS epidemic for educational planning in selected African countries: The demographic question.* AIDS Campaign Team for Africa, ACTAfrica. Washington, DC: World Bank.

———. 2002. *Education and HIV/AIDS: A window of hope.* Washington, DC: World Bank.

World Conference on Education for All. 1990. *World Declaration on Education for All* and *Framework for Action to Meet Basic Learning Needs.* Jomtien, Thailand: World Conference on Education for All, March 5–9. Available at http://www.unesco.org

World Education Forum. 2000. *The Dakar framework for action: Education for all; meeting our collective commitments.* Dakar, Senegal: World Education Forum, April 26–28. Available at http://www.unesco.org

World Summit for Children. 1990. *World declaration on the survival, protection, and development of children.* New York: World Summit for Children, September 30. http://www.unicef.org/wsc/declare.htm

ZOCS (Zambia Open Community Schools). 2001. *Walking the way forward with children.* ZOCS Annual Report 2001. Lusaka, ZOCS Secretariat.

4

Psychosocial Impact of the HIV/AIDS Epidemic on Children and Youth

Laurie Bauman with Stefan Germann

In this third decade of HIV/AIDS, the world community continues to stagger under the impacts of the pandemic, but no group carries a heavier burden than children. Worldwide, children affected by HIV/AIDS are disproportionately poor and malnourished. They are more likely to lack shelter, education, and health care. They are vulnerable to sexual abuse by adults. They are used for child labor in domestic or field work. In the developing world, as infants they may have acquired HIV infection from their mothers; if infected they typically die young, without access to life-prolonging treatment. In the United States and other developed countries, perinatal transmission has been dramatically reduced through the identification of HIV-infected pregnant women and administration of antiretrovirals during pregnancy and labor and after delivery.

Those who escape HIV infection, however, do not escape the impact of the disease. They may suffer the pain of the death of a parent. They may serve as caregivers to their ill parents – washing and feeding bedridden mothers or fathers – and often assume adult responsibilities for household maintenance. Older children may seek paid employment to support their family when no adult is well enough to work, and may raise their younger siblings in the place of their parents. When they are orphaned, they depend on the goodwill and resources of family, friends, or neighbors to take them in and care for them.

In the face of such economic and physical vulnerability, the psychological burdens of the HIV/AIDS epidemic may seem less important – less urgent, less compelling – but not to the children themselves. In their world the emotional demands of HIV/AIDS are heartbreaking, as these statements from children in New York (Gerstadt 2003), indicate.

Stefan Germann contributed several of the figures contained in this chapter and consulted on the material relating to Africa.

What if I'm in school and . . . she faints and I'm not there to help her?
She could be OK today but I worry the next day she won't get up from the bed.
If my mother were dead, I would want to go before her.
If my mom were to pass, me and my brother would be homeless. We'd be in a foster
home or something because none of our family members would take us.
She . . . I don't even want to say it . . . she is dying. I can't take care of myself. I need
someone to help me get older.
Sometime soon – not very soon – but soon – she will die and I won't have a mom
anymore.

Despite the urgency of children's needs, society and governments have
failed to acknowledge adequately children's anxiety, fear, mistrust, depression, anger, and guilt, and the impact of the stigma that pervades their lives.
Due to this failure, children often carry the burden alone – in silence and
in isolation – with no adult to guide them, yet they lack the cognitive and
emotional maturity and skills to cope. If we listen to their voices, we will
learn about their emotional, psychological, developmental, and behavioral
needs.

The effects of parental HIV/AIDS on children are complex and wide-
ranging (Bauman and Wiener 1994; Fanos and Wiener 1994; Geballe,
Gruendel, and Andiman 1995; Levine 1993; Levine and Stein 1994). Many
of these effects (increased poverty, lack of access to education and health
care, homelessness, and vulnerability to HIV infection) are addressed in
other chapters in this volume.

This chapter summarizes research and field experience concerning the
emotional burden of the HIV/AIDS epidemic for children who are HIV-
infected, whose parents are ill, or whose parents have died. The first section
describes the ways HIV/AIDS creates vulnerability to psychological distress. The second section identifies protective factors that can shield children from even the most traumatic events. The third section reviews the
ways psychosocial problems are manifested in children, how these vary
by age and maturation, and some of the possible consequences of childhood bereavement for social and psychological functioning in adulthood.
The fourth section describes the kinds of grassroots interventions that are
being tried worldwide to address children's vulnerability to psychosocial
problems from HIV/AIDS.

Throughout, the chapter addresses the different challenges HIV/AIDS
poses to children in the developed world and in the developing world, particularly in sub-Saharan Africa. The contributors to this chapter come from
very different worlds. One has conducted research for several years among
mothers with HIV/AIDS and their children in New York City. The majority
of these women are African American or Latina, are among the poorest in
the population, and have suffered the crushing consequences of drug mis-
use (their own, their partner's, or both) long before HIV/AIDS entered their
lives (See also Chapter 8). The other has for the past decade developed and
disseminated psychosocial support interventions for orphans and other

children made vulnerable by AIDS throughout Zimbabwe and Eastern and Southern Africa. Though a majority of the research literature on the topic of children affected by AIDS is from studies in the United States and other Western countries, the essential findings are relevant to other parts of the world.

No matter our different backgrounds, we both conclude that all children affected by HIV/AIDS carry a heavy psychosocial burden that must be acknowledged, understood, and ameliorated by the adults in their lives and in their communities, and by those in leadership positions. The responses will differ depending on the cultural, socioeconomic, and religious context and the scale of the epidemic in a particular setting. Although Western models are not directly applicable to other settings, they offer insights into the needs of children everywhere. Western practitioners and policymakers can gain valuable information from the developing world in terms of mobilizing family and community support for children and youth affected by HIV/AIDS.

In this chapter the term *psychosocial problems* (or distress) is used broadly to refer to (1) behavioral, psychological, and emotional problems that limit normal functioning or cause unhappiness for children or for the people around them; (2) psychiatric disorders that have been caused or exacerbated by HIV/AIDS, including depression, anxiety, post-traumatic-stress disorder, school phobia, and conduct disorder; and (3) limitations on the child's normal developmental opportunities and growth. In addition, HIV-infected children may experience cognitive problems and developmental delay.

HIV-RELATED RISK FACTORS FOR PSYCHOSOCIAL
PROBLEMS IN CHILDREN

Why does HIV/AIDS create a particular psychosocial burden for children? Knowing how the epidemic affects children can provide a blueprint for action in two ways: It can lead to the development of *preventive* interventions that can reduce exposure to and consequences of the known risks, and it can lead to the development of *supportive* programs that help children as they experience the inevitable challenges of HIV/AIDS.

Childhood Chronic and Terminal Illness

Children infected with HIV who live past infancy experience all the challenges that affected children do, but must in addition cope with the illness itself. In the developed world, studies of children with chronic health conditions of many kinds (such as cancer and neurological diseases) find higher rates of behavioral and emotional disorders than in their healthy peers. Factors that may increase this risk include characteristics of the disorder itself: Is it life-threatening? Does the disease or its treatment change the child's physical appearance? Does it interfere with learning? Does it require intrusive medical care? The severity of the symptoms and functional limitations also affect children's adjustment. Some research suggests that, among children with chronic health conditions, behavioral problems may be more severe among boys, children from poor families, those whose mothers have less formal education, and those from single-parent families.

Adults may reject HIV-infected children, causing them to feel unworthy or unloved. These children may become demoralized and depressed, and a lack of affection may lead to isolation, withdrawal, despair, and aggressive behavior. The physical effects of the disease include disability, pain, disfigurement, and fatigue, all of which can limit activities and can lead to depression. Cognitive effects include delayed motor development as well as speech and learning problems. In the care of a loving, resourceful family, with access to medical care and support of many kinds, HIV-infected children can lead happy and productive lives. Unfortunately the ideal situation is uncommon, with access to mental health services rarer still.

Children Affected by HIV/AIDS

Children who are not themselves infected with HIV still may be affected by HIV in many ways, mostly deriving from the one inescapable reality of living with HIV-infected parents. When a parent has a chronic and ultimately terminal illness, children's basic needs for love, trust, security, and parenting are threatened, and they are unlikely to experience anything like a normal childhood.

Figure 4.1, "Walking the Road," illustrates the progressive impact of HIV/AIDS from an African perspective. The University of Natal, South Africa, developed the "walking the road" model for community-based reflection on children's psychosocial needs. This tool is very useful and easy to use at the local level. It looks at the impact of HIV/AIDS on children from the time infection has entered the household. The analysis can be made with different age and gender variables to build possible impact scenarios. While the specifics differ in the American context, the general trajectory involves the arrival of new stressors, lack of predictability, and inadequate and dwindling resources.

Once the scenario in a given context is mapped out, an assessment can be performed of what support and resources are available at the community level to mitigate the negative impact AIDS has on children. This assessment helps to identify capacity gaps. By filling these gaps with adequate support responses, a continuum of care can be ensured at the community level.

Illness in a Parent

Parental chronic or terminal illness is a stressor that increases psychological risk for children (Garmezy 1983; Rutter 1979, 1987). Worry about the health

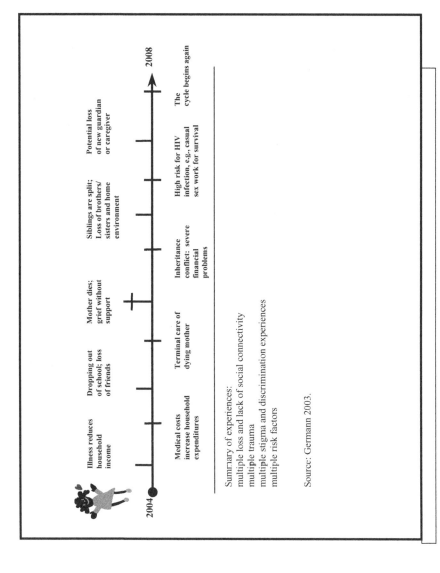

FIGURE 4.1. Walking the road: The impact of AIDS on children. (Adapted from Germann 2003.)

of ill parents results in anxiety, fear of abandonment, and chronic insecurity. Sometimes children resent their parent's illness, and their resentment leads to guilt feelings, anger, and a low tolerance for frustration. They feel, not without reason, that life is unfair and uncontrollable.

Older children are more vulnerable than younger children, and girls more vulnerable than boys, especially as they move from early to middle adolescence. One reason for girls' increased vulnerability to behavioral problems and distress may be that they have increased family responsibilities when a parent is ill.

The specific behavioral and psychological impact of parental HIV/AIDS on children is a neglected area of research, but it is clear that the course of the disease can be remarkably disruptive to children. Parents with AIDS exhibit noticeable physical changes, such as fatigue, disability, skin lesions, and wasting; they may also show behavioral and cognitive changes, such as memory loss or irritability. Thus, the parent – the person the child counts on for stability and predictability – becomes unpredictable and erratic. The child never knows whether today will be a good day or a bad day.

Periods of serious acute illness may require episodic hospitalizations. During these episodes, children may stay informally with family or neighbors, be placed in foster care, or be left without adult supervision. These uncertainties may interfere with healthy personality development (Nagler, Adnopoz, and Forsyth 1995) and result in elevated distress.

Studies in the United States suggest that, compared to children with healthy parents, children of parents with HIV/AIDS are more likely to be depressed and anxious ("internalizing" problems) and have more behavior and conduct problems ("externalizing" problems); poor social competence and less ability to pay attention have also been reported (Esposito et al. 1999; Forehand et al. 1998; Forsyth et al. 1996). A study in New York City (Bauman et al. 2002) reported that the rate of self-reported depression among 167 HIV-negative children of HIV-positive mothers was higher than U.S. norms. Mothers' ratings were higher than children's: Based on their report, 40 percent of their children had clinically significant symptoms. More sobering were the results of the analysis of psychological problems in eight-to-twelve-year-old children followed for two years (Bauman et al. 2003). In this study *every* child exhibited clinically significant behavioral and emotional symptoms; 88 percent exhibited problems more than once. Also in New York City, Gerstadt (2003) reported that 60 percent of children of single mothers with serious HIV/AIDS disease met criteria for a diagnosis of a mental disorder.

Parental Depression

Most parents with AIDS are themselves depressed. Silver et al. (2004) reported that over 70 percent of mothers had scores on a symptom checklist that indicated "high" symptom levels, and 55 percent had symptoms consistent with a diagnosis of major depressive disorder. Depressive symptoms may worsen as the implications of their HIV/AIDS become clearer. Parents manifest disabling symptoms, take multiple medications with serious side effects, and experience a decline in their health that may signal approaching death.

Parental depression often has serious implications for children. Generally, studies show that children and adolescents of depressed mothers, compared with peers whose mothers are not depressed, have higher rates of psychological diagnoses (particularly depression), have poorer behavioral, emotional, and academic functioning, and have lower self-esteem (Anderson and Hammen 1993; Weissman, Gammon, and John 1987). Adolescent children of depressed mothers are more likely to experience depression, substance abuse, and conduct disorder (Downey and Coyne 1990; Schwartz et al. 1990; Weissman et al. 1987). Children of HIV-positive mothers report more depressive symptoms than children of non-HIV-infected women (Biggar and Forehand 1998) and are more likely to be depressed when their mother is depressed (Bauman et al. 2002).

How does parental depression influence children's psychosocial functioning? First, depression affects parental behaviors and beliefs. Depressed parents generally have more punitive attitudes toward child rearing, inaccurate knowledge of child development, and less supportive relationships with their children. Second, parental depression affects the family environment in ways that compromise children's emotional security, resulting in more emotional outbursts and insecure parental attachment. Third, parental depression may limit children's relationships and contacts outside the home, thereby inhibiting the child from developing an adequate extrafamilial social support network. This inhibition is particularly true when children have been told not to talk about the parent's illness with others.

Parental Death

Death of a parent is one of the most devastating and powerful risk factors for psychosocial problems in children. Compared to children with living parents, children who have experienced a parent's death have twice the rate of psychiatric disorder (Rutter 1966) and more symptoms of depression, anxiety, and withdrawal (Felner et al. 1981; Sandler et al. 1988). Their school performance declines in the short term, and their disinterest in school persists one year later (Van Eerdewegh et al. 1982).

Most research on the effects of parental death on children has limited relevance to children whose parent dies of AIDS, however, even in the United States, for several reasons. Most studies (for example, on the effect of a parental death from cancer) have enrolled samples of children who are living with a surviving parent. Many parents with HIV/AIDS are single or the other parent has already died. Little is known about how loss of one's only custodial parent is related to psychological disturbance. Also, most research on grief in children has been conducted on Euro-American children, but almost 90 percent of women with HIV/AIDS in the United States are African American or Latina, and most children affected by HIV/AIDS worldwide are African or Asian. Overall, the literature on the impact of parental death from AIDS on children is sparse (Siegel and Gorey 1994).

Cumulative Loss

Children who have a parent living with HIV/AIDS may have experienced other losses in their young lives. Some have watched for months or years the deterioration and eventual death of the other parent or a cherished relative from AIDS. For them, one parent's illness presages what may happen to the other. Some have helped care for the ill parent or witnessed their pain, cognitive deterioration, and disability. Parental illness creates insecurity and personal vulnerability in children, who may question their strength to go through it again or their ability to cope. Some may openly or privately resent the burden the ill parent placed on their freedom to have fun, attend school, or socialize with friends – to just be normal.

Children also may have a sibling with HIV/AIDS. Being the healthy sibling of a child with a chronic illness can have advantages in terms of the development of responsibility, maturity, and an ability to empathize. But it can also cause jealousy because of the perception, and sometimes the reality, that the ill sibling gets disproportionate attention from parents. The well child can become angry at parents while at the same time understanding the need of the ill child for attention. If a brother or sister has died from HIV/AIDS, the surviving siblings must adjust to major loss, and may have difficulty coping with their feelings of sadness, survivor guilt, and resentment.

Problems of Children of Single Parents with HIV/AIDS

Many children affected by HIV/AIDS in the United States live in single-parent homes and face special challenges. First, they often have a special sense of vulnerability or lack a sense of security. Small children are unsure of their ill mother's ability to be a parent and to provide for them. Older children fear that their parent will die, leaving them in charge. Second, children may fear leaving their parent alone when they are in school. Their fear can result in generalized or separation anxiety, including refusal to go to school. In the New York City research, several children recounted terrifying experiences in which they came home from school to find their parent hospitalized or dead. Children may assume disproportionate feelings of responsibility for their parent's well-being, and feel that they have to be at home in case their mother needs help.

Third, children like being the center of attention, but having an ill parent may cause them to feel neglected when their ill parent gets most of the attention from other family members. Children and adolescents may act out or become oppositional in order to be noticed. Although this resentment is common, it is usually accompanied by fears for the parent's well-being and fear of parental death. Children rarely have the developmental ability to reconcile and understand these conflicting emotions without help.

Fourth, research has shown that children do best when life is structured and predictable – when there is a family routine. But, AIDS is an illness characterized by uncertainty. Periods of apparent health are punctuated by intermittent crises as parents sicken. Life feels like a roller coaster; planned outings are canceled, holidays ruined, good times missed. Without other adults to help care for the children and maintain some routine, the chaos resulting from parental illness will play itself out daily.

Parentification: Child Caregiving to Siblings or an Ill Parent

HIV / AIDS may change all family roles to accommodate the parents' need for care (Cates et al. 1990; Levine 1990, 1995). When a parent is chronically ill, children and adolescents often take on special responsibilities. Older children may provide direct care to parents, including toileting, bathing, feeding, assisting with transfer and mobility, and giving medications and emotional support. In extreme circumstances, children may become parentified, that is, assume the parent's role in the family system, caring for siblings, and maintaining the household.

Parentification sometimes includes the role reversal of the child acting as parent to the parent, as well as parent to siblings. Role reversal may be more problematic than caring for siblings because, if prolonged or intense, it may inhibit development and result in guilt and lowered self-esteem (Barnett and Parker 1998). Older children who are responsible for their younger siblings' care find that this does not mean simply an increase in time spent babysitting, but rather having the major or total responsibility for raising the children. They may supervise younger children's homework, bedtime, friendships, and extracurricular activities, monitoring their whereabouts. As a result, younger children may not receive the kind of parenting they need, or not be parented at all. Even if older siblings try to help, or there are older family members looking in, the day-to-day parenting that helps nurture children may be missing. Although their basic needs may be met, children may lack the sustained guidance of a parent as they grow and develop.

It might be assumed that children and youth in Africa and other poor regions are more often involved in the care of sick relatives and younger siblings and may have lower rates of psychosocial morbidity than their peers in the West. Data recently collected from a comparative study in Zimbabwe and the United States (Bauman, Foster, and Silver 2004) found that mothers in Mutare were sicker than mothers in New York, and that children in Mutare aged eight to sixteen spent more time providing personal care to mothers (seventeen hours a week) compared with New York children (thirteen hours). However, more children in New York helped mothers with feeding, dressing, and mobility, and more took care of siblings. On average, more children in Zimbabwe were significantly depressed than were children in New York (63 percent compared with 20 percent). In both samples, children with a lot of responsibility for chores were not more depressed unless they also felt unappreciated by their mothers. (It is possible, however, that the New York children, many of whom had already been removed from their parents' care on other occasions, may have underreported symptoms of depression to avoid investigation into their situations. More research is needed to clarify this concern.)

Some children (particularly girls) become confidantes to their ill parent and are called upon to provide emotional support to adults who are depressed, afraid, and insecure. In the United States, HIV-infected mothers asked to name their closest friend will sometimes name a young child. Bauman et al. (2001) found that offspring who provide emotional support to an ill parent have extremely high rates of depression, but their ill parents are unaware of the emotional cost to their daughters. Children who provide personal care and emotional support to ill parents may have concerns about the future, have a limited social life, and lack parenting themselves. Inhibited development and depression are both possible outcomes when children take on the parenting role (Wallace 1996). The burden of providing care to an adult is a potent stressor that exhausts even adults, and children often have no one to talk to about their situation.

If the parent is too ill to manage the household, children may take on this responsibility far beyond usual childhood chores. They may have to plan and shop for meals (not just prepare simple meals under instruction or a parent's direction); they may have to handle paying bills, such as rent; they may have to clean house, organize their time, do laundry, and so on. If the parent's illness has affected family income, children may feel it is their responsibility to work to provide for the family. In Africa and Asia, it is not uncommon for children to manage the family farm, work in factories, or turn to prostitution for income.

Among inner-city U.S. children, bonds between parents and children may have been tenuous prior to the onset of HIV/AIDS. Living with poverty, parental drug or alcohol abuse, and domestic violence, children often grow up "parenting their parents" (Pivnick and Villegas 2000). In developing countries, health services are often inaccessible or unavailable, which leaves the major responsibility for care to family, particularly women and children. Children become caregivers when there is no family member available, and the choice of which sibling is the primary caregiver is a function of gender (usually girls), older age, co-residence, inclination, and income-earning ability. Despite the negative impacts, parentification can have some positive results, such as increased maturity and coping skills, a close and rewarding relationship with the ill parents, a sense of being needed and valued, and, for some, the beginning of a career in nursing or other health care work.

Deficits in Parenting

Poor child adjustment to parental illness may be due to disruptions in the parenting role, which include reduced parental support for the child, fewer efforts at discipline, neglecting or ignoring the child, changes in family routines, and parental absence. A parent's chronic illness also disrupts the ability to parent directly, through increased partner conflict, or indirectly, through increased parental depression. Emotional distress related to HIV may grow and may take the form of guilt, uncertainty, mood fluctuations, and fear (Armistead and Forehand 1995).

Some of the effects of parents' inability to parent have different implications, depending on their children's developmental stage. Younger children may be less supervised and left alone more often because the ill parent cannot be available physically or emotionally. This parental unavailability may mean that the child fails to develop cognitive, academic, social, or emotional skills. In the United States, children may watch television for hours and miss out on sports, reading, and school activities. For adolescents, lack of supervision and monitoring may increase their risk for involvement in early sexual activity, cigarette use, alcohol and drug use, or involvement in gangs.

HIV/AIDS Disclosure and Psychosocial Problems in Children

Disclosure is one of the most complex and painful decisions parents must make: Should I try to keep the cause of my illness a secret? Do I tell my child I may die? If I disclose my HIV status to my children, will they be sad and worried? Will they tell others about my diagnosis? How do I answer when they ask, "Who will care for us?" There is little research on the effects of HIV disclosure on children's and adolescents' well being. In the United States about 35 percent of women with

HIV disclose their diagnosis to their children (Bauman and Silver 2001; Murphy et al. 1999). Older children are more likely to have been told the HIV diagnosis than younger children (Bauman and Silver 2001; Lee, Lester, and Rotheram-Borus 2002). Some studies find that HIV disclosure is associated with more behavioral symptoms in children (Lee et al. 2002; Lee and Rotheram-Borus 2002), and others do not (Bauman and Silver 2001).

The disclosure decision is complex. As Michael Lipson (1994, S63) points out, "Disclosure...would force into common awareness...the parent's own illness and potential death." Parents fear disclosing, but children usually suspect something is wrong and feel they cannot ask (Hackl et al. 1997). The argument for disclosure has two parts: disclosure can benefit the family, and withholding the HIV diagnosis can be harmful.

Disclosure can be helpful when children think or know that something is wrong; the uncertainty about the parent's illness can then be detrimental (Mischel 1981). When children repeatedly voice their fears or ask questions, it may be best to disclose; open communication allows the child to be part of future planning and can improve the parent-child relationship (Armistead and Forehand 1995). One widely used approach in both the developed world and Africa is the "memory box" (see Figure 4.2), a way for parent and child to construct a tangible record of their family and relationship and plan for the future.

Children in AIDS-affected households become vulnerable long before their parents die. In Uganda, memory box work was begun by a group of HIV-positive mothers. Over the past few years, many programs supporting children affected by AIDS have successfully used similar approaches.

Memory boxes and books enable people to record their own life stories. They include information about the parents, the family history, childhood stories, photographs, drawings, special family memories, and so on. The parent works with the children in putting together the memory book, using simple card boxes, string, used paper, and paint.

The process of creating a memory book or box empowers parents, enabling them to communicate better with their children; it includes the possible disclosure of their health status and can initiate the process of future planning together. It gives children a unique opportunity to ask questions about their parents' illness and to be involved in discussions about who will care for them after their parents die.

Engaging children in this way also provides them with information that strengthens their knowledge of HIV prevention and enables them to better withstand stigma and discrimination. Memory approaches are a simple yet powerful tool to support children affected by AIDS at the family level.

FIGURE 4.2. Memory approaches

Short-term consequences of disclosure for children may include depression, anxiety, and anger (Armistead and Forehand 1995), because they know their parent is dying and there is no cure. But the long-term benefits may be considerable for the child who then has the opportunity to engage in anticipatory grieving. Parkes and Weiss (1983) report that open discussion of death can be fulfilling and can increase cohesion among family members. This option may be more difficult in sub-Saharan Africa and in other cultures as well, where talking about death is taboo because it is feared it will bring about the death. The decision to disclose HIV/AIDS to adults or children must be made with sensitive understanding of the particular cultural context.

The argument for disclosure also points out that not telling – secrecy – can have negative consequences for children. When children are not told what is wrong with their parent, they may imagine scenarios worse than the truth. Younger children may feel that the problem is their fault (magical thinking). Also, children may actually know about the HIV diagnosis because they figured it out, overheard it, or were told by another family member and have no one to talk to about what it means or what will happen to them if their parent dies.

If the parent or other important adults have lied – denying the parent has AIDS, giving the illness a different name, reassuring the child that the parent will get better soon – the child, feeling betrayed, may grow to distrust all adults. Without trust the child lacks an essential part of successful child adjustment. Suspicion and fear can lead to anxiety, resentment, and acting out.

Finally, when parents do not disclose their HIV/AIDS status, succession planning is more difficult. Some parents with HIV fear they will lose custody of their children if someone finds out (Siegel and Gorey 1994), but making legal arrangements for a child's care and custody, at least in the United States, is best done prior to parental death.

The argument against HIV disclosure is also multifaceted. First, parents fear that their children cannot handle the diagnosis and will become depressed or act out; there is nothing they can do to change the situation, they argue, and coping with the knowledge is unnecessary until the parent is quite ill. Second, parents fear that children will want to know how they acquired HIV/AIDS, a discussion most want to avoid. Third, many parents feel that it will be too hard on them to discuss their illness and likely death, and they want to put it off for as long as possible. Fourth, many feel that younger children cannot handle this information, and will choose to disclose only to older children and tell them to keep the secret from younger siblings. The need to keep secrets within a family can hurt family relationships and create tension for older children, who need to deal with anticipatory grief and their worry about their future with no one to talk with (Hackl et al. 1997). Fifth, there are often real consequences to the larger community's learning about a parent's HIV diagnosis. Stigma from HIV, while perhaps lessening as the disease becomes more prevalent, is still powerful and cruel; families have experienced loss of income, housing, and community standing. Some people have even been physically assaulted after public disclosure. Therefore, when children are told about the parent's HIV they are usually instructed not to talk about it with anyone. This leaves them without a source of support and shifts the burden of secrecy from the ill parent to the child.

Does HIV/AIDS Stigma Affect Children's Adjustment?

The stigma of HIV/AIDS may be visited not only on the parent with AIDS but on the family members as well. Bereavement and successful grieving may be complicated by the effects of social stigma associated with HIV disease and secrecy (Esposito et al. 1999; Lipson 1996; Siegel and Gorey 1994). In the United States, children who know the diagnosis find out that many people believe that those with HIV/AIDS have brought their illness on themselves, a process involving labeling with words such as promiscuous, drug addict, or homosexual. They learn that many people believe HIV/AIDS is easily contagious. In Africa, distress and social isolation are common among children whose parent is HIV-infected; in addition, both before and after the death, children may feel shame, guilt, and rejection. Irrational fear of the speed of AIDS may deny children schooling and health care. Once the parent dies, children may be denied their rightful inheritance and property.

Other Risk Factors for Child Mental Health Problems

Parental HIV illness or death are more likely to be associated with psychological disturbance in children when they also have other kinds of chronic stress such as poverty, exposure to violence, previous loss, or a history of other deaths of loved ones. The effects are not cumulative but exponential: Children were found to be four times more likely to demonstrate psychiatric disorder when exposed to two stressors, and ten times more likely when exposed to more than five (Rutter 1979). Because children of parents with HIV/AIDS may experience many potent stressors for psychological disturbance independent of the parent's HIV illness, they may be especially vulnerable to psychological disorder.

In the United States, most children of parents with HIV/AIDS live in poor inner-city neighborhoods that are disproportionately affected by violence. Many young children and most adolescents know someone who has died, and they may have seen someone shot, stabbed, or killed. Children who live in situations of random violence have an increased risk of mental health problems and perceived vulnerability. In some sub-Saharan African countries, war and conflict are responsible for the deaths of many parents and the orphaning of thousands of children. Thus, many have already experienced grief and loss.

In the United States, children most affected by maternal HIV/AIDS are disproportionately found in communities already burdened by poverty, homelessness, illness, inadequate medical care, and a host of other interrelated social problems (Bauman and Wiener 1994; Groce 1995). In addition, about 70 percent of affected children come from households in which one or both parents used illegal substances. Parental drug addiction can have a direct influence on children's behavior and emotional health (Esposito et al. 1999; Mok, Ross, and Raab 1996; Robertson, Ronald, and Raab 1994. It can also have indirect effects through serious economic problems, abuse and neglect, poor parenting skills, and family dissolution and disruption.

Many children have experienced negligence, sexual and physical abuse, and homelessness, with most of these experiences attributed to parental drug use. Many have spent time in legally assigned foster care or more informal fostering arrangements with relatives or family friends, often with the children lacking clear notions about why and for how long they would be under foster care. Many chronic stressors have been found to affect children's mental health, and experiencing multiple life stressors will impact on predeath and postdeath adjustment from parental HIV/AIDS.

RESILIENCE AND PROTECTIVE FACTORS

According to research in the United States, most children who are affected by HIV/AIDS will have clinically significant levels of psychological disturbance at some time during the trauma; more than half will qualify for the diagnosis of a psychiatric disorder. Research has also shown, however, that *resilience*, the capacity for successful adaptation despite challenging or threatening circumstances, and *protective factors*, such as an easy-going disposition and the presence of supportive adults, can reduce the intensity and longevity of these symptoms (Masten, Best, and Garmezy 1990).

Whether a child confronts a societal problem (such as chronic poverty), an acute or chronic disaster (such as war or famine), or a traumatic event (such as maltreatment or parental illness), various individual and situational characteristics affect a child's ability to adapt. Successful intervention programs use these characteristics to identify children's strengths and vulnerabilities and to individualize services. One such program is Masiye Camp (see Figure 4.3). Similar camps, sometimes offering parent-child stays, have been created in the United States.

Through adventure-based experiential learning, the Salvation Army Masiye Camp program in Zimbabwe addresses psychosocial support issues in children. The program started in 1998 and is complementary to community-based home visitation programs in support of children affected by AIDS. In keeping with the African tradition of life initiation camps, every year over twelve hundred children participate in life-skills camps in the Matopos Hills National Park to enhance their resilience and coping capacity.

Tandi, a slender young girl, is an example of how activity and play-based psychosocial support through the camp experience can have a significant impact on children's resilience and coping capacity. During the first few days at camp, Tandi was withdrawn, sad, and very quiet. When her group went for the "Burma Bridge" (high ropes course) exercise, the instructor took the children to the top of a cliff, described the activity, and then asked who wanted to start. The group looked at how far away the ground was, then looked nervously at each other. Almost immediately Tandi's hand was in the air to volunteer. Swiftly her instructor, a volunteer youth and former camper, put the harness around her hips, ready to go. Her face tensed up as she drew a deep breath and took the first wobbling steps on the shaking "Burma Bridge" fifteen meters above the ground. Although starting out was difficult, she caught on quickly and traversed without a problem. A large smile spread over her face and she told the group: "I have done it, I can do it." After that experience, she behaved differently in the group, always volunteering a joke or a story. During the grief and bereavement session later in the week, she referred to her "Burma Bridge" experience as having helped her overcome some of the worries that affected her since the loss of her mother the previous year.

FIGURE 4.3. Masiye Camp

One factor that affects how children respond to the risks associated with HIV/AIDS is developmental age and stage. Older children, for example, are at increased risk because they may need to assume an adult role prematurely. Cultural beliefs can also affect the level of comfort and support children receive during times of crisis. Cultures have complex norms that govern the assistance provided to ill members, and informal rules about familial responsibilities concerning custody and caretaking of orphaned children. Children may find their ordeal considerably ameliorated if they experience love and support from their extended family and the larger community. To the extent that children live in communities already plagued by discrimination, poverty, violence, and demoralization, however, cultural resources may be lacking. In many developing countries, AIDS has already demanded extraordinary sacrifices from communities, particularly from grandparents, who often must care for multiple grandchildren from several of their dead children. Children may have an easier time coping with loss if they still have a healthy remaining parent who can help them grieve successfully.

Child Characteristics

Children who are old enough to have developed cognitive abilities and coping skills are better able than their younger siblings to understand the parent's illness and what it means for the family's future, and they can use previous experience and social and decision-making skills to adjust to the demands of HIV/AIDS. Children with strong intellectual ability and cognitive maturity (developmental age) are more likely to be classified as resilient.

Often, children who are resilient are attractive and appealing to adults (Werner 1993). Even as infants some children elicit positive attention from adults; they are described as active, affectionate, cuddly, good-natured, and easy to deal with. As toddlers they are more autonomous than their peers and show positive social orientation; as school children they show better reasoning and reading skills. Resilient children tend also to have "dispositional" protective factors. These include use of proactive (vs. reactive) coping strategies, high self-efficacy, and self-esteem. In elementary school, resilient children tend to get along well with other children and have many interests, activities, and hobbies. In high school, resilient children have inner control and a positive self-concept, and they are more responsible, achievement-oriented, assertive, and independent.

Family Characteristics

Parents and other caregivers are the most important and consistent protective factor for children under stress (Masten et al. 1990). In the New York City study (Bauman et al. 2002), the most important predictor of childhood mental health in school-aged children whose mothers have HIV/AIDS was an open, supportive relationship with their ill mothers. In addition, a strong positive relationship between child and new caregiver is an important protective factor after parental death. Parents who can function adequately under stress and who are consistent and responsive will facilitate successful coping and adaptation in their children. The strength of the attachment of parent and child is the best predictor of whether a child will develop self-reliance, the capacity for self-regulation, and positive self-regard (Carlson and Sroufe 1995). Children who are insecure in their attachment are vulnerable; they have experienced unavailable or inconsistent support from caregivers and are more likely to develop psychopathology in the face of major stresses. Among inner-city children, the quality of parent involvement was positively related to children's social competence (Reynolds, Weissberg, and Kasprow 1992). Other family factors that may provide buffers against the harmful effects of parent death include protective parenting styles, and family resourcefulness and adaptability.

Parents are the most important guides and partners in the construction of a child's personality: they are best aware of how their child copes with traumatic experiences and can provide emotional support and help in understanding such events (Bretherton 1993). In particular, open communication between an ill parent and a child may facilitate the child's long-term adjustment after parental death, especially when there was discussion of the likelihood that a parent might die and the parent was able to tolerate the child's expression of strong emotion, such as grief or anger.

Although the pivotal role of parents and social support in buffering trauma for children is well documented, there has been little attention to the impact of the loss of parental support. The illness and death of a parent combines the most traumatic risk factors for children's adjustment with the loss of their most powerful and important resource for coping – their parent's love and support.

Starting before the HIV/AIDS epidemic (especially during the crack cocaine epidemic of the 1980s and continuing to the present), a growing number of older people have become surrogate parents for children orphaned by these dual catastrophies. In a sample of three pediatric clinics in high-risk urban neighborhoods, Joslin and Brouard (1995) found that the parent was not the caregiver in 11 percent of families with children under twelve. Most often the caregiver was a grandmother over fifty-five, caring for more than one child. In addition to the stress on older people of caring for young children, many low-income, African American, and Latino grandparents are at greater risk for poor health in general. A New York City study found that half of the children went to live with grandmothers after parental death (Draimin, Hudis, and Segura 1992). Others have found a similar pattern of kinship caring, with grandparents the most common caregivers (Boland, Czarniecki, and Haiken 1992; Simpson and Williams 1993).

Clinical and longitudinal data are needed on how prolonged surrogate parenting in late life affects the health of older caregivers and the children in their care. The caregiver – child relationship is key to children's future adjustment. The caregivers' level of chronic stress and psychological health will influence child adjustment through a variety of mechanisms (Billings and Moos 1983; Holahan and Moos 1987; Rutter and Quinton 1984). Caregivers often take on the newly bereaved child with good intentions but rapidly learn that the transition to a new family structure is difficult, especially for teenagers. Building the new relationship is influenced by the quality and length of the previous relationship between the caregiver and child (if any), who else lives in the household, child characteristics and temperament, child psychological and emotional distress, and housing and financial problems.

The Humuliza program in Tanzania is addressing psychosocial support needs for orphans and vulnerable children in rural Kagera district. (The Humuliza program is sponsored by the Novartis Foundation for Sustainable Development and Terre des Hommes Switzerland.) In March 2000, during a workshop with teenage orphans, some participants agreed that they wanted to start their own orphans organization. They asked two program staff from Humuliza to support them in their endeavor as facilitators. The objectives of the orphans' organization were (1) to assist members in their schooling; (2) to work collectively in the community to increase the image of orphans; (3) to start up a youth bank for small credits and savings; and (4) to ensure mutual assistance in case of illness and death of family members. They choose the name Vijana Simama Imara (VSI), which means "youth standing firm" in Kiswahili. Contrary to the common view that organized orphans would become more stigmatized, interviewed adult community members have shown a positive reaction. People appreciate the orphans' active self-reliance, and praise their willingness to contribute to community development. And though they are still called orphans, without their organization they would continue to be ignored and marginalized. VSI frees them from their roles of being victims, giving them a stronger position in the community.

FIGURE 4.4. Vijana Simama Imara ("Youth standing firm"): Humuliza

External Social Support

Children benefit from having a social support network outside the immediate family. Children with at least one adult mentor or confidant are more likely to overcome adversity than children whose support is entirely from their family members (Masten et al. 1990; Rae-Grant et al. 1989; Rutter 1979; Werner and Smith 1982). When a parent is ill, psychologically disturbed, or incapacitated, other adults in a child's life – such as neighbors, teachers, ministers, youth workers, or elder mentors – can play caring roles. An example of such support, organized by youth themselves, is the "Youth Standing Firm" group in Tanzania (see Figure 4.4).

Community Strengths

Children in Africa have a very different relationship to their extended families and communities than children in industrialized Western cultures. Children in the United States who have a parent ill with AIDS often have no clear idea of who will take care of them after their parent dies, whereas children in Africa typically regard extended family members as parent figures who traditionally assume responsibility for their relatives' children. Thus a child in Africa may adjust to a foster parent who is a relative with greater ease than an American child would adjust to life with a foster parent who may or may not be a relative. Furthermore, households fostering orphaned children receive emotional, spiritual, and material support from neighbors and friends as part of the "community safety net" in many African societies. Children and families who receive such support from extended families and communities are more likely to be resilient in the face of adversity. However, much depends on the relationship with the new guardians, who may expect the children to be grateful and helpful as repayment for taking them in (Mann 2003).

Disruption and Change after Parental Death

Upheavals in a child's life after parental death create a "causal chain" that can culminate in long-term disorder. These upheavals can include the unavailability of a surviving parent who is too distraught to help a child, and displacement from the home. The upheaval is intensified when siblings are separated, especially for children whose older siblings were also their caregivers. Orphaned children are often relocated to a different community after parental death. As a result, they are separated from their friends and social supports and moved to an unfamiliar neighborhood and school; this experience is associated with increased risk for school failure and behavioral problems. It is clear that a protective factor for children recently orphaned is to keep as much of their life consistent and familiar as possible – keeping them with their siblings, in the same dwelling and school, with their same peer and adult support network, and surrounded by people who are familiar and supportive.

SYMPTOMS AND MANIFESTATIONS OF PSYCHOSOCIAL PROBLEMS

Evidence suggests that children affected by HIV/AIDS can exhibit the full range of emotional and behavioral symptoms – including poor school performance or attendance, conflicted or absent peer relationships, conduct problems, and depression and anxiety. This is as true in Africa as it is in the United States (Makame, Ani, and Grantham-McGregor 2002). For some, the type and severity of symptoms suggest a diagnosable psychiatric disorder. For others, symptoms are episodic, short-term, or mild. For those who aim to help troubled children, it remains hard to identify the ones who are most in need. Most children with serious psychological symptoms go unidentified and untreated, in large measure because it is difficult to recognize symptoms in children. Children (particularly those under age eight, for example) may not be able to describe or recognize their feelings. Nonetheless it is generally accepted among experts that children themselves are the best reporters of "internalizing" symptoms, such as depression and anxiety. Parents are often asked about their child's psychological and behavioral status, but they vary in their ability to describe symptoms accurately.

Bauman and Camacho (2000) reported that about one-third of mothers with AIDS in New York underestimate depression in their children. Some, especially those who are ill and cannot spend much time with their children, lack the opportunity for observation. Some children have reported that they do not share their feelings and fears with their ill mother in order to protect her. Those who say they have a poor relationship with their parent also withhold their feelings, keeping the adults in the dark. Some parents see their children's behavior through the distorting lens of depression: They may unwittingly project their own depressive symptoms on their child, or they may lack the capacity to recognize their child's depression. Aware that their condition is a burden, some parents tend to see only the positive behaviors and minimize any problems as being expected under the circumstances.

Teachers may be particularly helpful in identifying children who have behavior problems, but they tend to overlook "good" children who are sad, withdrawn, or anxious. Although children affected by HIV/AIDS might display any of a range of psychological symptoms, some are more likely than others, as we describe next.

Depression

Children of parents with HIV are likely to be depressed. Depressed children may bully a sibling, pick a fight at school, or suffer frequent, unexplained aches and pains. Almost all depressed children display their anger and depression through improper behavior at school or home. Depression in younger children is particularly hard to identify. Infants and toddlers may be diagnosed with failure to thrive or their speech or motor development may be delayed. They may have emotionless faces and minimal activity and be unresponsive or withdrawn, with either excessive or very little crying. Preschoolers may fail to control urine or bowel movements, and be reckless, aggressive, or destructive. School-aged children may perform poorly in school, fear going to school, have a poor self-image, and engage in antisocial behavior (stealing or lying, for example). Excessive worrying, guilt over minor mistakes, sleep disturbances, and undue fatigue are all signs of depression. Teenagers may exhibit depressive symptoms that mirror those found in adults.

Depression in children is diagnosed using the same criteria used for adults, including sadness or feeling blue, somatic symptoms such as appetite and sleep changes, lethargy or an inability to get going, and loss of interest or pleasure in life. Irritability is one symptom that may be more important in childhood and adolescent depression (Hammen and Rudolph 1996). It is very hard to differentiate depression in children from other disorders, particularly conduct disorders and some anxiety disorders, which often co-occur. Children often show both their internalizing problems and their externalizing symptoms with oppositional behavior, fighting with other children, or misbehavior, making it more difficult to identify internalizing depressive symptoms.

Anxiety

Symptoms of general anxiety include excessive worry, fear of going to new places or meeting new people, clinging to parents, unusual dependency, fear of separation from the parent, inability to sit still, and a range of somatic symptoms such as stomachaches, sweating, loss of appetite, sleep problems, nightmares, and hand tremors. Anxiety can be generalized or can focus on a specific place or thing, such as school phobia. Anxiety is particularly likely among children who are worried about their parent's health, fear leaving them alone, or fear being abandoned.

Externalizing and Conduct Problems

Children who are in emotional pain often misbehave. Their oppositional behaviors are more obvious to parents and teachers than sadness or worry and may be a way to identify depressed and anxious children. Some children, particularly older children, may demonstrate a variety of conduct problems such as being defiant and ignoring parental discipline, consistently ignoring family rules, getting into fights, stealing, being absent without permission from school, drinking alcohol, and using illegal substances. Repeated punishment rarely fixes the problem, and parents and schools may overlook the fact that these behaviors are symptoms of an underlying psychological problem.

Bereavement and Grief in Children

Children's bereavement reactions tend to differ from those of adults. Their grief can vary widely by developmental status, but some general reactions are well characterized. These include shock, denial of the loss, feelings of guilt (the child feels responsible for the death), anger (which may be targeted at the dead parent or others), somatic expressions of grief (stomach or other pains, headache, weakness, or breathlessness), depression, fear that they or others will also die, curiosity about the death and what happens after death, and copying, in which the child adopts behaviors or mannerisms of the dead relative.

In contrast to grieving adults, children often fluctuate between intensely feeling the grief of their loss and denying that it occurred. They may cry uncontrollably, then play happily. This alternating pattern may confuse and concern adults, but it is quite normal and reflects the immature ability of children to tolerate the emotional pain of their grief for more than short periods (Osterweis, Solomon, and Green 1984). Children are also more likely to try to maintain internal relationships with the dead parents – talking to them, seeing them reappear – as an attempt to bring them back to life (Arthur and Kemme 1964).

For most children, psychological problems after parental death are not just short-term grief reactions. Many children exhibit their first serious symptoms years after the loss (Rutter 1966). For example, Elizur and Kaffman (1982) reported that while depression had declined in children forty-two months after parental death, general behavior problems had not. Over half of children showed signs of severe psychological disturbance fully eighteen months after the death of a father. Grief and bereavement are culturally determined in part, and rituals around death, grieving, and burial are socially prescribed. The intimate psychological process of grief, however, may not be very different for African, Asian, or American children – sadness, fear, worry, guilt, and depression are all likely.

Effects in Adulthood

The death of a parent in childhood has been found to be a risk factor for adult depression (Lutzke et al. 1997; McLeod 1991). The critical factors associated with poor long-term adjustment are familial – an unstable, insecure family and psychopathology or maladjustment in the surviving parent or caregiver (Harris, Brown, and Bifulco 1986, 1990; Silverman and Worden 1992; Tennant 1988). It is essential to consider the complex chain of experiences, especially current adversity, that may link the loss of a parent in childhood to adult depression. The degree to which an adult experiences depression after parental death in childhood is dependent on the quality of childhood adjustment to parental loss and the adequacy of parenting; a supportive relationship with the surviving caregiver is a protective factor (Breier et al. 1988).

Little research has been done to document the consequences of losing both parents, particularly when the deaths occur sequentially. One possibility is "bereavement overload," a concept coined to apply to the elderly who experience many losses (Kastenbaum 1997); multiple deaths may later leave children vulnerable to life-long disruption (Apfel and Telingator 1995; Fanos and Wiener 1994). Figure 4.5 outlines some of the potential long-term consequences of the lack of psychosocial support for children affected by HIV/AIDS within an African context for individuals, families, and societies experiencing large numbers of parental deaths.

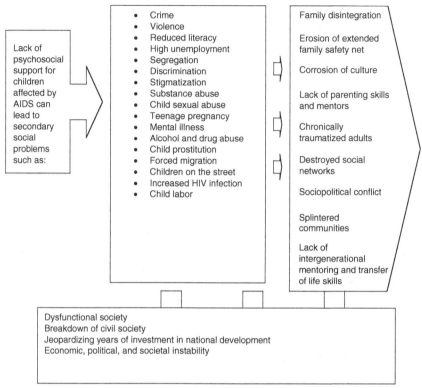

FIGURE 4.5. The lack of psychosocial support for children affected by HIV/AIDS has a cascading effect on social problems that affect them, their families and communities, and ultimately the entire society.

STRATEGIES FOR RESPONDING TO CHILDREN'S PSYCHOSOCIAL NEEDS

There are three main strategies for approaching the psychosocial needs of children affected by HIV/AIDS. First, we need to identify children – probably the minority – with chronic and serious psychiatric problems. Second, we should develop and evaluate interventions to prevent the adverse effects. Third, we need programs that will help children with clinically significant symptoms to adapt to the effects of HIV/AIDS. The reasons for these services are clear: Humanitarianism alone dictates that children in psychic pain receive assistance; children who cope successfully as children will be able to achieve normal developmental milestones and have a more normal childhood; and children who adjust successfully as children will be more likely to function successfully as adults.

Screening Children for Psychological and Behavioral Problems

Is screening a good idea? Is it even feasible? Some may question whether it is wise to screen large numbers of children for behavioral and emotional problems if there is no effective, accessible intervention available to help them. It is clear that no country, including the United States, has an adequate child mental health infrastructure, and that many children with full-blown psychiatric disorders remain untreated. Mental health resources are limited worldwide; even in the United States, inner-city families often wait long periods before receiving time-limited services.

Furthermore, mothers and children may dislike using formal psychological counseling, particularly because most professionals do not come from the same ethnic community as those affected by HIV/AIDS. However, it is important to recognize that there are many ways to assist children with emotional and behavioral problems that do not require professional mental health counselors, psychologists, or psychiatrists.

A second limitation of screening is that just about every child affected by HIV/AIDS will demonstrate clinically significant behavioral or emotional problems at some time. Clearly, one way to help children at risk is to provide a better infrastructure for all children – which would remove the stigma that results from identifying children affected by HIV/AIDS and reduce the likelihood that children with special needs will be overlooked. Examples of such programs might include universal access to education (such as the elimination of school fees in Africa), universal health care access (which is not guaranteed in the United States), home-based visiting programs of trained lay people and nurses, and school-based programs that enhance self-esteem and provide training in social and problem-solving skills.

Although improving the infrastructure is attractive, it is unlikely that we can mount a programmatic response to the mental health epidemic that would provide universal coverage. Until we can provide resources to all children, we will need to make triage decisions: Which children are in the most need? Which children need intensive one-on-one therapy? Which children would benefit from a home visitor, a peer who has the same problem, a support group, or an interested teacher? Which children need practical help (such as a caregiver) and which need monetary assistance? If we can classify the kinds of needs and match children with our scarce resources, we will be efficient without sacrificing efficacy.

Screening Tools. Identifying children with emotional and behavioral problems is best done by using *multiple reporters*, *multiple tools* (or measures), *over time*. It is vital that measures include parents, children themselves, teachers, and others who know the child well. Each person – child, parent, and teacher – has different insight into the child's world; if any one

TABLE 4.1. *Screening Tools for Child Emotional and Behavioral Problems*

Name	Symptoms Assessed	Age	Reporter(s)	References
Child behavior checklist (CBCL)	Full range	2–18	Parent	Achenbach and Ruffle 2000
Youth self-report (YSR)	Full range	11–18	Child	
Teacher report form (TRF)	Full range	5–18	Teacher	
Strengths and difficulties questionnaire (SDQ)	Full range	4–16	Parent	Goodman 2001
		11–16	Child	
		4–16	Teacher	
Children's depression inventory (CDI)	Depression	8–16	Child	
	Depression	8–18	Parent	Kovacs 1985

person acknowledges a problem, the child should be evaluated. Collecting information about the child from different reporters should be done using standardized, validated screening tools that ask about different kinds of externalizing and internalizing symptoms. Informal conversation can be helpful, but research suggests that many children with serious problems will go unidentified unless a systematic set of questions is used. Examples of some of the most accepted measures for this purpose are listed in Table 4.1. However, there is a pressing need for future research to establish whether these tools are valid and reliable across cultures. Most of them have been developed in the West, and thus may fail to capture cultural variation in the ways psychological symptoms are manifested, described, and interpreted.

It is important that children's mental health be assessed repeatedly – preferably every six months but certainly annually. The New York study of children aged eight to twelve found that about 40 percent of children might be identified as having a problem at any one point; over the two-year study, however, every child exhibited clinically significant symptoms, usually on both parent and child report, and many showed persistent symptoms. Any type of identification program must be sensitive and confidential, lest there be inadvertent disclosure of HIV/AIDS to the child or stigma when mental health problems are uncovered.

Should We Screen for Risk and Protective Factors? In addition to assessing children's symptoms, it is useful to assess children's strengths and capabilities as well. This is particularly helpful if there are several different types of intervention; matching children's needs to program strengths should increase program effectiveness. It may also help to identify children who are most at risk should resources be inadequate to meet the need: Those with clinical symptoms who also have other risk factors in the past or at present, or who lack resilience or protective factors such as a strong supportive caregiver, would be targeted for immediate attention.

Interventions to Meet Children's Psychosocial Needs

Grassroots and community-level responses to the HIV/AIDS pandemic have emerged to identify and address the countless needs of HIV-affected individuals and families. Many programs began as a way to address the concrete needs of those affected by HIV/AIDS, such as home health care and money for school fees or uniforms, or employment or business opportunities when families lost their breadwinner. However, in the process of working with families, the need for psychosocial support to children and families became clear, and many programs have added psychological support services.

Comprehensive Programs. Comprehensive programs have many advantages: They are more efficient, they avoid the problems that emerge from failed referrals to other systems of care, and they can offer services when and where they are needed. One example in Malawi is Scaling Up HIV/AIDS Interventions through Expanded Partnerships (STEP), formerly called Community-Based Options for Protection and Empowerment (COPE). STEP works with communities to prevent and mitigate the impact of HIV/AIDS by providing psychosocial support to families and children affected by HIV/AIDS, home-based care, fund-raising to pay for school costs and other needs, and increasing economic opportunities to vulnerable households. (See Chapter 1 for more details on the STEP/COPE experience.) Interestingly, there are no comparable programs in the United States.

Founded in 1995 by Susie Howe, the Bethany Project is a social welfare organization in the Zvishavane District of the Midlands Province, Zimbabwe. The Bethany Project is a community-based program that aims to enable orphans to have lives like other children. It works with community leaders and representative members to mobilize and train them to meet the psychological, physical, and spiritual needs of orphans, to identify sources of funds for material needs) (including payment of school fees) and to raise awareness of the rights of children and teach HIV prevention.

FOCUS (Families, Orphans, and Children under Stress) was established in 1993 by FACT (The Family AIDS Caring Trust) in Mutare, Zimbabwe. FACT, founded in 1987 by Dr. Geoff Foster, counsels people affected by AIDS and works closely with several community groups that provide regular visiting and material support to orphaned children. The program has expanded to include income-generating and microlending projects, advocacy and public awareness activities, and psychological assessment and support. In 2001, the separate programs of FACT, including the Home Care

Programme and the Orphan Programme, were integrated so that program volunteers offer holistic care for families, often establishing relationships with children before their parents die.

Targeted Behavioral Support Programs. There are few examples of programs that have been designed to provide emotional and behavioral interventions for children affected by HIV/AIDS. One exception is the Special Needs Clinic at New York-Presbyterian Hospital, one of the first specialized child psychiatry clinics of its type (Ng, Mellins, and Ryan n.d.). Founded in 1992, the clinic was initiated to address the mental health needs of children and families affected by the dual epidemics of HIV infection and substance abuse. The clinic staff believes that HIV infection affects the entire family; therefore, children and adolescents with HIV infection are treated in the same clinic as their siblings, parents, and legal guardians.

Succession Planning and Security. After the death of a parent, children need consistency and stability (Furman 1983; Nagera 1970; Osterweis et al. 1984; Rutter 1966). Children deserve a well-considered, carefully evaluated, realistic answer to the poignant question, "Who will take care of me?" (Bauman et al. 2000). If children's basic physical and emotional needs are not met, mourning may be inhibited because "anxiety leads them to deny the loss" (Siegel and Gorey 1994). Thus, a key intervention for bereaved children is to avoid disruption in the postdeath phase (Rutter 1966).

Researchers from Makerere University in Kampala, Uganda, together with Population Council/Horizons, designed an evaluation project to study the effectiveness of succession planning services being implemented by the Ugandan office of Plan, an international NGO. The succession planning program included assistance in choosing a guardian, preparing a will, helping parents disclose their HIV status to their children and discuss the future, preparing children for the loss of their parent (by creating memory books and acclimating them to the guardian, for instance, and by enabling parents and future guardians to generate income). Results showed that succession planning led to more disclosure and a greater likelihood of parents' choosing a guardian for their children, and may have led more parents to write wills (Population Council/Horizons 2003).

Project Care is offered by The Family Center in New York City and provides in-home succession planning services (See also Chapter 8). The program has three core principles: family-centered services, involving all people important to the child as early as possible; a coordinated and flexible multidisciplinary team approach that allows for tailoring of services to meet each family's unique needs; and a commitment to provide a continuity of services to families before and after the death of the parent (Bauman et al. 2002).

The Zimbabwe branch of Island Hospice, formed in 1979 to care for terminally ill cancer patients, offers home-based care and bereavement counseling for terminally ill parents and their families; at present, the majority of their patients are being treated for AIDS. Counseling is offered to children before the parent dies and continues after the death; follow-up with the new guardian is done if necessary. The main branch is in Harare, a city in which the extended family is often not as available as one would be in a rural setting. As a result, Island Hospice encourages custody planning and writing wills. Furthermore, disclosure of HIV/AIDS status to children is encouraged as part of the process.

Family Options is a permanency planning project created in 1997 by the Illinois Department of Children and Family Services in conjunction with a network of legal and social service providers. The project provides legal and social work permanency planning and other supportive services to families in which at least one parent has HIV or AIDS. Families are recruited from staff outreach at HIV clinics and community-based programs in the Chicago area. Family Options social workers make home visits to families to counsel them on a range of issues that lead them to make a permanency plan for their children. Many HIV-affected families, for example, may need assistance with substance abuse or mental health issues, and project staff have good relationships with other providers and can make referrals. A range of mental health services is provided directly by Family Options social workers, who help families deal with acceptance/denial of their illness, disclosure, family therapy, end-of-life issues, and facing mortality. Legal permanency plans primarily have involved guardianship, standby guardianship, and short-term guardianships, adoption, and standby adoption. Flexible permanency plans, such as standby and short-term guardianships, are sought for families so that they can retain custody of their children for as long as the parents are able to provide care, yet have the assurance that the caregiver of their choice will assume responsibility for children when needed.

In the United States, few parents with AIDS have a realistic custody plan in place for their children. Helping parents with AIDS plan for the future custody of their children is complex. Ensuring that caregiver arrangements are feasible and legal is immensely complicated and intricate. (See Figure 4.6 for some elements of a good custody plan.) Planning and executing long-term guardianship for children is complicated further by the complexity of the service systems that must be coordinated for the development of a feasible plan. Families and their social service providers must be able to negotiate both the legal and entitlement systems, at the same time meeting the changing psychosocial needs of the ill parent, children, and other family members.

Children's psychological health is most dependent on the presence of a loving caregiver after parental death and the assurance that their physical

1. Is the plan intended to be permanent?
2. Will children be placed in a household where neither the caregiver nor anyone else will subject them to abuse or neglect?
3. Has the parent discussed his or her serious illness with the proposed caregiver in realistic (not hypothetical) terms, and has the caregiver agreed to the plan?
4. Is the caregiver in good enough health to care for the children?
5. Can the caregiver support the children financially, with assistance if needed and available?
6. To the extent possible, have the children participated in and agreed to the custody plan?
7. Will the children be placed with siblings, or at least kept in contact with them?
8. Does the plan keep the children in familiar neighborhood and school surroundings, or if this is not feasible, is there a plan for an orderly transition?
9. Does the proposed housing meet basic standards of safety and privacy?
10. Are there any barriers to legalizing the plan (e.g., caregivers' previous felony conviction or previous record on child abuse/neglect)?

Source: Levine, Draimin, and Bauman 1995.

FIGURE 4.6. Elements of a Good Custody Plan

and emotional needs will be met (Bifulco, Brown, and Harris 1987; Garmezy 1983). Children need a secure, predictable environment and routine or the risk of anxiety increases (Osterweis et al. 1984).

Bereavement Support. Bereavement programs can be offered to children who have experienced loss of any family member or friend. The grief process in children is a series of psychological tasks (Baker, Sedney, and Gross 1992). Using this framework, individual and group-level support services can assist children to grieve and adjust. In the first stage, the child must understand what has happened. It is critical that a sense of personal security is maintained while this understanding is achieved. In the second phase, the child must rework the relationship to the lost person. This involves maintaining an inner attachment to that person but distinguishing between fantasy and reality. At this point the full emotional impact of the loss, including ambivalent feelings of love and anger, must be experienced and worked through. In the third phase, the child must evolve a new sense of personal identity that includes the experience of loss, and must start to invest in new relationships and developmentally appropriate activities.

It is critical for the child to have adult support in this process. Children need the encouragement of an adult to talk about the death of loved ones.

Otherwise, they are likely to avoid the grieving process and even deny the death (Becker and Margolin 1967; Rosenthal 1980). Children may also harbor false beliefs that their actions or neglect caused the death. For children whose parent died of HIV, it is important to avoid surrounding the cause of death with secrecy, which gives the child the impression that something shameful has happened (Siegel and Gorey 1994). In contrast, though, if the reason for the death is public, children may be teased or rejected by other children. Such stigma has been shown to cause psychological problems and poor school achievement (Rinella and Dubin 1988).

Adults hold myths and misconceptions about children's understanding of death. Instead of protecting children, myths tend to deny children opportunities to talk about their grief or to mourn with the help of a supportive adult. Misconceptions in turn are integrally tied to adults' lack of knowledge about what children of different ages understand about death, which is closely associated with developmental stage.

Young children may be unable to grasp the abstract concept of death, but they do understand and grieve a loss. By age seven or eight, however, children generally understand that death is final, and by age ten or eleven, they can understand the causes of death (Osterweis et al. 1984). Although children can understand death and do grieve, children do not mourn like adults. They may acknowledge loss of the parent in the real world but try to maintain a relationship with the dead parent in their inner world.

Adults need to encourage children to talk about their feelings of guilt, loss, anger, and sadness; such talk has been shown in many studies to enhance the adjustment of children to parental death (Black and Urbanowicz 1987; E. Furman 1983; Kliman 1973; Miller 1971; Nagera 1970). Fostering open communication is difficult, however, in families experiencing what Doka (1994) defines as "disenfranchised grief," that is, grief that cannot be openly acknowledged and socially supported. The stigma and secrecy that surround AIDS in families can be expected to have a negative impact on children's ability to mourn openly. Well children may worry that they have acquired AIDS from their parent and need to be reassured (Siegel and Gorey 1994).

Supporting New Caregivers. New caregivers are likely to be older family members, especially grandparents, responsible for the care of many children, grieving their own losses as well as responding to the children's grief and adjustment problems. An important component of many programs focuses on the material and psychosocial needs of these family members. For example, the Family Options Project in Chicago provides support, referrals, and linkages to services for new caregiver families. The project can ease a child's transition into a new family setting. Legal "aftercare" services include helping a standby guardian obtain guardianship of a child after the parent has died or become incapacitated. Attorneys also help new caregivers access benefits on behalf of the children now in their care. Assistance is also provided to new caregivers who wish to make their own permanency plans for the new children in their care.

Grandparents with custody of their grandchildren have become an organized advocacy force in the United States. Beyond HIV/AIDS and drug use, many grandparents have taken custody because of their child's mental illness and inability to parent. In the federally funded National Family Caregiver Support Program, the U.S. Administration on Aging allocated specific funds for programs that serve grandparents.

PUTTING KNOWLEDGE INTO PRACTICE: LESSONS LEARNED

The psychosocial burden of HIV/AIDS on children is large, but the available resources are not. It is likely that all children affected by HIV/AIDS will, at some point in their childhood, experience psychiatric symptoms serious enough to warrant a diagnosis. Most will experience sadness, paralyzing anxiety, anger, and isolation, and many will lack the assistance they need to cope successfully with the challenges. This is as true in Africa as it is in the United States. A study in the poor suburbs of Dar Es Salaam, Tanzania, for example, compared orphans and non-orphans. Orphans had markedly increased internalizing problems, as well as being more likely to go to bed hungry and be absent from school. A third of them had contemplated suicide in the past year (Makame et al. 2002).

In the absence of a sufficient mental health infrastructure to provide professional health care for children affected by HIV/AIDS, the focus must turn to community-based efforts that can use available resources combined with the expertise and research available on children and loss. The advantages of community-based programs are many, including the likelihood that they will be practical and sustainable, and that they will be congruent with the cultural and familial beliefs and expectations of the people served. We have described the ingenuity and creativity of just a few on-the-ground programs for children affected by HIV/AIDS. These are testimony to the ability of communities to define and meet their children's needs. These programs can be models for other communities, although it is vital that there be formal documentation and evaluation.

In addition to adopting models others have found helpful, it is important to develop more general principles that can help guide future program development. Based on the extensive research on children and stress, the psychiatric and psychological literature on childhood disorder and grief, and the model programs already in place, some lessons can be extracted:

1. Parents and families need support. Children live in families, and family-friendly policies and programs can make all the difference in the

ability of a family to meet the needs of a child with a mental health problem. These needs can be idiosyncratic, so home-based visiting programs are often well suited to help families identify problems and find solutions. Home-visiting programs generally use a peer model in which volunteer parents or grandparents agree to visit other parents to give advice or help out. Peer models can be very effective because they use the experiential wisdom of successful parents to help those in crisis.

2. Programs must avoid stigmatizing children. Some programs target for attention the children who are worst off (the triage model); some target children who are exposed to a stressor (for example, children affected by HIV/AIDS); and some are universal in approach (all children are eligible). Communities must decide which approach is best for their circumstances. However, programs that target children with behavior problems or who are affected by HIV/AIDS may add to, rather than subtract from, their burden. Mental illness is typically a stigmatizing condition, as is HIV/AIDS. Although it is laudable to target assistance to such children, programs may label children, add to their poor self-image, and isolate them from their community. Targeted programs must be offered in nonstigmatizing ways.

3. Programs that are open to all children have advantages. In universal programs children are not labeled deficient, needy, different, or problematic, nor do they require screening or the up-front expenses required to case-find and verify eligibility. Such programs focus on building resilience, providing access to resources, and teaching coping skills that are preventive. Universal programs also have disadvantages, however. The main one is that they may be more costly because all children are eligible: It is less expensive to serve fewer children. In resource-poor settings, a universal program may not be practical. Another disadvantage is that the needs of children with profound psychological distress are unlikely to benefit from universal programs because they need intensive counseling.

4. Prevention is worth the investment. It is easier and less costly for communities to provide prevention programs than treatment programs. By implementing programs that increase protective factors, communities can help make children stronger in facing challenges and less likely to have severe or prolonged periods of disability due to psychosocial problems. Prevention programs aim to build individual strengths through providing skills or resources, recognizing that:

- each child needs a trusted adult outside the family to provide support,
- children need information that is provided honestly and at their developmental level,
- children need their basic security needs for food and shelter met,
- children should attend school, and
- children benefit from learning decision making and social and communication skills.

Prevention programs may also build community-level strengths, for example through parenting classes, custody planning services to insure continuity, bereavement services, or paying school fees to insure universal access to education.

5. Children benefit from structure and predictability. Children need to be a part of the community and its rhythms and to live according to a clear routine. To the extent possible they should go to school, be part of cultural traditions, attend celebrations, share public grief, and experience what other children their age experience.

6. Every child needs an adult. Whether or not children have a strong relationship with a parent, they need an adult mentor outside the family whom they can trust and depend on. Research is clear that children who have a trusted adult friend do better in the face of hardship. Even communities with few resources can facilitate building and maintaining such ties as a powerful way to provide a safety net for children.

7. Children need child-based spaces. A community center open to all children is a wise investment. It provides a safe space for children to play and make friends. It is universal and does not stigmatize those in need, but it is an invaluable place to identify those children who are already in trouble or who are at risk. It is normalizing, and provides an opportunity to build trust between adults and children. Every community should have a place where children can go to seek advice and counsel.

8. Community adults can be trained to support children's psychosocial health. Adults who routinely come into contact with children (such as those in child-based spaces, teachers, sports coaches, or medical and health personnel) can be trained to recognize and intervene with youngsters who are showing symptoms of psychological disturbance. Training programs should teach counseling skills (such as listening for the feelings behind the words or actions, using "I" statements, helping a child clarify and [re]define the nature of a problem, and providing support) and explain childhood developmental ages and stages (what children of different maturity levels can understand), and how to distinguish normal and complicated bereavement reactions.

9. Adults trained to provide psychosocial support need access to professional expertise. Some children will have profound symptoms, including depression, suicidal ideas, and hostility. Lay adults will be more willing to become a community expert on child behavior when they have access to a "hot line" or monthly routine visits from a trained professional. A consultation model is relatively inexpensive because one professional can support many outreach workers.

10. Intervention programs must come from the community. Some communities have developed a board or working group of community leaders and parents to define children's needs for psychosocial care, support, and services. Such a board insures cultural congruence and political buy-in

and increases the likelihood that the community will invest resources in a sustainable way. Sometimes it is necessary to mobilize a community to acknowledge and address the problem of children's unmet psychosocial needs. Public education programs may be needed to increase awareness of adults about the problems children may have and the ways they can help.

11. Professionals and lay leaders need tool kits to use in identifying and caring for the most common forms of psychological problems in children. Such kits should include ways to determine the difference between a problem and a disorder (between sadness and depression, normal and complicated grief, and acting out and conduct disorder, for instance). It could also describe ways to help such children and when to call a professional if feasible.

12. Empowerment models build skills, increase self-confidence, and can provide a workforce. Being a helper is more empowering than being helped. Children and adolescents who are experiencing special challenges related to HIV can organize (as in the Humuliza program in Tanzania, Figure 4.4) to improve their standing in the community and increase successful coping through self-help strategies. Youth also can be trained through peer counseling and social skills programs to help other children like themselves. The act of helping others can help children work out their own problems: It can help them feel needed, esteemed, valued, and important to the community, and it can provide services to others who need support. A rolling system in which those who are served by this model in turn are trained to become the providers means a growing cadre of youth who have the ability to help.

References

Achenbach, T., and T. Ruffle. 2000. The Child Behavior Checklist and related forms for assessing behavioral/emotional problems and competencies. *Pediatrics in Review* 21:265–71.

Anderson, C., and C. Hammen. 1993. Psychosocial outcomes of children of unipolar depressed, bipolar, medically ill, and normal women: A longitudinal study. *Journal of Consulting and Clinical Psychology* 61 (3): 448–54.

Apfel, R., and C. Telingator. 1995. What can we learn from children of war? In *Forgotten children of the AIDS epidemic*, ed. S. Geballe, J. Grunedel, and W. Andiman, 107–21. New Haven: Yale University Press.

Armistead, L., and R. Forehand. 1995. For whom the bell tolls: Parenting decisions and challenges faced by mothers who are HIV seropositive. *Clinical Psychology: Science and Practice* 2 (3): 239–50.

Arthur, B., and M. Kemme. 1964. Bereavement in childhood. *Journal of Child Psychology and Psychiatry* 5:37–49.

Baker, J. E., M. A. Sedney, and E. Gross. 1992. Psychological tasks for bereaved children. *American Journal of Orthopsychiatry* 62 (1): 105–16.

Barnett, B., and G. Parker. 1998. The parentified child: Early competence or child-hood deprivation? _Child Psychology & Psychiatry Review_ 3 (4): 146–66.

Bauman, L. J., and S. Camacho. 2000. Discrepancies between child and maternal reports of child mental health. Poster presented at the annual meeting of the American Association for Public Opinion Research, Portland, OR, May.

Bauman, L. J., S. Camacho, E. J. Silver, J. Hudis, and B. Draimin. 2002. Behavior problems in school-aged children of mothers with HIV/AIDS. _Journal of Clinical Child Psychology and Psychiatry_ 7 (1): 39–54.

Bauman, L. J., G. Foster, and E. J. Silver. 2004. Children as caregivers to their ill mothers with HIV/AIDS. Poster presented at the 15th International AIDS Conference, Bangkok, Thailand.

Bauman, L. J., C. Levine, B. Draimin, and J. Hudis. 2000. Who will care for me? Planning the future care and custody of children orphaned by HIV/AIDS. In _Working with families in the era of HIV/AIDS_, ed. W. Pequegnat and J. Szapocznik, 155–88. Thousand Oaks, CA: Sage.

Bauman, L., L. Phuong, E. Silver, and R. Berman. 2001. Lean on me? Adjustment of children who provide support to their ill mothers with HIV/AIDS. Poster presented at the annual meeting of the Pediatric Academic Societies, Baltimore, May.

Bauman, L., and E. Silver. 2001. Disclosure of maternal HIV/AIDS to children. Poster presented at the annual meeting of the Pediatric Academic Societies, Baltimore, May.

Bauman, L., E. Silver, B. Draimin, and J. Hudis. 2003. Children of mothers with HIV/AIDS: Unmet needs for mental health services. Poster presented at the annual meeting of the Pediatric Academic Societies, Seattle, May.

Bauman, L. J., and L. Wiener. 1994. Priorities in psychosocial research in pediatric HIV infection. _Journal of Developmental and Behavioral Pediatrics._ Supplement 15(3).

Beardslee, W., and I. Wheelock. 1994. Children of parents with affective disorders: Empirical findings and clinical implications. In _Handbook of depression in children and adolescents_, ed. W. Reynolds and H. Johnston, 463–79. New York: Plenum.

Becker, D., and F. Margolin. 1967. How surviving parents handled their young children's adaption to the crisis of loss. _American Journal of Orthopsychiatry_ 37:753–7.

Bifulco, A., G. Brown, and T. Harris. 1987. Childhood loss of parent, lack of adequate parental care, and adult depression. _Journal of Affective Disorders_ 12 (2): 115–28.

Biggar, H., and R. Forehand. 1998. The relationship between maternal HIV status and child depressive symptoms: Do maternal depressive symptoms play a role? _Behavior Therapy_ 29:409–22.

Billings, A. G., and R. H. Moos. 1983. Comparisons of depressed and nondepressed parents: A social-environmental perspective. _Journal of Abnormal Child Psychology_ 11 (4): 463–85.

Black, D., and M. Urbanowicz. 1987. Family intervention with bereaved children. _Journal of Child Psychology and Psychiatry_ 28:467–76.

Boland, M., L. Czarniecki, and H. Haiken. 1992. Coordinated care for children with HIV infection. In _Children and AIDS_, ed. M. Stuber, 161–81. Washington, DC: American Psychiatric Press.

Breier, A., J. R. Kelsoe, P. D. Kirwin, A. Beller, O. M. Wolkowitz, and D. Pickar. 1988. Early parental loss and development of adult psychopathology. *Archives of General Psychiatry* 45:987–93.

Bretherton, I. 1993. Theoretical contributions from developmental psychology. In *Sourcebook of family theories and methods: A contextual approach*, ed. P. G. Boss, W. J. Doherty, R. LaRossa, W. R. Scumm, and S. K. Steinmetz, 275–301. New York: Plenum Press.

Carlson, E. A., and L. A. Sroufe. 1995. Contribution of attachment theory to developmental psychopathology. In *Developmental psychopathology*, ed. D. Cicchetti, and D. J. Cohen, vol. 1, *Theory and methods*, 581–617. Hoboken, NJ: John Wiley & Sons.

Cates, J., L. Graham, D. Boeglin, and S. Tielker. 1990. The effect of AIDS on the family system. *Families in Society: The Journal of Contemporary Human Services* 7 (4): 195–201.

Doka, K. 1994. Suffer the little children: The child and spirituality in the AIDS crisis. In *AIDS and the new orphans: Coping with death*, ed. B. O. Dane and C. Levine, 33–42. Westport, CT: Auburn House.

Downey, G., and J. Coyne. 1990. Children of depressed parents: An integrative review. *Psychological Bulletin* 108:50–76.

Draimin, B. H., J. Hudis, and J. Segura. 1992. *The mental health needs of well adolescents in families with AIDS.* New York: Human Resources Administration.

Elizur, E., and M. Kaffman. 1982. Children's bereavement reactions following death of the father: II. *Journal of the American Academy of Child Psychiatry* 21 (5): 474–80.

Esposito, S., L. Musetti, M. Musetti, R. Tornaghi, S. Corbella, E. Massironi, P. Marchisio, H. Guarechi, and N. Principi. 1999. Behavioral and psychological disorders in uninfected children aged 6 to 11 years born to human immunodeficiency virus-seropositive mothers. *Journal of Developmental and Behavioral Pediatrics* 20 (6): 411–17.

Fanos, J., and L. Wiener. 1994. Tomorrow's survivors: Siblings of human immunodeficiency virus-infected children. *Journal of Developmental and Behavioral Pediatrics* 15 (3): 243–6.

Felner, P., M. Ginter, M. Boike, and E. Cowen. 1981. Parental death or divorce and school adjustment of young children. *American Journal of Community Psychology* 9:181–91.

Forehand, R., R. Steele, L. Armistead, E. Morse, P. Simon, and L. Clark. 1998. The family health project: Psychosocial adjustment of children whose mothers are HIV infected. *Journal of Consulting and Clinical Psychology* 66 (3): 513–20.

Forsyth, B., L. Damour, S. Nagler, and J. Adnopoz. 1996. The psychological effects of parental human immunodeficiency virus infection on uninfected children. *Archives of Pediatrics and Adolescent Medicine* 150:1015–20.

Furman, E. 1983. Studies in childhood bereavement. *Canadian Journal of Psychiatry* 28:241–7.

Garmezy, N. 1983. Stressors of childhood. In *Stress, coping, and development in children*, ed. N. Garmezy and M. Rutter, 43–66. New York: McGraw-Hill.

Geballe, S., J. Gruendel, and W. Andiman. 1995. *Forgotten children of the AIDS epidemic.* New Haven: Yale University Press.

Germann, S. 2003. Psychosocial needs and resilience of children affected by AIDS: Long-term consequences related to human security and stability. Power Point presentation, at the World Bank OVC Conference, Washington, DC, May 14.

Gerstadt, C. 2003. Discrepancies in the reporting of the mental health of children who have mothers with HIV/AIDS. *Dissertation Abstracts International* 63: 8-B.

Goodman, R. 2001. Psychometric properties of the strengths and difficulties questionnaire. *Journal of the American Academy of Child and Adolescent Psychiatry* 40:1337–1345.

Groce, N. 1995. Children and AIDS in a multicultural perspective. In *Forgotten children of the AIDS epidemic*, ed. J. G. S. Geballe and W. Andiman, 95–106. New Haven: Yale University Press.

Hackl, K. L., A. M. Somlai, J. Kelly, and S. C. Kalichman. 1997. Women living with HIV/AIDS: The dual challenge of being a patient and a caregiver. *Health and Social Work* 22 (1): 53–62.

Hammen, C., and K. D. Rudolph. 1996. Childhood depression. In *Child psychopathology*, ed. E. J. Mash and R. A. Barkley, 153–95. New York: Guilford Press.

Harris, T., G. W. Brown, and A. Bifulco. 1986. Loss of parent in childhood and adult psychiatric disorder: The role of lack of adequate parental care. *Psychological Medicine* 16 (3): 641–59.

———. 1990. Loss of parent in childhood and adult psychiatric disorder: A tentative overall model. *Development & Psychopathology* 2 (3): 311–28.

Holahan, C., and P. Moos. 1987. Risk, resistance, and psychological distress: A longitudinal analysis with adults and children. *Journal of Abnormal Child Psychology* 96:3–13.

Joslin, D., and A. Brouard. 1995. The prevalence of grandmothers as primary caregivers in a poor pediatric population. *Journal of Community Health* 20 (5): 383–401.

Kastenbaum, R. 1997. What is the future of death? In *Death and the quest for meaning: Essays in honor of Herman Feifel*, ed. S. Strack, 361–80. Northvale, NJ: J. Aronson.

Kliman, G. 1973. Facilitation of mourning during childhood. In *Perspectives on bereavement*, ed. I. Gerber, A. Wiener, and A. H. Kutscher. New York: Irvington Press.

Kovacs, M. 1985. The children's depression inventory (CDI). *Psychopharmacology Bulletin* 21:995–8.

Lee, M., P. Lester, and M. Rotheram-Borus. 2002. The relationship between adjustment of mothers with HIV and their adolescent daughters. *Clinical Child Psychology and Psychiatry* 7 (1): 71–84.

Lee, M., and M. Rotheram-Borus. 2002. Parents' disclosure of HIV to their children. *AIDS* 16 (16): 2201–7.

Levine, C. 1990. AIDS and changing concepts of family. *Milbank Quarterly* 68 (1): 33–59.

———, ed. 1993. *A death in the family: Orphans of the HIV epidemic*. New York: United Hospital Fund.

———. 1995. Orphans of the HIV epidemic: Unmet needs in six U.S. cities. *AIDS Care* 7 (suppl. 1): S57–S62.

Levine, C., B. Draimin, and L. Bauman. 1995. Is this custody plan viable? Ten questions to consider. *The Source: Newsletter of The National Abandoned Infants Assistance Resource Center*, Fall. Reprint no. 30.

Levine, C., and G. Stein. 1994. *Orphans of the HIV epidemic: Unmet needs in six U.S. cities*. New York: The Orphan Project.

Lipson, M. 1994. Disclosure of diagnosis to children with human immunodeficiency virus or acquired immunodeficiency syndrome. *Journal of Developmental and Behavioral Pediatrics* 5 (3): S61–S65.

————. 1996. Telling: Discussion of HIV and death with children and adolescents. *Pediatric AIDS HIV Infection* 7:239–42.

Lutzke, J., T. Ayers, I. Sandler, and A. Barr. 1997. Risks and interventions for the parentally bereaved child. In *Issues in clinical child psychology: Handbook of children's coping; Linking theory and intervention*, ed. S. Wolchik and I. Sandler, 215–43. New York: Plenum Press.

Makame, V., C. Ani, and S. Grantham-McGregor. 2002. Psychological well-being of orphans in Dar Es Salaam, Tanzania. *Acta Paediatrica* 91 (5): 459–65.

Mann, G. 2003. *Family matters: The care and protection of children affected by HIV/AIDS in Malawi; A CPSC case study*. Stockholm: Save the Children Sweden.

Masten, A., F. Best, and N. Garmezy. 1990. Resilience and development: Contributions from children who overcome adversity. *Development and Psychopathology* 2:425–44.

McLeod, J. D. 1991. Childhood parental loss and adult depression. *Journal of Health and Social Behavior* 32 (3): 205–20.

Miller, J. 1971. Children's reactions to the death of a parent: A review of psychoanalytic literature. *Journal of the American Psychoanalytic Association* 19:697–719.

Mischel, M. 1981. The measurement of uncertainty in illness. *Nursing Research* 30:258–63.

Mok, J., A. Ross, and G. Raab. 1996. Maternal HIV and drug use: Effect on health and social morbidity. *Archives of Diseases of Childhood* 74:210–14.

Murphy, L. B., K. Koranyi, L. Crim, and S. Whited. 1999. Disclosure, stress, and psychological adjustment among mothers affected by HIV. *AIDS Patient Care and STDs* 13:111–17.

Nagera, H. 1970. Children's reaction to the death of important objects: A developmental approach. *Psychoanalytical Study of the Child* 25:360–400.

Nagler, S., J. Adnopoz, and B. Forsyth. 1995. Uncertainty, stigma, and secrecy: Psychological aspects of AIDS for children and adolescents. In *Forgotten children of the AIDS epidemic*, ed. J. G. S. Geballe and W. Andiman, 71–82. New Haven: Yale University Press.

Ng, W. Y. K., C. A. Mellins, and S. Ryan. n.d. The mental health treatment of children and adolescents perinatally infected with HIV. *Topic of the Month*. http://www.hivfiles.org/topic.html.

Osterweis, M., F. Solomon, and M. Green. 1984. *Bereavement: Reactions, consequences, and care*. Washington, DC: National Academy Press.

Parkes, C., and R. Weiss. 1983. *Recovery from bereavement*. New York: Basic Books.

Pivnick, A., and N. Villegas. 2000. Resilience and risk: Childhood and uncertainty in the AIDS epidemic. *Culture, Medicine, and Psychiatry* 24:99–134.

Population Council/Horizons. 2003. Succession planning in Uganda: Early outreach for AIDS-affected children and their families. Washington, DC. Available at http://www.popcouncil.org/horizons

Rae-Grant, N., H. Thomas, D. Offord, and M. Boyle. 1989. Risk, protective factors, and the prevalence of behavioral and emotional disorders in children and adolescents. *Journal of the American Academy of Child and Adolescent Psychiatry* 28 (2): 262–8.

Reynolds, A., R. Weissberg, and W. Kasprow. 1992. Prediction of early social and academic adjustment of children from the inner city. *American Journal of Community Psychology* 20 (5): 599–624.

Rinella, V., and W. Dubin. 1988. The hidden victims of AIDS: Healthcare workers and families. *Psychiatric Hospital* 19:115–20.

Robertson, J., P. Ronald, and J. Raab. 1994. Deaths, HIV infection, abstinence, and other outcomes in a cohort of injecting drug users followed up for 10 years. *British Medical Journal* 309:369–72.

Rosenthal, P. 1980. Short-term family therapy and pathological grief resolution with children and adolescents. *Family Process* 19:151–9.

Roth, J., R. Siegel, and S. Black. 1994. Identifying the mental health needs of children living in families with AIDS or HIV infection. *Community Mental Health Journal* 30 (6): 581–93.

Rutter, M. 1966. *Children of sick parents: An environmental and psychiatric study.* London: Oxford University Press.

———. 1979. Protective factors in children's responses to stress and disadvantage. In *Primary prevention in psychopathology*, ed. M. Kent and J. Rolf, 49–74. Hanover, NH: University Press of New England.

———. 1987. Continuities and discontinuities from infancy. In *Handbook of infant development*, 2nd ed., ed. J. D. Osofsky. Hoboken, NJ: Wiley.

Rutter, M., and D. Quinton. 1984. Parental psychiatric disorder: Effects on children. *Psychological Medicine* 14 (4): 853–80.

Sandler, I., J. Gersten, F. Reynolds, C. Fallgren, and P. Ramirez. 1988. Using theory and data to plan support interventions. In *Marshalling social support: Formats, processes, and effects*, ed. B. H. Gottlieb, 53–83. Newbury Park, CA: Sage.

Schwartz, C., D. Dorer, W. Beardslee, P. Lavori, and M. Keller. 1990. Maternal expressed emotion and parental affective disorder: Risk for childhood depressive disorder, substance abuse, or conduct disorder. *Journal of Psychiatric Research* 24:231–50.

Siegel, K., and E. Gorey. 1994. Childhood bereavement due to parental death from Acquired Immunodeficiency Syndrome. *Developmental and Behavioral Pediatrics* 15 (3): S66–S70.

Silver, E., L. Bauman, S. Camacho, and J. Hudis. 2004. Factors associated with psychological symptoms among mothers with late-stage HIV/AIDS. *AIDS and Behavior* 7 (4): 421–31.

Silverman, P. R., and J. W. Worden. 1992. Children's reactions in the early months after the death of a parent. *American Journal of Orthopsychiatry* 62 (1): 93–104.

Simpson, B. J., and A. Williams. 1993. Caregiving: A matriarchal tradition continues. In *Until the cure: Caring for women with HIV*, ed. A. Kurth, 200–11. New Haven: Yale University Press.

Tennant, C. 1988. Parental loss in childhood. *Archives of General Psychiatry* 45:1045–50.

Van Eerdewegh, M., M. Bieri, R. Parrilla, and P. Clayton. 1982. The bereaved child. *British Journal of Psychiatry* 140:23–9.

Wallace, B. 1996. *Adult children of dysfunctional families: Prevention, intervention and treatment for community mental health promotion.* Westport, CT: Praeger.

Weissman, M., G. Gammon, and K. John. 1987. Children of depressed parents: Increased psychopathology and early onset of major depression. *Archives of General Psychiatry* 44:847–53.

Werner, E. 1993. Risk, resilience, and recovery: Perspectives from the Kauai Longitudinal Study. *Development & Psychopathology* 5 (4): 503–15.

Werner, E., and R. Smith. 1969. Loss, rage, and repetition. *Psychoanalytic Study of the Child* 24:432–60.

———. 1982. *Vulnerable but not invincible: A study of resilient children.* New York: McGraw-Hill.

5

Human Rights and Children Affected by HIV/AIDS

Sofia Gruskin and Daniel Tarantola

HIV/AIDS epidemics around the world have drastically changed children's lives. Millions of children have been infected with HIV and have died of AIDS, and many more are affected as HIV spreads through their families and communities. The epidemics have an impact on adolescents as well as younger children, and increase the marginalization of children living in particularly difficult circumstances.

To effectively support these children, and to fulfill their potential for growth and development, many approaches are needed: economic, educational, psychosocial, and health care, along with community mobilization. Essential to the effectiveness of these approaches, and as a necessary approach in its own right, is attention to human rights – the focus of this chapter. In November 1989, the United Nations General Assembly approved the first human rights document to focus specifically on the rights of children – the Convention on the Rights of the Child (CRC) (United Nations 1989).

Although the HIV/AIDS epidemics were not a motivating factor in creating the CRC, the document's timing was fortuitous because the devastating impact of the pandemic on the lives of children was becoming more apparent. Within a few years, 191 states signed on to the legal obligations of this document, which became effective in September 1990; today only Somalia and the United States have not ratified it. Some countries have agreed to be bound to the CRC's provisions only insofar as the convention does not contradict their customs and traditions. Nonetheless, none of these reservations has been considered to violate the object and purpose of the treaty.

All countries that have ratified the CRC are bound by its provisions. They must report regularly to the eighteen-member Committee on the Rights of the Child (the treaty-monitoring body serviced by the United Nations Office of the High Commissioner for Human Rights), describing the ways they are and are not in compliance with the treaty provisions.

Their legal obligations include showing constant improvement in their efforts to respect, protect, and fulfill the rights in question.

Implementation of the CRC is guided by four principles: nondiscrimination; best interests of the child; life, survival, and development; and participation of the child in decision making. Integrating the rights of the child into the policy and program responses to HIV/AIDS does not mean a one-size-fits-all approach. The child rights issues that come into play, as well as what is effective, within one setting with one population might not be so in a different setting with another. The central focus in all settings should be on meaningful implementation of the underlying principles, as well as children's genuine participation in the formulation and implementation of HIV/AIDS strategies, programs, and policies. Action, rather than rhetoric, must prevail.

The CRC defines a child as any human being below the age of eighteen years, unless a country's laws define adulthood at a younger age (Art. 1). It further defines government responsibilities for protecting children and ensuring that they are no longer just the object of decisions affecting them, but participants involved in these decisions as their capacity to do so grows (Van Bueren 1995).

Fulfilling children's rights is directly relevant to reducing their risk of HIV infection, as well as to ameliorating the long-term impact of HIV on their lives, their families, and their communities. This chapter raises some questions and maps some issues pertaining to the rights of the child in the context of HIV/AIDS, drawing on the perspectives offered by the CRC and other relevant human rights documents. It does not focus exclusively on children orphaned by AIDS, because the issues raised here must be considered holistically. Furthermore, because other chapters in this volume deal extensively with the economic, educational, and psychosocial impacts of HIV/AIDS on children and their families, this chapter highlights the ways in which stigma and discrimination exacerbate these serious consequences. Human rights are not separate from the need to ensure children a safe and supportive environment; they are integral to the fulfillment of these basic requirements. Because other chapters focus on the roles of community-based organizations and international aid groups, as well as religious communities, this chapter with its emphasis on human rights emphasizes the essential role of government in fulfilling these rights for children.

The chapter begins with an introduction to the contexts in which HIV/AIDS permeates the lives of children and then sets out the human rights obligations of governments under the CRC and other relevant human rights documents. After proposing an approach that integrates these perspectives, this chapter draws attention to some critical questions in relation to age and gender for ensuring the relevance of HIV/AIDS policies and programs to the lives of children. It concludes with the implications

of the rights of the child for policy and programmatic responses to
HIV/AIDS.

CHILDREN'S RIGHTS IN THE CONTEXT OF HIV/AIDS

Every day around the world sixteen hundred children are born with perinatally transmitted HIV infection (Global Strategies for HIV Prevention
2003); 95 percent of them live in the developing world (USAID, UNICEF,
and UNAIDS 2002). In addition, an unknown number of children acquire
the virus from unsafe blood and blood products and unsterile needles
(from medical injections performed inside and outside the formal health
care setting and injection drug use), and through sex, including sexual
abuse. Except for perinatal infection, the modes of HIV transmission are
the same for children and adults. However, because they occur in children,
who depend on adults, each must be considered from a more complex
perspective.

The complicated relationship of children to adult support and decision
making is often hidden by a tendency to regard children as homogeneous,
regardless of sex, age, and evolving intellectual capacity. In reality, differences in sex, age, and the social, economic, cultural, and political context
in which children live must be taken into account in any policy or programmatic response to the HIV/AIDS epidemics. From a child rights perspective, HIV/AIDS illuminates how cultural norms and legal precepts
facilitate or constrain the capacity of children to decide on issues central
to their health and well-being. From a health perspective, the relationship
between childhood and HIV/AIDS emphasizes the evolving capacity of
boys and girls to participate, at different stages of their physical and intellectual development, in decisions relevant to the future course of their lives.

These perspectives are crucial not only to promoting and protecting
children's rights, but also to stimulating a dynamic understanding and
response to the HIV/AIDS epidemics, as well as to the broader context
of child health and development. Attention to the rights of the child is a
priority in and of itself, but it can also help governments to conceptualize
how HIV exists within a society and to design, implement, and evaluate
relevant policies and programs – as well as allocate resources – in a manner
that comprehensively focuses on children (Tarantola and Gruskin 1998).

Consideration of the rights of the child in the context of HIV/AIDS rec-
ognizes both the public health responsibilities of governments and their
human rights obligations under the CRC and other binding human rights
documents. Over twenty years of experience have shown that it is essential
to integrate rights into the policy and program responses to the epidemics.
This principle has largely been accepted in adult programs for HIV prevention and care; it is equally true for mitigating the impact of HIV/AIDS
on the lives of children orphaned and otherwise affected by HIV/AIDS.

CHILDREN CONFRONTING HIV/AIDS: INFECTED, AFFECTED, AND VULNERABLE

As the pandemic evolves, its impact is increasingly being felt by children in the developing world and in marginalized communities in the industrialized world. Infected by HIV, affected by the loss of parents and family members, and vulnerable to HIV infection, infants, young children, and adolescent girls and boys are confronting new challenges to their health and development.

Children Living with HIV/AIDS

Girls and boys with HIV suffer the physical consequences of infection through stunted growth, disability, increased morbidity, and premature death. Furthermore, their condition creates psychological stress and may expose them to stigma and discrimination. This societal response not only violates their rights and increases their susceptibility to the health effects of the virus, but decreases the quality of their lives and jeopardizes their growth and development. Discrimination on the basis of real or perceived HIV status can impact on children's families and communities and on the services available to them, including entitlements to educational, health, and social services. For children and adolescents already infected with the virus, discrimination on the basis of their diagnosed or presumed HIV status may result in the denial of their rights to equal access to health care, treatment, education, and social programs.

Children with HIV/AIDS are often heavily discriminated against in the formal and informal educational systems (Carr-Hill et al. 2002). In some countries, where the health system's overall capacity is already strained, children with HIV have been routinely denied access to basic health care (UNAIDS 1996). Infected children living in difficult circumstances may find themselves experiencing stigma and discrimination on the basis of their social and economic marginalization, as well as their HIV status. At its extreme, discrimination against HIV-infected children may result in their abandonment by their family, community, or society.

While the number of children infected around birth can be estimated, there is an unacceptable gap in data on the incidence of infection among children as they grow into adulthood. There is an acute lack of information on how, when, and to what extent girls and boys become infected through early sexual activity, sexual abuse, substance use, or exposure to unsterile blood, blood products, and skin-piercing instruments (Tarantola and Schwartländer 1997). There is also insufficient research on children living with HIV/AIDS to guide the design of care and support programs for them.

As a first step in fulfilling their obligations to children in the context of HIV/AIDS, governments should design prevention, care, and treatment programs in the light of appropriately collected information. Governmental obligations extend to ensuring that all children, including those living with HIV/AIDS, have access to health services, treatment, education, and social programs. The quality and, indeed, length of life of children living with HIV can be improved if the coping capacity of the family is enhanced, either by increasing its ability to support itself or through direct social support. Some governments have achieved considerable progress in this direction; others have yet to respond adequately, if at all, to rising needs.

Affected Children

Children are affected when their close or extended family, their community, and, more broadly, the structures and services that exist for their benefit are strained by the consequences of the HIV/AIDS pandemic. The most devastating impact on children occurs when their immediate family environment and support system is weakened by the sickness, disability, and premature death from AIDS of one or both of their parents. The emotional impact of such a trauma, including living through the deprivation of parental support and loss of childhood, can create serious obstacles to a child's development.

Furthermore, as a result of the reduced ability of infected parents and extended families to sustain their livelihood, children may have to leave their homes, drop out of school, find jobs, or seek a life on the streets. When communities or services are not well informed and otherwise prepared, the disclosure of the HIV-infected status of one or both parents may exacerbate the stigma associated with HIV/AIDS, resulting in their child's being marginalized or discriminated against. For these children, their stigmatization and social isolation may be accentuated by discrimination resulting in a decrease in or loss of access to education, health, and social services. Education and access to services for these children are necessary for their own sakes, but they are particularly salient in the context of the HIV/AIDS epidemics, because children must acquire the skills to reduce their risk of becoming infected and many must support themselves prematurely if their parents die.

Children affected by HIV need support to continue their education, provide care to other family members, and grow through adolescence and adulthood without stigma or any other disadvantage. While it is now recognized that the extended family, with the support of the surrounding community, is the best source of care for orphans, the next generation of orphans will have fewer older adults left to care for them, thus the number of older children caring for their younger brothers and sisters will only increase. Assistance must be provided to affected families so that, to the maximum extent possible, children can remain within existing family structures and receive needed care. Additional support will likely be needed if these children are to have adequate access to food, education, vocational training, services, and care.

At the same time, paradoxically, it is also important to avoid singling out HIV-affected children for special attention, ignoring similar problems faced by other children within a community. Directing assistance only to children orphaned by AIDS can increase the stigma and discrimination they face, create hostility toward them (due to the perception they are unfairly being privileged), and undermine any sense of community responsibility to respond to their needs.

Governments must strive to prevent and alleviate the impact of HIV/AIDS on these children. This entails guiding, facilitating, mobilizing, and at times providing support for affected families so that, to the maximum extent possible, children remain within existing family structures and receive needed care. It also includes ensuring that children who find themselves without family are given care through alternative systems, and that all children are protected against all forms of abuse and exploitation.

Vulnerable Children

Children are vulnerable to HIV/AIDS by the simple fact that they are born, grow up, and become sexually active in a world that has added the risk of acquiring HIV infection to many of the already risky situations that mark their childhood (Levine, Michaels, and Back 1996). Social, cultural, economic, and other factors determine the degree of risk that a child will be exposed to HIV infection or deprived of access to treatment, care, and support if infected. Children's capacity to reduce this risk depends on their degree of awareness and ability to avoid behaviors and situations that risk exposure to HIV. Behaviors and risks are influenced by the social environment in which children live and the availability of, and access to, services intended for their benefit. In many countries, children's vulnerability to HIV/AIDS is increased because they are denied access to information and to sexual and reproductive health services, and even when these are made available to them, they are seldom designed to meet children's specific needs. Girls' culturally influenced lack of control over sexual encounters greatly increases their vulnerability.

Vulnerability and risk of HIV infection are even more acute for children in exceptionally difficult circumstances (Santa Barbara 1997). Poverty, sex discrimination, and the difficulties faced by children in need of special protection – whether institutionalized, living in the streets, or involved in armed conflicts or substance use – reflect the neglect or violation of the rights of children and increase their vulnerability to HIV infection, which fuels the epidemics. In addition to the direct consequences of physical or mental abuse, negligent treatment, exploitation, survival on the street, inadequate alternative systems of protection, violence, and displacement, children's vulnerability to HIV and the impacts of AIDS are amplified.

Every governmental effort toward realizing the conditions necessary for children's harmonious, safe development is a step toward reducing their vulnerability to HIV/AIDS. Reducing vulnerability includes building an economic, social, and political environment in which children and their families are safe and can support themselves and make informed choices.

THE ADVENT OF THE RIGHTS OF THE CHILD

Recognition of the vulnerability of children has in recent years generated increasing governmental attention and commitment to promoting and protecting their rights. International human rights documents ranging from the United Nations (1966) International Covenant on Civil and Political Rights to the CRC contain legally binding provisions specifically detailing the human rights of children, and nearly every article in the general human rights instruments apply equally to children and to adults. While none of the human rights treaties contains specific elaborations of rights in the context of HIV/AIDS, the treaty-monitoring bodies have, to varying degrees, expressed their commitment to explore the implication of HIV/AIDS for governmental obligations under their treaties (Gruskin, Hendriks, and Tomasevski 1996). In particular, in 2003 the United Nations Committee on the Rights of the Child adopted the General Comment on HIV/AIDS and the Rights of the Child, which provides comprehensive guidance to governments on how to take into account the rights of the child within their prevention, care and treatment, and impact-mitigation efforts in the context of HIV/AIDS (United Nations Committee on the Rights of the Child 2003). The General Comment states that its objectives are:

.... 4. (a) To identify further and strengthen understanding of all the human rights of children in the context of HIV/AIDS;
(b) To promote the realization of the human rights of children in the context of HIV/AIDS, as guaranteed under the Convention on the Rights of the Child...;
(c) To identify measures and good practices to increase the level of implementation by States of the rights related to the prevention of HIV/AIDS and the support, care and protection of children infected with or affected by this pandemic;
(d) To contribute to the formulation and promotion of child-oriented plans of action, strategies, laws, policies and programmes to combat the spread and mitigate the impact of HIV/AIDS at the national and international levels.

Political commitments in the programs of action adopted at recent international conferences have also stated governments' responsibility for ensuring the rights, health, and well-being of children and reducing the impact of HIV/AIDS on individuals and communities. Formal commitments were made in the United Nations World Summit for Children (1990), the United Nations World Conference on Human Rights (1993), the United Nations International Conference on Population and Development (1994), the United Nations World Summit for Social Development (1995), the United Nations Fourth World Conference on Women (1995), the First World Congress against Commercial Sexual Exploitation of Children (1996), the United Nations Millennium Summit (2000), the United Nations Special Session on HIV/AIDS (2001), and the United Nations General Assembly Special Session on Children (2002). In addition, formal declarations were made at regional conferences, including the African Summit on HIV/AIDS, Tuberculosis, and Other Related Diseases (2001) in Abuja, Nigeria, and the African Union Ministerial Conference on Human Rights in Africa (2003), in Kigali, Rwanda.

UNAIDS and UNICEF have emphasized the rights of the child in relation to HIV/AIDS in all aspects of their work. Children Living in a World with AIDS was the theme of the World AIDS Campaign for 1997, and in 1998 it was Force for Change: World AIDS Campaign with Young People. The theme of the World AIDS Campaigns for 2002 and 2003 was Stigma and Discrimination, with the slogan "Live and Let Live." The Office of the United Nations High Commissioner for Human Rights and UNAIDS issued and updated its *International Guidelines on HIV/AIDS and Human Rights* (1998, 2002) that included specific attention to children and young people.

Despite these commitments, there has been a chasm between the rhetoric and the reality. The pandemic and rights violations both continue to grow. Moving beyond the rhetoric to the applicability of the human rights framework to the design and evaluation of HIV/AIDS policies and programs could go a long way toward reducing the impact of the pandemic on the lives of children. The four general principles of the CRC provide the lens critical to any analysis and action in relation to the rights of the child in the context of HIV/AIDS. These general principles of the CRC should guide consideration of all laws, policies, programs, and practices relevant to children and HIV/AIDS.

THE CRC'S FOUR GENERAL PRINCIPLES

The four general principles of the CRC are useful for conceptualizing the complex nature of the rights of children, who are at the same time both rights-holders and active agents in their own lives, but also vulnerable and in need of special protection. These principles are set forth as ordinary articles in the CRC, but they acquired a special status during the first session of the United Nations Committee on the Rights of the Child (1991). The Committee determined that these rights should be used as the lens through which realization of all rights in the CRC are analyzed, implemented, and evaluated. This concept is unique to the CRC; no other human rights treaty contains rights that are meant to be discussed both in and of themselves, and as a means of analyzing governmental progress toward implementation of other rights. A brief summary of the content of the four general principles follows:

- Nondiscrimination (Art. 2) requires that all children are protected from discrimination of any kind. Children are protected on the same grounds laid out in other human rights instruments, but additional general protections are specified based on ethnic origin, disability, and refugee status, as well as the status of parents or legal guardians. Confronting the stigma that remains attached to HIV/AIDS, children may benefit from specific protections from discrimination, for example, based on disability or in relation to their own or their parent's real or perceived health status. Irrespective of their citizenship, background, or circumstances, they are entitled to fundamental protection and care by governments if their family is unable to provide these.
- The Best Interests of the Child (Art. 3) makes the child's interests a primary consideration, on equal footing with the interests of parents, families, communities, and the state. The CRC explicitly identifies the few instances when it considers the best interests of the child not to be the primary consideration. For example, the temporary or permanent deprivation of children from their family environment, and the separation of children from adults in situations where they are deprived of their liberty (except when it is considered in the child's best interests not to do so), as well as determining who has primary responsibility for the upbringing and development of the child (par. 9, 18, 20, 21, 37) may be situations where there can be genuine disagreement about what is in the "best interests of the child." As a general principle, the child's best interests are equal to the interests of others, but do not trump them. It is understood that this concept is flexible, so as to respond to the evolving capacities of the child, living conditions, cultural norms, and expectations. The concern for the best interests of the child is of paramount importance in devising and implementing relevant HIV/AIDS prevention, care, and research programs.
- Life, Survival, and Development (Art. 6) is understood as the precondition for realization of all other rights. It concerns children's rights to benefit from economic and social policies that will allow them to survive into adulthood and to develop in the broadest sense of the word, as well as the right not to be killed arbitrarily at the hands of the state (Hammarberg 1995). The large-scale impact of HIV/AIDS epidemic hampers governments' capacities to fulfill these rights but in no way absolves them of their responsibility to do so. The reality of the limited capacities of governments with inadequate resources creates an

implied obligation and compelling interest of wealthier states to provide assistance beyond their own borders.

- Participation (Art. 12) concerns the child's right to express an opinion and have it heard, considered, and given due weight. This is perhaps the most radical provision of the CRC, in that it requires adults who normally wield power in affairs concerning children to make it possible for children to express their views, and it obliges them to consider children's views with respect to all matters, whether within the family or the broader community. The child's right to express an opinion and have it heard must be given due weight in devising and implementing relevant HIV/AIDS policies and programs. Central in all settings is the avoidance of rhetorical attention to children, coupled with their genuine participation in the formulation and implementation of HIV strategies, programs, and policies.

GOVERNMENTS AT THE FOREFRONT: RESPECT, PROTECT, AND FULFILL RIGHTS

The four general principles of the CRC have direct implications for addressing HIV/AIDS and its impacts on children. The interplay of these principles should guide governments with respect to any actions they take that may impact on child health and development. This broad set of governmental obligations may go far beyond policies and programs that are directly and consciously targeted at children. For example, a governmental decision concerning the reallocation of public space may result in restricting a socially secure environment in which children were able to play, thereby relegating them to unsafe gathering sites. From an HIV perspective, this suppression of conditions favorable to the enhancement of social skills in children may increase the likelihood of their engaging in unsafe behaviors that, in turn, may expose them to a higher risk of acquiring HIV infection. While from a rights perspective, the right of the child to rest and leisure (Art. 31) is the only right directly applicable, recognition of the four general principles can help mediate this process and lead to a decision best for all concerned.

Likewise, attention to HIV/AIDS may bring increased focus to realization of certain rights otherwise guaranteed under the human rights framework. For example, from a CRC perspective, a government's obligations under Art. 7 require that systems be in place to ensure the registration of every child at or shortly after birth. From an HIV perspective, realization of this right is critical later in life for children who have been orphaned by HIV/AIDS: Experience has shown these children have difficulty in accessing needed services, even if they are available, without this proof of identity once their parents have died.

States are responsible for not violating people's rights directly as well as for ensuring the conditions that enable them to realize their rights as fully as possible. This is understood as an obligation on the part of governments to respect, protect, and fulfill rights such as the right to an adequate standard of living (Eide 1995). This obligation includes the states' responsibility to ensure that neither they themselves nor nonstate actors – ranging from families and communities to pharmaceutical companies – neglect or violate the rights of children in the context of HIV/AIDS. Governmental obligations are taken to relate to every right, every person – adult or child – and every action taken. The following example considers three obligations governments have regarding the right any children infected, affected, or vulnerable to HIV/AIDS has to education.

Respect. Governments must refrain from directly violating rights. For example, for children infected with HIV, the right to education would be respected if access to primary school education were ensured. In contrast, this right would be violated if a government barred children from attending school on the basis of their HIV status. (See Figure 5.1 for an example of a successful challenge to this kind of discrimination.) For children affected by HIV, the extent to which governments respect the right

In January 2004 the Kenyan High Court approved an agreement between the Ministry of Education and the Nyumbani Children's Home that permits HIV-positive children in the home to attend government schools. While their HIV status was not named as the issue, previously the Ministry had refused to admit these children on the grounds that there was no room or that the children did not have birth certificates.

The landmark decision was important for children's rights in several ways. Most important, it affirmed the principle of nondiscrimination. In September 2003 the Chambers of Justice, a Nairobi-based human rights organization, petitioned the Ministry on behalf of the orphanage to admit the children, arguing that the Constitution of Kenya, the United Nations Convention on the Rights of the Child, and the Universal Declaration of Human Rights all prohibit discrimination. This explicit reference to international agreements is a second important aspect of the case.

In December 2003 the children of the Nyumbani Home filed suit against the Ministry, and the case was heard before Justice Martha Koome early in January 2004. In this expedited hearing the judge allowed more than thirty children to attend, which affirmed the principle of children's participation in decisions affecting them. The parties reached an amicable agreement, and the Director of City Education was ordered to begin the process of admitting the children of school age to public schools.

Source: Canadian HIV/AIDS Legal Network; www.aidslaw.ca

FIGURE 5.1. A Judicial Victory for HIV-Positive Children in Kenya

to education may be reflected in a government's choice in sustaining or closing a primary school in a community hard-hit by HIV/AIDS, or in eliminating financial and other barriers to attendance. For children vulnerable to HIV, respect of the right to education means that, for example, the government must provide and not withhold education to incarcerated children.

Protect. The government is responsible for preventing rights violations by private, nonstate actors including individuals, groups, and organizations. If a violation does occur, the government must ensure that there is a legal means of redress that people know about and can access. For infected children, protecting the right to education would impose an obligation on the government to take action against a private school that excluded children on the basis of their HIV status. A situation concerning children affected by HIV could include orphans who have lost both their parents to AIDS and whose surviving relatives want to remove them from primary school to work in a factory. Their right to education would be protected if the government ensured that these children were able to pursue their primary education, through whatever means appropriate, for example by waiving school fees or providing other means of support to the family. The vulnerability of adolescents to HIV infection can increase if they are denied access to accurate reproductive and sexual health education. Protecting the right to education of adolescents in the context of HIV requires governments to ensure that conservative groups are not successful in opposing such education (United Nations International Conference on Population and Development 1994, par. 4.76).

Fulfill. Governments have a duty to take administrative, budgetary, legislative, judicial, and other measures toward the full realization of rights. Governments must fulfill the right of children infected with HIV to gain an education by enacting laws that ensure that, for example, vocational education be developed that is "available and accessible to children with HIV" on an equal basis with other children. Governments must work to fulfill the right to education of children affected by HIV/AIDS by taking measures to ensure that the economic strains on HIV-affected communities do not result in children being withdrawn from school. The vulnerability of children to HIV/AIDS can be exacerbated if governments fail to fulfill their obligations to develop educational programs realistically targeted to the needs of all children within a society.

An agenda for governmental action must recognize the convergence of the three situations (infected, affected, and vulnerable) that confront children in a world with AIDS and the three levels of government obligation (respect, protect, and fulfill) that exist for every right. This approach would incorporate the promotion and protection of the rights of children into the diversity of responses needed to bring the pandemic under control and mitigate its impact. Table 5.1 summarizes governmental obligations to

TABLE 5.1. *Governmental Obligations with Respect to Children's Rights in the Context of HIV/AIDS*

	Children Infected with HIV/AIDS	Children Affected by HIV/AIDS	Children Vulnerable to HIV/AIDS
Respect	Government to refrain from directly violating the human rights of children living with HIV on the basis of their HIV status.	Government to refrain from directly violating the rights of children affected by HIV/AIDS.	Government to refrain from directly violating the human rights of children that impact on vulnerability.
Protect	Government to prevent rights violations by nonstate actors against children living with HIV/AIDS, and to provide some legal means of redress.	Government to prevent violations by nonstate actors that would increase the burden of HIV/AIDS on affected people, and to provide some legal means of redress.	Government to prevent rights violations by nonstate actors that may increase children's vulnerability to HIV/AIDS, and to provide some legal means of redress.
Fulfill	Government to take administrative, judicial, and other measures toward realization of the rights of children living with HIV/AIDS.	Government to take administrative, legislative, judicial, and other measures toward the realization of the rights of children affected by HIV/AIDS.	Government to take administrative, legislative, judicial, and other measures toward the realization of the rights of children in order to minimize their vulnerability to HIV/AIDS.

children's rights in the context of HIV/AIDS. The four general principles of the CRC should be understood as applicable to any analysis of each of the issues presented.

Attention to the rights of the child can in this way help to identify when governmental actions are abusive – whether intentionally or unintentionally. Recognition of human rights in the design, implementation, and evaluation of governmental policy can point the way toward actions that are not only necessary but, in public health terms, most effective (Gruskin and Tarantola 2001). The proactive approach by the governments of the world that is emerging in response to the UN Special Session (2002) goals for reducing the impact of HIV/AIDS on orphans and vulnerable children is an example of the positive action that governments can take to fulfill children's rights as well as not to harm them or deny their rights.

IS THERE AN AGE FOR CHILDHOOD AND AN AGE FOR HIV?

The age range used to define "children" and the age groupings used to analyze HIV epidemic trends and define population subsets targeted for prevention and care are inconsistent. The CRC defines children as every individual under the age of eighteen. For the purpose of epidemiological surveillance, newborns to fourteen-year-olds are considered children, and until 2004 fifteen-to-eighteen-year-olds were included in the fifteen-to-forty-nine-year-old "adult" category (USAID et al. 2002, 2004). The arbitrariness of this grouping categorized boys and girls in the under-fifteen age group as children, regardless of the age at which they become sexually aware, initiated, and active. The assumption inherent in this grouping appears to be that children over fifteen are as likely to be sexually active as anyone nineteen and older, and thus equally at risk of acquiring HIV (or other sexually transmitted diseases through sexual contacts.

Indeed, retrospective analysis of reported AIDS cases for which age-specific information is available suggests that the majority of all HIV infections acquired by adults do occur in the fifteen-to-twenty-four-year-old age group. While age-specific information is possible to collect in research and prevention projects conducted in well-defined study populations, few national epidemiological surveillance systems have the capacity to collect and analyze data with the degree of accuracy required to make such an analysis meaningful to policy and program design or evaluation.

Ideally, HIV incidence data (the proportion of those infected over a given period, usually a year) should be collected by single-year age groups to provide information that reflects the dynamics of HIV spread. Incidence data are commonly derived from annual differences in prevalence – that is, the proportion of children to young adults in a specific age category who are infected at a given point in time (UNAIDS and WHO 1998). This extrapolation would be possible for younger age groups whose exposure to HIV is likely to be recent, but becomes increasingly problematic as they grow older because the age at which they became infected can no longer be ascertained.

The aggregation of age groups into the children and adult categories for epidemiological purposes at the national and global levels also influences the ways in which health and social services are delivered. For example, a fourteen-year-old with an STD (sexually transmitted disease) may be referred to pediatric services, then, only a few months later (having reached the age of fifteen) to an adult STD clinic. In most cases, neither setting is sufficiently equipped to meet this young person's needs. Because epidemiological information is used to target and monitor services and programs, from a rights perspective using the zero-to-fourteen and fifteen-to-forty-nine age groupings obscures the relevant developmental, psychological, sexual, and societal factors that affect children's lives differently than adults'.

The collection of information on children in a manner consistent with the CRC would recognize that those under eighteen are children, and could bring into focus sexual and epidemiological factors that have not received sufficient attention. For example, the fact that children under eighteen have not yet attained "the age of majority" in a particular country could help underscore HIV/STD infection trends that may be due to sexual abuse or other rights violations. This, in turn, would call for targeted HIV prevention and care interventions combined with human rights protections, which to date have not been sufficiently recognized.

The issue of inconsistency of age groupings is further compounded by the different age cut-offs at which countries recognize the legal "age of consent" for consensual sex, as these may affect the degree to which children feel comfortable coming forward for needed services or openly discussing relevant behaviors and practices with health service providers. In many countries, there may be a difference between the age of consent for females and for males; and, in countries where same-sex activity is legal, there may be a difference in legal age depending on whether the person is engaging in sexual activity with a person of the same or different sex. (For a list of relevant legislation of all 181 Interpol member states, see Interpol n.d.)

The arbitrariness of these cut-off ages to the analysis of sexual behaviors and HIV/STD trends is pertinent to those working on HIV/AIDS. The arbitrariness of these legal cut-off ages is also pertinent to those more directly concerned with promoting and protecting the rights of the child in the interpretation of epidemiological trends, with determining the extent to which the rights of the child are fulfilled, and ultimately with putting into place effective HIV/AIDS prevention, care, and treatment programs.

The inconsistency in age groupings and in program targeting will probably remain for years to come, yet, it is essential that studies be conducted to explore the dynamics and determinants of HIV/STD infection and the situations and behaviors leading to infection in children from birth through age eighteen. Estimates of the number of children born with perinatally acquired HIV infection are usually extrapolated from HIV prevalence rates among pregnant women. However, little is known about the number of children who become infected through breast-feeding in their first years of life and even less through unsterile skin-piercing medical or other practices, blood transfusion, sexual contacts, or injection-drug use as they grow older. The invisibility of adolescents caught between childhood and adulthood, in terms of both their social status and their physical development, is detrimental to the protection of the rights of the child and to the development of effective HIV/AIDS strategies realistically targeted to their needs (UNDAW, UNICEF, UNFPA, and ECA 1997).

STILL IGNORING GENDER?

Societal and cultural norms defining gender roles for boys and girls add another layer of complexity to factors influencing vulnerability to HIV infection, as well as to the probability of receiving adequate care and support once infected. Epidemiological data from countries where heterosexual transmission of HIV predominates show that teenage girls have higher rates of HIV infection than boys of the same age (Nunn et al. 1994). In South Africa, for example, there are twice as many young women aged fifteen to twenty-four living with HIV as there are young men of the same age. In Kenya and Mali, the ratio is even more stark – 4.5 to 1 (UNAIDS 2004: 6).

As adolescent girls and boys grow through early adulthood this difference tends to shrink, so that by their mid-thirties, about as many men as women live with HIV infection (Family Health International 1996). The differential in HIV incidence in younger age groups has been attributed to patterns of sexual partnership (younger females having sexual contact with older males who are more likely than younger ones to be HIV-infected), the biological and physiological vulnerability of younger girls to HIV infection, and societal and cultural norms defining male and female gender roles that may make it extremely difficult for young women to insist on safer sex practices with their sexual partner.

Data from many countries has shown not only that girls tend to acquire HIV infection at an earlier age than boys, but also that once HIV infection has set in, discrimination may be more extreme as gender and HIV-related discrimination compound one another. To date, differentials determined by sex or gender roles in relation to HIV/STD infection in children and young people are not systematically considered in the collection and analysis of HIV/STD epidemiological data, nor are they sufficiently studied or built into the design of HIV/STD prevention programs targeted toward this population.

The need for the collection and analysis of epidemiological and other HIV/AIDS-related information specific to adult men and women, separately, is increasingly recognized. The same still cannot be said reliably for children (UNAIDS 2004). There remains insufficient attention to the fact that information is generally collected on children younger than fifteen without differentiation by sex. This lack of sexual differentiation generally may disaggregate obscure indications that might be relevant not only to the natural history of HIV infection but to prevention and care needs as well. One does not know, for example, how gender factors influence the relative risk of becoming infected through various routes of transmission during childhood, and how gender may influence patterns of access to and quality of care provided to boys and girls once HIV infection has set in. In countries where the HIV/AIDS pandemic has become mature, some fifteen-to-sixteen-year-old girls seen at antenatal clinics for their first pregnancy are already infected with HIV, but no information is available about the cause of this infection, whether it involves sex or other modes of transmission, nor whether once diagnosed these young girls continue to access needed care and support (Fylkesnes et al. 1997). Many young people have little access to information about HIV/AIDS and prevention methods (Family Health International 2000; UNICEF, UNAIDS and WHO 2002).

From the perspective of HIV/STD prevention and care, policies and programs must recognize the different needs – and the expression of these needs – among boys and girls. From the perspective of human rights, however, whether boys and girls should be treated differently in HIV prevention and care (and more broadly in the context of their health and development) raises the specter of gender-based discrimination. For example, in a number of places contraception is denied to young girls but provided to young boys, with the explicit rationale that access might prompt girls to be sexually active. This practice can be understood as discrimination against girls. Despite moral and cultural myths, all available information shows that access to contraception is no more likely to encourage girls to become sexually active than it is to prompt boys (UNFPA n.d.).

Each of the major human rights documents prohibits discrimination on the basis of sex when such distinctions result in a people being treated unfairly and unjustly on the basis of their sex. The prohibition of discrimination does not mean that differences should not be acknowledged, only that different treatment must be based on reasonable and objective criteria. Therefore, applying different approaches to information collection, analysis, and use in policy and programs affecting girls and boys should be based on the valid recognition of gender-related differentials in risk and vulnerability and attempts to minimize the influence of prescribed gender roles and cultural norms.

Different treatment of girls and boys in the context of HIV prevention and care, and more broadly as concerns their health and development, is commonplace throughout the world. Recognition of the ways in which assumptions about gender roles may impact on the design of prevention strategies and care is critical to bringing the pandemic under control. In this regard, the gender-based roles predominant in each situation should be carefully considered and directly addressed. Girls are often the ones who drop out of school first because they are expected to care for an ill parent and to assume additional household tasks, or simply because boys' education is valued more highly.

SO WHERE DO WE GO FROM HERE? PROGRAMMING EFFORTS

HIV/AIDS policies and programs are generally designed for adults, with scant attention to their effectiveness for children and adolescents. In part because of the rhetorical focus on children's rights in recent years, a number of efforts to integrate them into HIV/AIDS programming have taken place. Unfortunately, there appears to have been little consistency in methodology or approach in the range of efforts understood to be "rights-based." Attention to the potential for partnerships and multisectorality have driven some efforts, while others have been more focused on helping governments to fulfill their commitments in relation to the CRC. Still others have been more focused on ensuring the participation of children and their communities in the design of HIV-related programs. (See Figure 5.2 for examples of programs in which children, including those who are orphaned or affected by HIV/AIDS, provide care to people living with HIV/AIDS in their communities.)

The right of children to participate in decisions and activities affecting them can be implemented within families as well as through community or national programs. Many HIV/AIDS prevention programs targeted at young people involve them as peer educators. Young volunteers in programs such as the "Improvement of Health and Life Skills of Young People" organized by the Thai Ministry of Health assist in home visits and social activities for children in the community who are HIV-positive or whose family members are ill. Some of the volunteers are themselves orphans or children affected by HIV/AIDS. The program was started by Mathurot Songkaew, a twenty-two-year-old woman whose uncle died of AIDS and whose aunt is living with the disease. Her young cousin was ostracized by her schoolmates' parents. One of the goals of the program is to reduce stigma and discrimination.

In Zambia, an intervention study by the Horizons Program, in partnership with Care International and Family Health Trust, found that young people had much to contribute to community-based care and support activities. They may also have adopted more self-protective behaviors such as condom use. Some participants felt that the program was beginning to make a difference in reducing community stigma. An evaluation of the program concluded that involvement of community leaders at the outset is essential, the range of needs that youth caregivers can be expected to meet must be clearly established, and ongoing monitoring and training are essential to strengthen capacity and improve services.

Source: for Thailand, Prudence Borthwick, UNICEF (personal communication, December 9, 2004; for Zambia, www.popcouncil.org/pdfs/horizons/zmbcythfnl.pdf.

FIGURE 5.2. Children's Participation in HIV/AIDS Care Programs

While many of these initiatives are to be lauded on their own merits, this inconsistency has resulted in confusion among policymakers and programmers not fully familiar with human rights frameworks, as to which rights or how rights can actually improve their efforts to minimize the impact of HIV/AIDS on the lives of children. This inconsistency has even allowed for claims that attention to rights in the context of programming is in conflict with the well-being of children, and that a "child welfare" or "family survival" approach may be more useful. The following is an attempt to set out a few common principles in the hopes that they may shed light on these debates, as well as help guide comprehensive integration of the rights of the child in future HIV/AIDS programming efforts.

Conceptually, the first issue involves reducing the gaps between children who for civil, political, economic, social, or cultural reasons, are more vulnerable to HIV infection and its consequences, and children who enjoy better health and better services. The respect, protection, and fulfillment of human rights – civil, political, economic, social, and cultural – is necessary not only because they are the binding legal obligations of governments under international law, but because they are critical to mitigating the impact of HIV/AIDS on children and adolescents. Attention to the rights of the child brings a deliberate focus to both the underlying determinants of HIV infection and the ways in which HIV/AIDS-related policies, programs, and services are delivered. There is clear attention to the four guiding principles of the CRC – nondiscrimination, best interests of the child; life, survival, and development; and participation – in helping to determine priority interventions at each phase of policy and programmatic work. There is also deliberate attention to transparency, accountability, and functioning norms and systems to promote and protect HIV/AIDS-related rights, of both children and their communities.

Operationally, a rights-based approach brings attention to the legal and political context of HIV/AIDS programming. This attention addresses if and how (beyond ratification of the CRC) human rights norms and standards have been incorporated by a government in any actions that impact on HIV/AIDS. Is there a system to promote and protect HIV/AIDS-related rights? Has the country adopted a child-rights-centered approach to HIV/AIDS? Is there a comprehensive, multisectoral, national child-centered HIV/AIDS policy, strategy, and plan of action? Drawing this one step further requires attention not only to whether relevant laws, policies, or plans appear appropriate in the ways they are written, but also what documented realities show about the effects of how they are being implemented. (See Figure 5.3 for the UN Committee on the Rights of the Child's policy recommendations.)

Government-supported policies and programs can reduce discrimination, but often they inadvertently condone or ignore it. Attention to the rights of the child requires that national level indicators with appropriate

In 2003, the United Nations Committee on the Rights of the Child issued a General Comment (No. 3) on "HIV/AIDS and the Rights of the Child," which concluded with several policy recommendations for States parties:

"(a) To adopt and implement national and local HIV/AIDS-related policies, including effective plans of action, strategies, and programmes that are child-centered, rights-based and incorporate the rights of the child under the Convention [on the Rights of the Child]....

"(b) To allocate financial, technical and human resources, to the maximum extent possible, to supporting national and community-based action....

"(c) To review existing laws or enact new legislation with a view to implementing fully article 2 of the Convention [the right to nondiscrimination], and in particular to expressly prohibiting discrimination based on real or perceived HIV/AIDS status....

"(d) To include HIV/AIDS plans of action, strategies, policies and programmes in the work of national mechanisms responsible for monitoring and coordinating children's rights and to consider the establishment of a review procedure, which responds specifically to complaints of neglect or violation of the rights of the child in relation to HIV/AIDS....

"(e) To reassess their HIV-related data collection and evaluation to ensure that they adequately cover children as defined under the Convention, are disaggregated by age and gender ideally in five-year age groups, and include, as far as possible, children belonging to vulnerable groups and those in need of special protection....

"(f) To include in their reporting process under article 44 of the Convention, information on national HIV/AIDS policies and programmes, and to the extent possible, budgeting and resource allocations at the national, regional, and local levels.... The Committee requests States parties to provide a detailed indication in their reports of what they consider to be the most important priorities within their jurisdiction in relation to children and HIV/AIDS, and to outline the programme of activities they intend to pursue over the coming five years in order to address the problems identified...."

FIGURE 5.3. The UN Committee on the Rights of the Child's Policy Recommendations

benchmarks be developed in relation to HIV and the rights of the child to facilitate monitoring at the national and international levels. Disaggregation of data is key, because it can help to show the degree to which the rights and health of all children within a population are being progressively realized.

Disaggregation is important not only with respect to HIV-specific data, but also in relation to the effects of discrimination on the availability, acceptability, accessibility, and quality of health systems among different groups of children within a population. Attention to the rights of the child asks that national-level health information be disaggregated according to the attributes on which discrimination is often based – including of course age and sex, but also such factors as prior health status, disability, and social status. Ideally, one could move from there toward looking at how these intersect with one another. For example, moving from a needed focus on gender inequality and age to how these intersect with other forms of discrimination (ethnicity, religion, political affiliation) in relation to HIV status, and to the access to health systems and services that exist within the population. This information ultimately would be relevant to capturing and addressing the differences in vulnerability among children in a population, and could help point to differences between government unwillingness and government incapacity, as they relate to both access and interpretation of any data that are collected.

At a programmatic level, attention to human rights requires transparency and accountability, and leads to concrete questions about the factors that figure into public health processes: Who represents whom? Who decides? What were the processes used for setting priorities and allocating resources? Who do these decisions impact and in what ways? For example, effective HIV/AIDS prevention requires that governments not limit children's access to contraceptives and other means of maintaining sexual and reproductive health, and that governments not censor, withhold, or intentionally misrepresent health-related information, including sexual education and information. Effective HIV/AIDS prevention means giving careful attention to sexuality as well as to the behaviors and life circumstances of children, even if they do not conform to the societal determination of what is acceptable under prevailing cultural norms for a particular age group. Competent programs acknowledge the realities of young people's lives, address sexuality, and provide voluntary HIV-testing and counseling that does not require parental consent. Evidence has shown that young people are more likely to use friendly and supportive services that are geared to their needs, that ensure their opportunity to participate in decisions affecting their health, and that are accessible, affordable, confidential, nonjudgmental, and do not require parental consent (Family Health International 2000). These services are fundamental to the rights of the child, but also – by protecting the rights and the health of adolescents – they are necessary to bring the HIV pandemic under control.

The collection and analysis of data from a rights and health perspective by necessity brings attention to the degree to which children have been able to participate in the decisions that affect their health. As rights holders, children have a right to participate (in accordance with their evolving maturity) in the development of HIV/AIDS policies and programs. In all cases children and their communities must be at the center of the response to HIV/AIDS – in other words participants in assessing needs and defining strategies. A supportive and enabling environment requires that children be able to receive support for their own initiatives and to participate at both community and national levels in HIV policy and program design, implementation, mechanisms, coordination, monitoring and review. (See Figure 5.4 for an example of children participating in legislative review and advocacy.)

Resources and other constraints can make it impossible for any government to fulfill all rights relevant to mitigating the impact of the HIV

In South Africa, one of the most significant pieces of legislation concerning children's rights is the Children's Bill, introduced in 2003 to revise the Child Care Act of 1983. The Children's Bill is intended to put into practice Section 28 of the 1994 Constitution and Bill of Rights, which established children's rights to a basic package of social and economic benefits and services. The rights of children in the context of HIV/AIDS are among the most critical issues addressed by the bill. Many organizations are involved in efforts to enact the bill, including the Children's Institute of the University of Cape Town.

To bring the voices of children to the political process, the Institute brought together a group of twelve young people between the ages of twelve and seventeen, selected by partner organizations in various regions. A capacity-building program of participatory workshops and other activities gave the young people information and skills to debate the bill's provisions and to form opinions about what additional stipulations might be needed. These leaders could then talk to other children about the bill, design posters and t-shirts, talk to decisionmakers about their concerns, and write radio dramas, rap songs, and poems. The group decided to call themselves *Dikwankwetla – Children of Action* and their slogan is "Children are the future; give them their rights."

The Children's Bill has not yet been passed, and while these young people and their adult colleagues have more work to do, their engagement in this advocacy effort continues to be of use in a number of ways.

Source: "Child Rights in Focus," Children's Institute Newsletter, November 2004; http://web.uct.ac.za/depts/ci/enews.

FIGURE 5.4. Children as Advocates for their Rights

epidemics on children's lives immediately and completely. In practical terms, governments need more than just good policy. They require financial resources, trained personnel, facilities, supplies, equipment, community mobilization, and a sustainable infrastructure, as well as other structures and resources that may not be immediately available. Realization of rights is understood to be a matter of progressive realization, of making steady progress toward a goal. In resource-poor countries, while support from the international community is critical, HIV/AIDS programs must nonetheless be driven by local people, local needs, and local priorities with sufficient attention to the views of affected children in decision-making processes and structures.

CONCLUSION

The synergistic relationship between the promotion and protection of human rights and sound public health policies and programs is increasingly being recognized. Far more attention is also being given to the meaning and implications of the rights of children to their health and development, as well as to the roots and consequences of the HIV/AIDS epidemics.

However, to translate this awareness into effective actions will require the sustained involvement of young people and the combined efforts of governments, intergovernmental and nongovernmental institutions, the private sector, and communities. Attention to human rights can and should be better used to stimulate government accountability for what is being done – and not done – for children living in a world with AIDS. Much work lies ahead to establish and promote the links between the rights of the child and child health and development – with respect to HIV/AIDS as well as other diseases and health conditions. Empirical knowledge and experience acquired through community-based work, linked to policy- and program-based research, will be necessary to better shape the governmental and other responses necessary for the survival and developmental needs of children.

ACKNOWLEDGMENT

The authors gratefully acknowledge the research assistance of Alyssa Wigton.

References

African Summit on HIV/AIDS, Tuberculosis, and Other Related Diseases. 2001. *Abuja declaration on HIV/AIDS, tuberculosis, and other related diseases*. OAU/ SPS/ABUJA/3. Abuja, Nigeria: Organization of African Unity. http://www. un.org/ga/aids/pdf/abuja_declaration.pdf

African Union Ministerial Conference on Human Rights in Africa. 2003. *Kigali declaration*. MIN/CONF/HRA/Decl.1 (1). Kigali, Rwanda: African Union.

Carr-Hill, R., K. J. Katabaro, A. R. Katahoire, and D. Oulai. 2002. *The impact of HIV/AIDS on education and institutionalizing preventive education*. Paris: International Institute for Educational Planning and UNESCO.

Eide, A. 1995. The right to an adequate standard of living, including the right to food. In *Economic, social, and cultural rights: A textbook*, ed. A. Eide, C. Krause, and A. Rosas, 00–00. Dordrecht: M. Nijhoff.

Family Health International. 1996. *The status and trends of the global HIV/AIDS pandemic: Final report*. Arlington, VA: Family Health International.

———. 2000. *Meeting the needs of young clients: A guide to providing reproductive health services to adolescents*. Arlington, VA: Family Health International.

First World Congress against Commercial Sexual Exploitation of Children. 1996. *Declaration and agenda for action*. Stockholm: First World Congress against Commercial Sexual Exploitation of Children, August 27–31. http://www. csecworldcongress.org/PDF/en/ Stockholm/Outcome_documents/Stockholm %20Declaration%201996_EN.pdf

Fylkesnes, K., K. Kasumba, Z. Ndhlovu, and R. Musonda. 1997. The making of HIV epidemics: What are the driving forces? *AIDS* 11(suppl. B): S23–S32.

Global Strategies for HIV Prevention. 2003. *A call to action to prevent HIV infections of newborns*. San Rafael, CA: Global Strategies for HIV Prevention. http://www.globalstrategies.org/resources/call_to_action_newborns.html

Gruskin, S., A. Hendriks, and K. Tomasevski. 1996. Human rights and responses to HIV/AIDS. In *AIDS in the world II*, ed. J. M. Mann and D. Tarantola, 326–40. New York: Oxford University Press.

Gruskin, S., and Tarantola, D. 2001. HIV/AIDS, health, and human rights. In *HIV/AIDS prevention and care programs in resource-constrained settings: A handbook for the design and management of programs*, ed. P. Lamptey, H. Gayle, and P. Mane, 661–78. Arlington, VA: Family Health International.

Hammarberg, T. 1995. Children. In *Economic, social, and cultural rights: A textbook*, ed. A. Eide, C. Krause, and A. Rosas, 336–79. Dordrecht: M. Nijhoff.

Interpol. (n.d.) Legislation of 181 Interpol member states on sexual offences against children. http://www.interpol.int/Public/Children/SexualAbuse/NationalLaws

Levine, C., D. Michaels, and S. D. Back. 1996. Orphans of the HIV/AIDS pandemic. In *AIDS in the world II*, ed. J. M. Mann and D. Tarantola, 278–86. New York: Oxford University Press.

Nunn, A. J., J. F. Kengeya-Kayondo, S. Malamba, J. A. Seeley, and D. W. Mulder. 1994. Risk factors for HIV-1 infection in adults in a rural Ugandan community: A population study. *AIDS* 8:81–6.

Santa Barbara, J. 1997. The psychological effects of war on children. In *War and public health*, ed. B. S. Levy and V. W. Sidel, 168–76. New York: Oxford University Press.

Tarantola, D., and S. Gruskin. 1998. Children confronting HIV/AIDS: Charting the confluence of rights and health. Health and Human Rights 3 (1): 60–86.

Tarantola, D., and B. Schwartländer. 1997. HIV/AIDS epidemics in sub-Saharan Africa: Dynamism, diversity, and discrete declines? AIDS 11 (suppl. B): S15.

UNAIDS (Joint United Nations Programme on HIV/AIDS). 1996. *HIV/AIDS and children*. Geneva: UNAIDS.

———. 2003. *AIDS epidemic update*. Geneva: UNAIDS and WHO, December. Available at http://www.unaids.org

———. 2004. *2004 Report on the global HIV/AIDS epidemic*. Geneva: UNAIDS and WHO, July. http://www.unaids.org/bangkok2004/GAR2004_Execsumm_en_pdf

UNAIDS and WHO (World Health Organization). 1998. *Improving estimates: Report on the global HIV/AIDS epidemic*. New York: UNAIDS.

UNDAW (United Nations Division for the Advancement of Women), UNICEF, UNFPA (United Nations Population Fund), and ECA (United Nations Economic Commission on Africa). 1997. *Report of the expert group meeting on adolescent girls and their rights, Addis Ababa, Ethiopia, 13–17 October 1997*. EGM/AGR/1997/Rep.1, par. 22. Addis Ababa: UNDAW, UNICEF, UNFPA, and ECA.

UNFPA (United Nations Population Fund). n.d. *Issue in brief: Supporting adolescents and youth*. http://www.unfpa.org/issues/briefs/adolescents.htm

UNICEF, UNAIDS, and WHO. 2002. *Young people and HIV/AIDS: Opportunity in crisis*. New York: UNICEF. http://www.unicef.org/publications/pub_youngpeople_hivaids_en.pdf

United Nations. 1966. *International covenant on civil and political rights*. UN General Assembly Res. 2200A(XXI), UN GAOR, 21st sess., supplement no. 16, at 49, UN Doc. A/6316. New York: United Nations.

————. 1989. *Convention on the rights of the child*. UN General Assembly Res. 44/25, UN GAOR, 44th sess., 41st plen. mtg., annex, UN Doc. A/RES/44/25 (December 12). Geneva: United Nations. http://www.unchr.ch/html/menu3/b/k2crc.htm

United Nations Committee on the Rights of the Child. 1991. *General guidelines*. CRC/C/5, par 14. New York: UNCRC.

————. 2003. *General comment no. 3, HIV/AIDS and the rights of the child*. CRC/GC/2003/1. New York: UNCRC.

United Nations Fourth World Conference on Women (Beijing Conference). 1995. *Action for equality, development, and peace*. UN Doc. A/CONF.177/20/Rev.1 (96.IV.13). Beijing: Beijing Conference, September.

United Nations General Assembly Special Session on Children. 2002. *A world fit for children*. UN Doc. A/RES/S-27/2. Geneva: United Nations.

United Nations International Conference on Population and Development. 1994. *Programme of action*. UN Doc. A/CONF.171/13, par. 4.76. Cairo: UNICPD, September 5–13.

United Nations Millennium Summit. 2000. *United Nations millennium declaration*. UN Doc. A/RES/55/2. Geneva: United Nations.

United Nations Office of the High Commissioner for Human Rights and UNAIDS. 1998, reprinted 2001. *International guidelines on HIV/AIDS and human rights*. UNCHR res. 1997/33, UN Doc. E/CN.4/1997/150. http://www.ohchr.org/english/issues/hiv/guidelines.htm.

————. 2002. Revised Guideline, on access to prevention, treatment, care and support. UNAIDS/02:49 E. http://www.ohchr.org/english/issues/hiv/guidelines.htm.

United Nations Special Session on HIV/AIDS. 2001. *Declaration of commitment on HIV/AIDS*. Geneva: United Nations, June.

United Nations World Conference on Human Rights. 1993. *Vienna declaration and programme of action*. UN Doc. A/CONF.157/23. Vienna: UN World Conference on Human Rights, June 14–25.

United Nations World Summit for Children. 1990. *World declaration on the survival, development and protection of children*. New York: United Nations World Summit for Children.

United Nations World Summit for Social Development. 1995. *Report of the World Summit for Social Development*. UN Doc. A/CONF.166/9. Copenhagen: UN World Summit for Social Development, March 6–12.

USAID (United States Agency for International Development), UNICEF, and UNAIDS (Joint United Nations Programme on HIV/AIDS). 2002. *Children on the brink: A joint report on orphan estimates and program strategies*. Washington: TvT Associates/The Synergy Project, USAID. http://www.unicef.org/publications/pub_children_on_the_brink_en.pdf

————. 2004. *Children on the Brink 2004: A joint report of new orphan estimates and a framework for action*. New York: UNICEF. Available at http://www.unicef.org/publications/index_22212.html.

Van Bueren, G. 1995. *The international law on the rights of the child*. Dordrecht: M. Nijhoff.

6

Religion and Responses to Orphans in Africa

Geoff Foster

> The bread in your cupboard belongs to the hungry man; the coat hanging unused in your closet belongs to the man who needs it; the shoes rotting in your closet belong to the man who has none; the money which you hoard in the bank belongs to the poor. You do wrong to everyone you could help but fail to help.
>
> – Saint Basil the Great, fourth century

For centuries, religious groups have proven their sustainability and resilience through their continuous presence in societies. Members of religious organizations have demonstrated their commitment to respond to human need based on the teachings of their faith, and they do so voluntarily and over long periods. They have continued to respond in the face of conflict, natural disaster, political oppression, and disease. Faith-based organizations (FBOs), addressing the universal need for community and spiritual life, endure for the long term when others tire, drop out, or shift energies to other crises. As HIV/AIDS continues to create a "caring deficit," eroding the capacity of communities to care for those affected, religious organizations will be crucial in responding to the impact of the disease and in promoting a caring mentality and sustaining hope.

During the past decade, religiously motivated individuals and organizations throughout Africa have developed responses to care for growing numbers of children affected by HIV/AIDS. The strength of religion in Africa is fundamental to the resilience of its responses to orphans and vulnerable children. It is difficult to overemphasize the importance of faith on this continent where religion is ubiquitous. From the educated elite to the urban slum-dweller and the village peasant farmer, the vast majority (99.5 percent) of Africa's 750 million people have a religious connection, proportionately greater than any other region of the world (Adherents.com Database). Religion features at important milestones of a majority of the population, including birth, marriage, death, and regularly in between.

Some two million churches, mosques, and traditional gatherings blanket the continent (Barrett 2001). Religious bodies offer the most extensive, best-organized, and most viable network of community organizations. In many countries, over one-third of the health and education infrastructure is run by religious organizations, making faith-based social sector networks second only to government in providing service, and often providing higher quality services than secular or government institutions, with more motivated staff and fewer political constraints. Faith-based institutions have established structures and channels of communication at every level of society. Religious infrastructure connects villages, districts, and regional centers and provides mechanisms to organize people, mobilize action, and channel information and resources. Congregations convene adherents weekly and many leaders speak with credibility and authority. FBOs have experience in creating interactive information sharing among peer groups, especially with youth and women.

The association between poverty and HIV/AIDS means that organizations that work with the poor have an advantage in responding to the epidemic. Religious groups have a theological commitment to work with the poor, the sick, the underprivileged, and with vulnerable children. They are able to champion the needs of the marginalized, bucking political and economic forces favoring the rich and powerful. In remote rural situations and conflict zones, faith-based groups are often in evidence, assisting the social and spiritual development of the poor and oppressed. And for people in urban areas, including those living in slums or shanty towns who are detached from their rural homes and clans, the religious community acts as a surrogate for the extended family and community of village neighbors (Shorter 1975).

This chapter summarizes the teachings of major religions that motivate believers to respond to the plight of orphans. It provides examples of religious responses to vulnerable children and outlines factors that spur their initiatives. It also reviews the limits of these responses, including beliefs of religious groups that at times have hampered development of effective HIV/AIDS responses and have contributed to the increasing dimensions of the crisis. Strategies are suggested for agencies seeking to strengthen faith-based responses to orphans and vulnerable children.

TEACHINGS OF MAJOR RELIGIONS ON ORPHANS

The major religions share common ground in areas of social concern by upholding values such as respect for life, the sacredness of human beings, concern for the marginalized, and the importance of community. Religious teachings encourage the commitment of both financial and human resources to support the underprivileged. The Bible, Quran, and Vedas (Hindu primary texts) instruct believers to protect and care for orphans. In the Judeo-Christian tradition, over forty Biblical references mention widows and orphans: they are protected by God himself and believers are urged to do likewise:

God defends the cause of the fatherless and the widow, and loves the alien, giving him food and clothing.

(Deuteronomy 10:17–18)

Defend the cause of the weak and fatherless; maintain the rights of the poor and oppressed. Rescue the weak and needy; deliver them from the hands of the wicked.

(Psalm 82:3–4)

Religion that God our Father accepts as pure and faultless is this: to visit and look after orphans and widows in their distress.

(James 1:27)

Christian practices are based on the example of the early church in establishing community-based support programs for the poor. Around A.D. 40, the leaders of the Jerusalem church supervised daily distribution of food to destitute widows and orphans (Acts 6:1–6). The apostle Paul instructed church leaders on the functioning of an order of older widow deaconesses responsible for identifying and supporting orphans and widows. Believers should support their own relatives, enabling the church to help others in the community:

If any woman who is a believer has widows in her family, she should help them and not let the church be burdened with them, so that the church can help those widows who are really in need.

(I Timothy 5:16)[1]

The Islamic Scriptures warn against exploitation and encourage acts of charity toward orphans:

Give orphans the property that belongs to them. Do not exchange their valuables for worthless things or cheat them of their possessions, for this would be a grievous sin. . . . Those who unjustly eat up the property of orphans eat up a fire into their own bodies; they will soon be enduring a blazing fire!

(Sura 4:1, 10)

They ask you, Muhammed, what they should spend in charity. Say: whatever wealth you spend, that is good, for the parents and children and orphans and those in want and for wayfarers. And whatever you do, that is good – Allah knows it well.

(Sura 2:215)

It is righteousness to believe in God and . . . to spend of your substance, out of love for Him, for your kin, for orphans, for the needy . . . and practice regular charity; to fulfill the contracts which you made; and to be firm and patient in suffering and

---

[1] Other references include Deuteronomy 14:28–29; Psalms 27:10; 68:5–6; Proverbs 23:10–11; Hosea 14:3; Mark 10:13–16; I Timothy 5:9–15.

I know a man named Bac Sieu in Thua Thien Province in Vietnam, who has been practicing generosity for fifty years. With only a bicycle, he visits villages of thirteen provinces, bringing something for this family and something for that family. . . . Our orphanages, dispensaries, schools, and resettlement centers were all shut down or taken by the government. Thousands of our workers had to stop their work and hide. But Bac Sieu had nothing to take. He was truly a "bodhisattva," working for the well being of others. I feel more humble now concerning the ways of practicing generosity.

"The war created many thousands of orphans. Instead of raising money to build orphanages, we sought people in the West to sponsor a child. We found families in the villages to each take care of one orphan and then we sent $6 every month to that family to feed the child and send him or her to school. Whenever possible, we tried to place the child in the family of an aunt, an uncle, or a grandparent. With just $6, the child was fed and sent to school, and the rest of the children in the family were also helped. Children benefit from growing up in a family. Being in an orphanage can be like being in the army – children do not grow up naturally. If we look for and learn ways to practice generosity, we will improve all the time.

Thich Nhat Hanh is a Buddhist monk who founded the Van Hanh Buddhist University in Saigon, Vietnam.

Source: Nhat Hanh n.d.

FIGURE 6.1. Support to Orphan Families in Vietnam by a Buddhist Monk

adversity and throughout all periods of panic. Such are the people of truth, the God-conscious.

(Sura 2:177)[2]

Muslims who look after orphans will receive an eternal reward, according to the words of the Prophet Muhammad:

"I and the caretaker of the orphan will enter Paradise together like this (raising by way of illustration his forefinger and middle finger jointly, leaving no space in between)."

(Saheeh Al-Bukhari)

Other world faiths uphold similar precepts (Figure 6.1). The Hindu and Bahai scriptures both teach that believers should be nonjudgmental and demonstrate a selfless spirit toward the disadvantaged:

He is liberal who gives to anyone who asks for alms, to the homeless, distressed man who seeks food. . . . He is no friend who does not give to a friend, to a comrade who comes imploring for food. Let him leave such a man – his is not a home – and

---

[2] Other references include Sura 2:83, 22; 17:7; 4:2–3, 36; 59:7; 89:15–20; 90:4–17; 107:1–7.

rather seek a stranger who brings him comfort.... For wealth revolves like the wheels of a chariot, coming now to one, now to another.

(Rig Veda 10.117.1–6)

O Lord of the home, best furnisher of resources for orphans and vulnerable children are you. Grant us the strength from you for a healthy domestic life.

(Hindu prayer)

The poor in your midst are My trust: guard My trust, and be not intent only on your own ease.

(Bahai Scriptures)

INFLUENCE OF TRADITIONAL RELIGIONS

Close to half the population of Africa have a primary allegiance to Christianity and over one-third are adherents to Islam. Studies suggest that less than 10 percent of Africans are followers of traditional religions (Adherents.com Database). This small figure belies the influence of traditional belief on African culture. For most of the twentieth century, a majority of Africans espoused traditional religions. Even now, many Christian and Muslim Africans hold traditional beliefs alongside their other religious doctrines, and among those who abandon traditional religious practices, the influence of traditional belief on their cultural, family, and community values remains.

Traditional religions play a distinctive role both in explaining the ultimate sources of supernatural power and authority that sanction public morality, and in reinforcing philanthropic responses to vulnerable children. They continue to shape the structure of African societies, and in large measure account for the strength of Africa's extended families and communities.

By promoting the ideal of a peaceful and harmonious existence, traditional religions reinforce the widespread practice of fostering deceased relatives' orphans. Families in traditional societies typically involve a large network of connections among people in relationships that include multiple generations, extend over wide geographical areas, and are based on reciprocal rights and duties. The extended family has been – and still is – the traditional social security system. Its members are responsible for protecting the vulnerable, caring for the poor and sick, and transmitting social values. When relatives die, the extended family support network ensures that children are cared for. In the past – and still to a considerable extent today – the sense of duty and responsibility of African extended families has been almost without limits. Even though a family may not have sufficient resources to care for existing members, orphans are taken in nonetheless. This practice has been the basis for the assertion that, traditionally, there is no such thing as an orphan in Africa (Foster 2000). According to traditional belief, to neglect caring for a member of the family is to risk incurring the wrath of the ancestors, invisible members of the clan who are superior to human beings.

At the community level, the mechanism that keeps many African households from destitution consists of material relief, labor, and emotional support provided by neighbors. The community safety net is underpinned by traditional beliefs and practices. In many African countries, chiefs are responsible for promoting traditional religious values. In response to the orphan crisis in rural Zimbabwe, traditional leaders revived a grain-saving scheme known as "the chief's field." In this practice, community members contribute labor in the field of the chief, and the produce is given to households in need. Traditional leaders decide which needy families should benefit. Grain-saving schemes form an important source of community support to AIDS-affected households, and help mitigate the impact of an adult lost to AIDS (Mutangadura 2000). In Tanzania, there is a tradition of social support groups; members assist one another in routine ways by helping to cultivate one another's fields and contributing labor, money, or food to one another at times of special need, such as sickness and funerals (Mukoyogo and Williams 1991). These supportive actions are part of a clearly understood system of solidarity: It ensures that, if affected by similar adversity, individuals will receive the same assistance that they provide to others.

The sense of community connectedness, though strongest in rural villages, extends to modern African cities. A visitor to Africa is soon struck by the frequent use of "we" and "ours" in everyday speech. People living away from their communities remain loyal to their extended families and villages. City-dwellers generally return to their rural homes from time to time to join in cultural events. For traditional Africans, the community is basically more sacred than secular (Ejizu n.d.). Ostracizing an individual who has flagrantly disobeyed the community's values is thought to be one of the severest forms of punishment. The offender is not allowed to share in community life; there are no visits to the family, no exchange of greetings, and no trade with the ostracized. Serious moral breaches affect not only individuals, but are believed to destabilize the well-being of the whole community. In cases such as murder or incest, the moral pollution must be cleansed through religious ceremonies or else the whole community risks suffering disaster. In such ways, traditional religious beliefs maintain a sense of harmonious living and strengthen the responses of extended families and communities to protect and support vulnerable children in their midst.

In Africa, cultural values are often passed on through oral tradition, especially through an extensive heritage of proverbial folklore and wisdom. Traditional African culture reinforces the practice of caring for vulnerable children as illustrated by proverbs from the Shona of Zimbabwe and Mozambique (Hamutyinei and Plangger 1987): "What has befallen me today will befall you tomorrow." This proverb reminds community members that all are subject to the same fate. Consequently, it bolsters the principle of reciprocity: Through caring for others, community members endorse mechanisms that ensure assistance for their own children should they be affected by similar adversity. Another saying, which resembles the well-known African proverb "it takes a village to raise a child," reminds community members that everyone is responsible for raising children: "The child of the mother is the one in the womb but once born everybody plays with it."

Traditional religious beliefs and practices thus buttress the extended family and community safety nets, and reinforce the notion of providing care and support to orphans and neighbors. The lessening importance of traditional religion has left enormous gaps in the social structure, particularly in areas of interpersonal and societal relationships. Fortunately, the forces that precipitate and sustain radical change on the continent, such as Christianity, Islam, and Western sociopolitical systems and culture, now largely provide new frameworks for community living and harmony in much of Africa (Ejizu n.d.). (See Figures 6.2 and 6.3.)

RELIGIOUS ORGANIZATIONS RESPONDING TO ORPHANS

Many development practitioners are unfamiliar with social development activities implemented by congregations and religious coordinating bodies. *Congregation* refers to the basic community-level religious gathering, such as the local church in the Christian faith, the mosque in the Muslim tradition, the synagogue in Judaism, the assembly in the Bahai faith, or the temple in the Hindu religion. Congregation HIV/AIDS initiatives are administered by individuals who see the response as part of the ministry of their local religious group. Most congregations belong to faith communities administered by religious coordinating bodies (RCBs) that organize, support, and supervise congregations, mainly in relation to their spiritual ministries. Since the advent of HIV/AIDS, some RCBs have appointed HIV/AIDS coordinators, set up their own projects, or started supporting the HIV/AIDS activities of their congregations. It is difficult for outsiders to comprehend how RCBs function, given their bewildering religious terminologies and distinctive structures, which range from congregational to several-tiered hierarchies. RCB names include muftiates, dioceses, parishes, synods, unions, conferences, circuits, associations, fields, supreme councils, national spiritual assemblies, and brigades.

Faith-based responses to orphans and vulnerable children are widespread throughout Africa. In the past, Christian and Muslim missionary involvement in orphan support led to the establishment of residential institutions for vulnerable children. With the advent of AIDS, most

UMWO is a self-help body established in the mid-seventies when Muslim families started settling in Umoja estate near the city center. The area is in one of the poorer parts of Nairobi and is surrounded by other very poor areas. The main reason for its inception was to build a mosque to start madrassa (religious) classes for children and to bring unity and development among the Muslim residents of the estate. Buildings on the site consist of a large mosque, imams' living quarters, and two classrooms for evening classes, adult learning, and a madrassa class. UMWO organizes collections for the poor and housing for needy Muslim families. It is led by an elected committee of twelve members, who run the affairs of the Mosque and the activities of the community.

UMWO receives support from Orphan Aid, a British Muslim charity, to assist the education and welfare of children, especially orphans. The community believes one of the most pressing needs is the lack of proper Islamic education for children in Umoja. Parents who cannot afford schooling are forced to send their children to non-Muslim schools, where they are taught secular and non-Islamic concepts. In the case of orphans, very few receive any education at all. This is the start of a vicious cycle since in the short term they are forced into child labor and sometimes into illegal activities. In the long term they have little chance of securing a job, and, because they have not been exposed to Islamic education, they often do not develop as full Islamic individuals.

Orphan Aid held a series of face-to-face meetings with the Umoja committee and agreed to help fund a junior school with ten classrooms to accommodate 350 children. This school offers Islamic and secular education for Muslim children and so stimulates their intellectual, moral, emotional, and social development, as well as providing them with a foundation of Islamic education. The school caters to the most needy children and orphans who are provided with additional support as required. At least 120 places are provided for orphans with ongoing costs paid for by Orphan Aid.

Source: Umoja Muslim Welfare Organization n.d.

FIGURE 6.2. Umoja Muslim Welfare Organization (UMWO), Kenya

congregations responding to the orphan crisis have not created new institutions: A survey of FBO activities found over 85 percent of recent initiatives were community-based (Foster 2004).

In most countries with severe epidemics, congregations started initiating responses to children affected by AIDS during the 1990s. Recently, the trickle of responses has become a flood. A survey of churches in Namibia found over half had a full-fledged or developing HIV/AIDS response; only 13 percent – mostly small independent churches – had no response whatsoever (Yates 2003). A study of responses in six countries found most congregations had initiated support activities, with over half established in 1999–2002. The study interviewed 690 FBOs that involved

This facility houses forty-five children, almost all under the age of two. It was established by Catholic sisters in response to growing numbers of maternal deaths and situations where families were unable to afford artificial milk or provide orphaned babies with appropriate nutrition. Most babies are admitted from the surrounding area, after screening by the Department of Social Welfare (DSW). Babies are fed, receive free medical treatment, and a stimulating play environment provided by women from the surrounding rural community. The unit has an innovative approach to family reunification. Relatives who bring babies for admission must agree to the following responsibilities:

1. To visit the unit monthly (DSW provides transport permits);
2. To bring food or money to the value of 2,000 Tanzanian shillings (about US $2), which is waived if the family is destitute; and
3. To take the children back into their families when they reach two years of age. Almost all children are reunited with their families. Occasionally this is not possible, and then the unit finds a foster family.

FIGURE 6.3. Igogwe Mission Hospital Orphanage, Mbeya, Tanzania

some 9,000 volunteers supporting over 156,000 orphans and vulnerable children, mostly through community-based initiatives incorporating spiritual, material, educational, and psychosocial support. Congregation members usually initiate activities without significant external facilitation or financial support, depending instead on resources raised from within local communities. Though many congregation responses are small, supporting fewer than a hundred children, the cumulative impact of thousands of such initiatives is considerable (Foster 2004).

THE VALUES BUILT INTO FAITH-BASED RESPONSES

Community studies suggest that FBOs are one of the few sources of external support for orphan households other than the extended family (Mutangadura 2000). The number of congregations throughout Africa becoming involved in supporting orphan households is growing daily. What accounts for the remarkable proliferation by FBOs of activities in response to the orphan crisis?[3]

While Christian and Muslim sacred scriptures encourage believers to protect and support orphans, this factor does not adequately explain the explosion of faith-based orphan initiatives. These same religious texts also

---

[3] Much of the following, including unascribed quotations, is based on data from a study of FBO responses to orphans and vulnerable children in Eastern and Southern Africa for the World Conference of Religions for Peace (Foster 2004).

instruct believers to care for people who are sick and to protect the poor, but it is uncommon to see churches or mosques establishing support groups, advocating for the rights of people living with HIV/AIDS, or engaging in activities that effectively and realistically address HIV transmission and associated behaviors. The profusion of faith-based orphan initiatives contrasts with a relative dearth of congregation-led initiatives that directly address HIV/AIDS. Value-based belief systems that are characteristic of religious organizations help explain these differences.

A religious leader in Kenya explained his reason for not becoming involved in orphan support, saying: "Our congregation is spiritual and against immoralities like adultery and pre-marital sex. By supporting orphans and people with AIDS, we would be encouraging sin." Though this response is uncharacteristic and represents an extreme viewpoint, nonetheless it illustrates one way in which moral beliefs can influence religious responses. From a value-based perspective, most religious people, on one hand, view orphans as innocent victims of the epidemic who did nothing to deserve their predicament. On the other hand, they frequently view their dead or dying parents as being guilty, directly or by association, of having brought catastrophe upon themselves. Consequently, religious groups are less likely to provide support to adults known to be suffering from HIV/AIDS, especially those deemed responsible for having acquired HIV infection outside marriage.

Complicating the innocent victim viewpoint is the widespread misperception that if a mother dies of AIDS, any orphans she leaves behind are almost certain to have HIV infection.[4] The perception of a double misfortune contributes to the innocent victim ethos and acts as a powerful motivating force to religious groups.

Volunteers who set up orphan support programs recognize AIDS as the cause of increasing parental deaths observed in their communities, yet often fail to directly address HIV/AIDS issues. Their involvement with orphans centers on poverty-related issues, such as the provision of food, clothing, and educational support, and children's psychosocial, spiritual, and cultural needs. Stigma and sexuality are the main sticking points that prevent congregations from expanding their focus beyond orphans and directly addressing HIV/AIDS topics.

While home care programs that deal with people suffering from AIDS frequently expand their scope to address the needs of orphans, it is less

---

[4] The author surveyed forty data collectors in 2002–3 in several African countries during training for the FBO response study in Eastern and Southern Africa. The average estimate for the positive HIV status of children orphaned by AIDS reported by the respondents was over 50 percent, with a range of 40 to 100 percent. In fact, fewer than 4 percent of children orphaned by AIDS are HIV-positive (Hunter 2000). The overestimates of the number of HIV-infected orphans are a consequence of the widespread use of the stigmatizing and misleading term "AIDS orphan."

common for congregations to expand the scope of their orphan initiatives to include the provision of home care to adults with AIDS. One obstacle is that religious groups associate people living with AIDS with sinful, extramarital acquisition of HIV infection. This lack of responses is doubly unfortunate, because sick adults who are housebound fail to receive home care, and children caring for dying parents fail to receive support until they become orphans, even though studies suggest that the social, economic, and psychological impacts of AIDS on children are most severe before children are orphaned (Gilborn et al. 2001; Poulter 1997; Sengendo and Nambi 1997).

Furthermore, many faith-based orphan programs fail to incorporate HIV prevention activities into their initiatives or address issues of vulnerability. In the past, religious groups have opposed HIV prevention programs, believing that they encourage immoral sexual behavior. Leaders have been unwilling to support risk reduction strategies, such as the provision of condoms, that involve recognizing sexual activity outside marriage because this might imply dilution of religious moral standards. Religious groups have focused almost exclusively on abstinence and faithfulness – behaviors that undoubtedly have contributed to the decline in HIV prevalence rates in countries such as Uganda and Senegal (Green 2002). By doing so, however, many FBOs restrict discussion concerning the reality and circumstances surrounding extramarital sexual behavior. Religious leaders repeatedly emphasize the association of HIV infection with sinful behavior. This has the consequence of strengthening the innocent–guilty paradigm and reinforces discrimination and stigma against people living with HIV/AIDS, including women or men whose only sexual partner has been a spouse.

Volunteers involved with orphans are frequently aware of the prevalence of sexual abuse and exploitation, especially among teenage orphan girls. It is rare for religious leaders, however, to break the silence concerning child abuse or to realistically address sexual behavior issues by providing orphans with appropriate information and life skills. Many religious people believe that such information will lead to young people's experimenting with premarital sex, and most are uncomfortable talking about topics involving sexuality. Providing religious groups with appropriate training can give them the confidence to engage more effectively in HIV prevention and may also reduce their opposition to risk-reduction strategies.

Change is taking place, and religious leaders are beginning to acknowledge past mistakes by adopting both pragmatic approaches to HIV prevention and more compassionate responses toward those affected. Undoubtedly, the increased death rate among adults in their prime has influenced leaders' attitudes. A pastor from Homa Bay, Kenya, confided, "This disease has affected us very much. Half my flock are orphans or widows. I have two hundred orphans and vulnerable children and fifty widows in my church." Priests, pastors, and imams are now painfully aware of the prevalence of death in young adults. Increasingly, they are called upon to care for the terminally ill and conduct funeral services for members of their own congregations and families. They can no longer overlook the reality that parishioners and youth group members have had sexual relationships outside marriage. It is becoming increasingly untenable to maintain that AIDS is simply a problem "out there," which will not breach the confines of the church or mosque. This realization is a wake-up call that has led many religious leaders and their congregations to establish orphan support activities. The challenge for external agencies is to help faith-based groups go further to overcome their moral prejudices, move beyond orphan programming, and tackle HIV/AIDS mitigation and prevention activities more directly and effectively.

STRATEGIES FOR EXPANDING THE RESPONSES OF RELIGIOUS GROUPS

The current state of faith-based orphan support activities in Africa is characterized by lack of knowledge, coordination, and partnerships among organizations at different levels. There are myriad small-scale, idiosyncratic congregation responses to the orphan crisis at the community level that are largely unknown and unsupported by outsiders. RCBs support churches and mosques in their religious activities, but many are unaware of their congregations' orphan responses. Nongovernmental organizations (NGOs) establish orphan support programs by mobilizing communities and volunteers, often without ascertaining whether congregations are implementing children's initiatives with which they might partner. Resource and development organizations fund NGOs to establish orphan support projects without realizing that these may inadvertently undermine community initiatives. Given the importance of spirituality as a motivating factor – and the existence of religious structures as conduits for information, resources, and programming – the extent to which development agencies have overlooked FBOs as partners in development programming is surprising.[5] A coordinated response to orphan support demands partnerships between policy and resource organizations and the religious sector. Figure 6.4 describes the activities and funding of an NGO network in Zimbabwe.

Many organizations engaged in scaling up HIV/AIDS programs are aware that religious organizations have established effective HIV/AIDS

---

[5] Some reasons faith-based responses are sidetracked are discussed in Kurt Alan 2000.

Zimbabwe Orphans through Extended Hands (ZOE), a Christian NGO, has helped local churches to establish orphan support responses since 1993. During a ZOE workshop, the characteristics of nineteen member organizations were documented. Most lead churches in this network are Pentecostal or independent. Most responses were established after pastors or their wives saw children in need going hungry, without school fees, lacking adequate clothing, lacking spiritual or parental guidance, or exploited, abused, raped, or pregnant.

Initiatives were based in both urban and rural areas. Most responses involved volunteers from other churches in the surrounding area. Each response involved on average three other churches and thirteen volunteers. Support was provided by each initiative to an average of 182 orphans and vulnerable children.

Regular visiting was the most common activity (see graph). The provision of material, educational, and spiritual support also featured prominently. As congregation responses developed, many started training volunteers and broadening their focus to involve psychosocial support and income-generating activities. Longer-established initiatives involved more volunteers and provided support to a greater number of needy families. The main challenges facing initiatives were the adverse economic and political situations and the overwhelming nature of the AIDS epidemic.

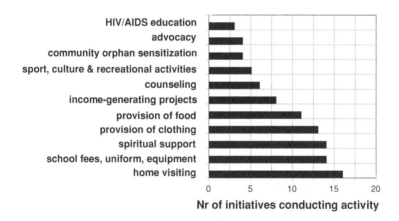

Most initiatives were self-resourced and few received external funding, with support for the preceding year averaging around one hundred dollars per initiative. Yet almost all initiatives wanted to increase their area of coverage, the number of children supported, the services they provided, and the number of volunteers. To do so, they required training in areas such as administration, psychosocial support, volunteer management and income generation, and financial support.

Source: Foster, Webster, Stephenson, and Germann 2002.

FIGURE 6.4. Congregation Responses in Zimbabwe

interventions, but few have sought to partner with faith-based groups. This failure may be a consequence of the idiosyncratic nature of religious groups, their difficulty meeting reporting requirements, and concern about the use of public funds for proselytizing. Another reason is that sacred and secular organizations hold divergent standpoints on sexual behavior. A WHO regional director stated: "The churches are impossible to work with because they have so many agendas that are actively hostile to HIV prevention" (Paterson 2002).

Secular agencies with a public health perspective have by and large failed to understand the value-based views of religious organizations and vice-versa. It is as though the two groups were speaking different languages. Policymakers often fail to appreciate that the public pronouncements of senior religious leaders about HIV/AIDS may differ from their private sentiments and be at odds with the practice of pastoral workers at the grassroots level. As a result of negative perceptions or lack of understanding, secular agencies either fail to mobilize religious groups as partners in HIV/AIDS work, or end up alienating them. In response, religious leaders incensed by the seeming disregard by public health agencies for the promotion of moral values resort to active opposition. FBOs withhold vital information about HIV prevention and in some cases disseminate untruths. Instead of seeking partnerships, religious groups establish and resource their own HIV/AIDS activities, often with scant regard for accepted best practices or national policy.

In recent years, however, there has been evidence of increased cooperation, with both sides recognizing the need to strengthen their partnerships and address HIV/AIDS more effectively. FBO responses to the orphan crisis can be strengthened in the following six ways:

OBTAIN THE ENDORSEMENT OF RELIGIOUS LEADERS. Religious leaders occupy strategic positions of influence. Their statements and actions influence the attitudes and practices of whole nations, not just their own religious groupings. When leaders urge others to care for people with AIDS, they help break down discrimination. When clerics expound the scriptures and uphold the care of orphans, believers go out and start support programs. Some leaders have promoted a theological basis for risk-reduction strategies, based on their religion's teachings. International and national agencies need to support such efforts by engaging with religious leaders to lessen their opposition to public health strategies and to promote HIV/AIDS programming.

During 2002, the World Conference of Religions for Peace organized an Africa-wide consultation involving more than one hundred senior religious leaders representing thirty countries and numerous religions as part of the Hope for the African Child Initiative. During the consultation, leaders acknowledged that religious organizations had been reluctant to speak openly about HIV/AIDS and as a result had contributed to the silence and stigma surrounding the disease. The meeting drafted a consensus statement (African Religious Leaders Assembly on Children and HIV/AIDS 2002) that was later circulated and read to thousands of congregations during their worship services. The statement acknowledges past mistakes and encourages believers to support orphans and people living with HIV/AIDS: "Through our silence and denial," a Ugandan Muslim leader at the consultation is quoted as saying, "we have contributed increased stigma and exclusion of people living with HIV/AIDS and their families; we are here to launch a continent-wide jihad on AIDS."

One of the most powerful contributions that religious leaders can make in combating the spread and impact of HIV/AIDS is to speak with one voice to condemn discrimination and a lack of caring responses for people living with HIV/AIDS.

APPRECIATE THE RESILIENCE OF COMMUNITY COPING RESPONSES. Those lacking local knowledge have a tendency to view community efforts as weak and floundering, and then to step in with prescribed external remedies to rescue the population from misery and desperation. Viewing the poor or disadvantaged as victims in need of rescue is especially congruent with the interventionist approaches of external organizations. Most people do not understand the ways in which community members provide a safety net to households in need, and fail to appreciate the resilience of communities. External agencies are unaware of the valuable orphan support activities carried out by congregations. RCBs frequently do not know about the orphan support activities of their own congregations. Local religious leaders fail to appreciate the value of activities carried out by their own church members. As 90 percent of HIV/AIDS care workers in Africa are women of faith, there appears to be an important gender perspective to this lack of knowledge (African Religious Leaders Assembly on Children and HIV/AIDS 2002).

Even volunteers tend to underrate the importance of the services they provide. When asked for instances of effective orphan support during a recent FBO survey, some volunteers mentioned a nearby children's home, others a donor-funded NGO project – overlooking their own activities and achievements. Programs that attract external funds, receive overseas visitors, or are featured in the media are perceived to be of greater consequence than the nonsensational visiting, material, and psychosocial support provided by volunteers on a daily basis. Externally driven orphan programs that are deemed successful may actually undermine the motivation of volunteers and diminish struggling community responses. It is the very ordinariness of community coping mechanisms that lead to them being undervalued, which contributes to the weakening of the safety net (Foster 2002b).

DOCUMENT AND EVALUATE CONGREGATIONAL ORPHAN SUPPORT ACTIVITIES. Many orphan support programs implemented by congregations and RCBs exemplify best practices, but few have been documented. Most religious people involved in orphan support activities do not have the time, inclination, or skills to detail their activities, and the development community has largely ignored the contributions of FBOs to social change. A review of leading development journals found scant references in the preceding fifteen years to topics of spirituality or religion, with two of the three journals containing no articles at all on the subject (Kurt Alan 2000). Documentation of faith-based orphan responses enables policy, resource, and technical support organizations to construct appropriate legislative environments and provide much-needed assistance.

Though the cumulative impact of thousands of congregation initiatives is considerable, measuring the scale of the response by religious groups is extremely difficult. Many groups do not keep records of the number of children supported, the number of home visits conducted by volunteers, or even the number of school fees paid. Without data, outsiders are unable to understand the nature of congregation initiatives, let alone determine whether these responses are effective. It would be unwise, however, to conclude that congregation responses have little impact based on lack of demonstrability to outsiders. In other areas of development, community-initiated activities are frequently more effective and sustainable than projects implemented by external agencies. External organizations such as RCBs and NGOs need to appreciate the essential support provided by congregations to orphan initiatives, and build the capacity of congregational responses through documentation and the provision of external assistance. Figure 6.5 describes a Seventh Day Adventist self-help group in Kenya.

ENABLE CONGREGATION RESPONSES TO DEVELOP. Volunteers often start responding to orphans on a limited basis, supporting households from their own congregation. Many responses expand to provide support to other orphan households in their communities. One initiative in Zimbabwe started with 4 volunteers supporting 187 orphans; three years later, 30 volunteers supported 467 children in 221 households. Established initiatives involve more volunteers, more vulnerable children, and a broader range of services than newer initiatives. Most congregation responses want to improve their services and expand their coverage but are constrained by lack of resources and limited organizational capacity (Foster et al. 2002). Initiatives reach a point where they cannot expand without external assistance.

The potential of the religious sector in supporting orphans has not been realized. There are more than a quarter of a million congregations in the

In 2001 the Mosando Seventh Day Adventist Church in Kisii established an initiative that involves 46 volunteers and supports 1,842 orphans and vulnerable children. These members are mostly women who are referred to as "mothers." The mothers are assigned specific families living nearby whom they visit at home at least once a week to talk, pray, and share a meal. The mothers are confidantes of the children, who consult them in times of need. These arrangements give children a sense of security, protection, love, belonging, and attention. Committee members meet regularly with mothers, guardians, and children to discuss issues and plan the way forward. Initiatives include:

- Land use: Orphan-owned land is used to produce food for orphans' own consumption and for sale to meet basic needs. By communally using the land for food production, the group encourages orphans to use their land to sustain themselves instead of going to the streets to beg.
- Microfinance: The group runs a low-interest loan scheme to pursue income-generating activities for orphans and widows.
- Bamako Initiative Pharmacy: One group runs a pharmacy that sells drugs and treated mosquito nets at low prices to orphans and widows.
- Clubs: The group also has active orphan and widow social clubs that enable members to meet and share experiences, problems, and solutions.
- Advocacy: The group advocates for orphans' and widows' rights, such as land ownership and access to family property.
- Spiritual care: The group offers spiritual care and nurturing of orphans and widows.

FIGURE 6.5. Omongina Self-help Group, Kenya

AIDS belt of Eastern and Southern Africa, more than enough to support the region's 12 million orphans. Kenya alone has over 80,000 congregations throughout the country. If every congregation helped 20 orphans, each of Kenya's 1.6 million orphans would be supported. At this stage in the crisis, most congregations have yet to establish structured orphan support responses, and represent an untapped pool of potential resources for HIV/AIDS and orphan programming. However, religious organizations require a great deal of capacity building and support if they are to expand their orphan programs. One group that has done this is described in Figure 6.6.

ENABLE RCBS TO STRENGTHEN CONGREGATION RESPONSES. RCBs are well placed to support congregation responses compared with secular and religious NGOs. RCBs already supervise faith-related activities of congregations, and they can use the same mechanisms to support congregations' HIV/AIDS and orphan activities. In terms of community development, RCBs have a considerable "multiplier" advantage over NGOs. Most NGOs

With more than one in five adults HIV-positive, Namibia has the third highest HIV prevalence of any country in the world. Catholic AIDS Action, established in 1998, was the first national faith-based response to the epidemic in Namibia. It promotes home-based care, orphan support, AIDS awareness, behavior change, and income generation. The church-based nature of Catholic AIDS Action gave it certain unique advantages. For a start, many Namibians can be reached through the Catholic Church's 91 parishes and 300 "small Christian communities." One in four Namibians is Catholic and church attendance is high. Throughout the country, the Catholic Church has an extensive human infrastructure of local congregations led by deacons, elders, catechists, and other lay church leaders, under the guidance of parish priests. Many communities also have access to a church school, health clinic, or hospital, usually run by religious Sisters and other skilled professional staff.

Catholic AIDS Action quickly established offices in five regional sites, and by early 2002 had ten offices spread out in eight of Namibia's thirteen regions. Over one thousand trained home-based care volunteers are the backbone of Catholic AIDS Action at the community level; they assist over sixteen hundred sick clients and five thousand orphans. The volunteers are the organization's most precious asset, and they are by no means all Catholics: Many belong to Namibia's Lutheran Church and other denominations. The volunteers have a particular responsibility for monitoring the general health and well-being of orphans and vulnerable children. Whenever the program has items such as blankets, school uniforms, and sweaters available for distribution to orphans, the volunteer groups are responsible for selecting the children in their area who are most in need of assistance. By 2003, Catholic AIDS Action was providing periodic support to sixteen thousand registered needy children around the country. This support may include blankets, school uniforms, bursaries, and meals from a soup kitchen. Staff and volunteers also provide orphans and vulnerable children with psychosocial support, especially in crisis situations such as cases of child abuse or neglect. Often this involves collaboration with government ministries, NGOs, and traditional healers.

Source: Byamugisha et al. 2002; Foster 2004.

FIGURE 6.6. Catholic Aids Action, Namibia

probably have no more than a dozen or so active partnerships with community groups. Many RCBs have a hundred or more congregations in their network, some of the largest reach thousands of congregations. RCBs therefore occupy a strategic position in terms of scaling up responses.

Some RCBs, mostly "mainline" faith communities, have appointed coordinators and broadened existing job descriptions to support congregation responses. Many smaller RCBs have limited resources and cannot redeploy staff in this way. Interreligious networking organizations can play an important role in encouraging and assisting smaller RCBs to establish their own HIV/AIDS responses or combine with others. Strengthening community-level responses must be the cornerstone of any support strategy for orphans in Africa. The following types of support for FBOs are needed:

- *Program support.* At the congregation level, training and exchange visits can help volunteers to develop skills in areas such as needs assessment, planning, monitoring, income generation, psychosocial support, and HIV prevention. Some RCBs require considerable technical assistance to enable them to deliver program support to congregations they supervise.
- *Organizational development.* As well as skills to improve the quality of their programs, congregations need help in strengthening their organizations. Training is required in areas such as governance, financial systems, administration, and volunteer management.
- *Funding.* The most effective and targeted material support to assist orphans is currently provided by community groups such as congregations. This support involves the community safety net, which frequently involves the poor helping the destitute. But there are limits to the number of households and amount of support that can be provided by communities themselves. Financial resources are needed to supplement the assets being expended by volunteers and congregations on destitute orphan households. RCBs are appropriate organizations for channeling financial support to congregations. In addition, resources are needed to fund the programs of RCBs to enable them to provide technical and financial support to congregations.

External agencies have a timely opportunity to partner with RCBs and to strengthen faith-based community responses to orphans. The value of such partnerships goes beyond funding, as RCBs require assistance in developing technical support skills such as training and mentoring. If they are able to provide technical support and small grants to congregations, RCBs could enable a massive expansion in the number of vulnerable children receiving appropriate support.

ENSURE THAT FUNDING REACHES AFFECTED COMMUNITIES. Many congregations are looking for sources of external financial support to supplement their own contributions. Yet current development funding mechanisms are inadequate because they rarely lead to "trickle down." "Water, water everywhere, but not a drop to drink" is the cry of many groups desperately looking for small injections of capital to help expand their initiatives. Relatively large amounts of money are being given as grants to international organizations for orphan programs, but little is spent at the grassroots level based on the priorities of affected communities. Because of their own constraints, donors generally do not provide grants directly to community groups, and the bulk of civil society grant making is provided to established NGOs. A British Christian donor that in the past has supported congregations recently decided (because it receives thousands of unsolicited requests) that it will reject new funding proposals. Fresh sources of funding need to be mobilized to support religious groups. Some FBOs have received modest amounts of support from congregations and philanthropic organizations in the North and the oil-producing countries of the Arab world; but, by and large, religious groups in these parts of the world have not responded generously to the hardships of orphans and other vulnerable children in Africa. There is need for innovative mechanisms to channel resources and technical support to community groups through intermediaries such as RCBs and community foundations (Foster 2002a).

CONCLUSION

Between 1990 and 2005 in the most severely affected countries, the number of orphans will more than triple and the number of children who have lost both parents will increase by a staggering 900 percent (USAID, UNICEF, and UNAIDS 2002). Until now, surprisingly few of Africa's thirty-four million orphans have slipped through the safety net and ended up living as street children or in unsupported child-headed households (Foster 2000; Foster et al. 1997). This reflects the strength of Africa's extended families and communities, with the latter acting as a kind of "extended-extended family." But the situation is rapidly changing: As a result of the impact of AIDS, both the extended family and community safety nets are unraveling. Vastly increased numbers of children are being put at risk of situations of extreme deprivation, vulnerability, and exploitation.

This outcome is not inevitable, however. Faith-based community initiatives are proliferating across Africa in response to the orphan crisis, led by an army of religiously committed and motivated volunteers. These dedicated and selfless acts of caring deserve to be supported by policymakers and resource organizations. Our task as outsiders is to ensure that our actions and words do not make matters worse for Africa's children, and to make certain that we understand and reinforce faith-based, community-owned orphan support initiatives.

ACKNOWLEDGMENTS

It would not have been possible to write this chapter without insights provided by numerous colleagues. Thanks are due to staff, volunteers, and researchers involved with the Family AIDS Caring Trust's Families, Orphans and Children Under Stress (FOCUS) program who developed and documented a model of community care that has been replicated by groups throughout Africa. I am deeply indebted to the research teams in six countries who in 2002–03 were part of the World Conference of Religions for Peace and UNICEF-initiated Faith-Based Organization Orphans and Vulnerable Children (FBO OVC) documentation study. And finally, thanks to Andrew Tomkins, Glen Williams, Heidi Verhoef, Kate Harrison, and Kerry Olsen for their helpful comments on early drafts.

References

Adherents.com Database. http://www.adherents.com

African Religious Leaders Assembly on Children and HIV/AIDS. 2002. *Final declaration*. Nairobi, Kenya: World Conference of Religions for Peace, June 9–12. http://www.wcrp.org/RforP/Press%20Releases/NEWS_NAIROBI ASSEMBLY_MAIN.html

Barrett, D. R. 2001. *World Christian encyclopaedia*. Oxford: Oxford University Press.

Byamugisha, C. G., L. Y. Steinitz, G. Williams, and P. Zondi. 2002. *Journeys of faith: Church-based responses to HIV and AIDS in three southern African countries*. St. Albans, UK.: TALC.

Ejizu, C. I. n.d. African traditional religions and the promotion of community-living in Africa. http://www.afrikaworld.net/afrel/community.html

Foster, G. 2000. The capacity of the extended family safety net for orphans in Africa. *Psychology, Health, and Medicine* 5:55–62.

———. 2002a. Supporting community efforts to assist orphans in Africa. *New England Journal of Medicine* 346 (24): 1907–9.

———. 2002b. Understanding community responses to the situation of children affected by AIDS: Lessons for external agencies. In *One step further: Responses to HIV/AIDS*, ed. A. Sisask, 91–115. SIDA Studies no. 7. Geneva: United Nations Research Institute in Social Development. Available at http://www.unrisd.org

———. 2004. *Study of the response by faith-based organizations to orphans and vulnerable children*. New York: World Conference of Religions for Peace and UNICEF. http://www.unicef.org/aids/FBO_OVC_study_summary.pdf

Foster, G. , C. Makufa, R. Drew, and E. Kralovec. 1997. Factors leading to the establishment of child-headed households: The case of Zimbabwe. *Health Transition Review* 7 (suppl. 2): 155–68. http://htc.anu.edu.au/pdfs/Foster1.pdf

Foster, G., J. Webster, P. Stephenson, and S. Germann. 2002. Supporting community initiatives is crucial to scaling up orphan support activities in Africa. Abstract MoPeF4099, 14. International Conference on AIDS, Barcelona.

Gilborn, L. Z., R. Nyonyintono, R. Kabumbuli, and G. Jagwe-Wadda. 2001. *Making a difference for children affected by AIDS: Baseline findings from operations research in Uganda*. Washington, DC: Population Council.

Green, E. 2002. The impact of religious organisations in promoting HIV prevention. *SafAIDS News* 10 (1): 9–12. Available at http://www.safaids.org.zw

Hamutyinei, M. A., and A. B. Plangger. 1987. *Tsumo-shumo: Shona proverbial lore and wisdom*. Gweru, Zimbabwe: Mambo Press.

Hunter, S. 2000. *Reshaping societies: HIV/AIDS and social change*. Glens Falls, NY: Hudson Run Press.

Kurt Alan, V. B. 2000. Spirituality: A development taboo. *Development in Practice* 10:31–43.

Mukoyogo, M. C., and G. Williams. 1991. *AIDS orphans: A community perspective from Tanzania*. Strategies for Hope Series No. 5. London: ActionAid.

Mutangadura, G. B. 2000. Household welfare impacts of mortality of adult females in Zimbabwe: Implications for policy and program development. Paper presented at the AIDS and Economics Symposium, IAEN Network, Durban, July 7–8.

Nhat Han. n.d. *The Second Precept: Generosity* http://www.ncf.carleton.ca/ip/sigs/religion/buddhism/introduction/precepts/precept-2.html

Paterson, G. 2002. The role of the church in combating HIV/AIDS. *SAfAIDS News* 10 (3): 13–14. Available at http://www.safaids.org.zw

Poulter, C. 1997. *A psychological and physical needs profile of families living with HIV/AIDS in Lusaka, Zambia*. Research Brief no. 2. Lusaka: UNICEF Lusaka.

Sengendo, J., and J. Nambi. 1997. The psychological effect of orphanhood: a study of orphans in Rakai district. *Health Transition Review* 7 (suppl.): 105–24.

Shorter, A. 1975. *African Christian theology*. London: Geoffrey Chapman.

Umoja Muslim Welfare Organization (UMWO). n.d. http://www.orphan-aid.org.uk/orphandet/umoja.htm

USAID (U.S. Agency for International Development), UNICEF, and UNAIDS (Joint United Nations Programme on HIV/AIDS). 2002. *Children on the brink 2002: A joint report on orphan estimates and program strategies*. Washington, DC: TvT Associates/The Synergy Project, USAID. http://www.unicef.org/publications/pub_children_on_the_brink_en.pdf

Yates, D. 2003. *Situational analysis of the church response to HIV/AIDS in Namibia: Final report*. Windhoek: Pan African Christian AIDS Network.

7

Making the Right Choices in the Asia-Pacific Region

Protecting Children and Young People from HIV and Its Impacts

Tim Brown and Werasit Sittitrai

The situation of orphans and vulnerable children in Asia and the Pacific, in particular children affected by AIDS, has received far less study and attention than has the situation in Africa. HIV/AIDS epidemics in the Asia-Pacific region began much later and have not yet risen to sub-Saharan Africa levels. As a consequence, the overall number of children orphaned by AIDS is much lower, below the threshold of most policymakers' concerns. The current low prevalence, however, also means that the most effective method of reducing the problems of children orphaned and affected by AIDS in the region is primary prevention of HIV infection. If countries respond effectively now, the problems of most children who would be affected by HIV in the absence of strong national responses can be averted. Acting now will also keep the magnitude of the problem small enough that available resources and institutions will be better able to address it.

Even with low prevalence, however, the number of affected children in Asia is substantial, owing to the fact that the region has over half the world's population and almost four times as many children (1.2 billion) as sub-Saharan Africa (350 million) (USAID, UNICEF, and UNAIDS 2004: 9). Almost two million Asian children have already lost at least one parent to AIDS, and many more have been or will be directly affected by the epidemic. Millions more children in the region are rendered vulnerable through poverty, prostitution, child labor, and trafficking.

In addition to highlighting the needs for care and support of orphaned and vulnerable children in Asia and the Pacific, this chapter emphasizes primary prevention as a major strategy. Even if the proportion of affected children is kept low in Asian-Pacific settings, though, much more needs to be learned about delivering effective care and support and scaling up programs to meet the growing needs of these children.

DIVERSITY IN THE EPIDEMICS OF THE ASIA-PACIFIC REGION

HIV came later to Asia and the Pacific than to the rest of the world; major epidemics became apparent only in the early 1990s. HIV epidemics in the countries of the region are diverse in nature and varied in intensity. A few regions, including Cambodia, Myanmar, Thailand, and several states in India, have serious HIV epidemics. Others have only recently experienced rapidly emerging epidemics, for example China, Indonesia, Papua New Guinea, and Vietnam. Still other countries, such as Japan and the Philippines, have reported comparatively little HIV to date.

Epidemics in this part of the world have been driven largely by sex work, injection-drug use, and male-male sex. It is now clear that variations in the percentage of men using sex-work services largely explain the differences in the rate of epidemic growth and severity among the countries in the region. In those countries and areas where as many as one-fifth of adult males use paid sexual services (Cambodia and Thailand, for example), the epidemic has grown explosively. In those areas where only one-tenth or one-twentieth of men pay for sex, the epidemics develop inexorably but more gradually. After a decade or more the epidemics enter a rapid growth phase, often fueled by interactions between injection-drug use and sex work.

Recent research conducted by the East–West Center and its collaborators has found that even in the lower risk countries of Asia, HIV epidemics may ultimately reach 3 to 5 percent of the adult population unless greatly expanded prevention programs are put in place. In localized higher risk areas the prevalence may rise as high as 15 to 20 percent, as it did in Northern Thailand (Brown and Peerapatanapokin 2004; Mason et al. 1995). Strong national responses to HIV in the region can turn things around, however. Effective interventions to prevent HIV transmission in sex work, injection-drug use, and male-male sex exist, and epidemics in the region have proven particularly amenable to appropriate and large-scale application. Both Thailand and Cambodia launched extensive and intensive prevention campaigns in the early 1990s, and within a few years prevalence declined in every major HIV surveillance population (Phalla et al. 1998; Phoolcharoen et al. 1998).

Given the late development of Asian epidemics, their comparatively low HIV levels, and the strong influence of sex work and injection-drug use, it might seem that Asian-Pacific epidemics would have comparatively little impact on children. Even with low prevalence, however, approximately 223,000 children in the region are estimated to be living with HIV, and approximately 43,000 children died of AIDS in 2002 (UNAIDS 2002).

Most infections occur through a chain of transmission that starts with men contracting HIV through sex-work services or sharing injecting equipment. These men bring HIV home to their families, leaving many children living with HIV, others orphaned, and many more affected by illness, stigma, and death. In the most severely affected areas in the region, 2 to 3 percent of all pregnant women are HIV-positive, and many of them will transmit HIV to their newborns. With Asia's large populations, such numbers add up quickly.

When AIDS ultimately claims parents' lives, children are orphaned. (Following epidemiologic convention, an orphan has been defined as a child under age fifteen who has lost one or both parents. Children are defined as being under the age of majority – usually eighteen unless otherwise noted – and youth are between the ages of fifteen and twenty-four.) These youngsters often live in societies that still discriminate strongly against those with HIV infection and their offspring. For orphans, HIV has a double impact, resulting not only in parental loss but also in increased vulnerability to HIV through worsened economic and health status, inadequate social support in their new families or institutional living arrangements, and stigma and discrimination. An estimated 28 percent of the roughly one million orphaned children in Thailand have lost a parent to AIDS, despite national adult prevalence levels below 2 percent (USAID, UNICEF, and UNAIDS 2002). UNAIDS estimates that over 1.8 million children under age fifteen in the Asia-Pacific region have lost one or both parents to AIDS, and this number is expected to rise to 4.3 million by 2010. Should there be extensive epidemic spread in one of the larger countries of the region, these numbers may prove to be serious underestimates.

Increasing numbers of children in marginalized circumstances are vulnerable. In Asian-Pacific countries some disadvantaged children – the poor, street children, and child prostitutes, in addition to orphans – are at heightened risk of sexual abuse or exploitation or are sometimes forced to use sex to survive. Trafficking in children, both for sex work and for labor, remains a major problem in several countries. Estimating the number of these children is difficult, but there is no doubt about their extreme vulnerability to HIV.

The number of youth at risk of HIV infection is steadily increasing as patterns of sexuality and drug use evolve. These changes are occurring while the number of youth in the region has grown rapidly, from 284 million in 1960 to 615 million in 2000 (United Nations Population Division 2001) and the age at marriage has risen steadily. Between 1950 and 1990, the number of single women in the region increased by a factor of 4 – the combined impact of a doubling of the size of the youth population and a doubling of the percentage of single young women among them (Westley and Choe 2002).

CHILDREN ORPHANED AND AFFECTED BY AIDS IN ASIA
AND THE PACIFIC

Our knowledge about children orphaned and affected by AIDS in Asia and
the Pacific comes from only a few countries – those most severely affected.
As was observed early in Africa, even within these countries there is significant microgeographic variation; some provinces or districts are very
heavily affected by HIV, while others are not (Barnett and Blaikie 1992).
As a result, there are localized areas, such as Chiangmai and Chiangrai
provinces in Thailand and Sangli district in Maharashtra, India, where
HIV prevalence has risen to substantial levels of 5 to 10 percent (Brown
and Sittitrai 1995; Verma et al. 2002). Anecdotal reports are also available from affected families in Yunnan, one of the most heavily affected
parts of China (China HIV/AIDS Socio-Economic Impact Study Team
2002).

One must therefore be cautious about generalizing too broadly in a
region as diverse as Asia and the Pacific. With this acknowledgment of limitations, what follows summarizes what is known about children orphaned
or affected by HIV/AIDS in the Asia-Pacific region. In a review of the
impacts of HIV and AIDS on children in Asia, Wijngaarden and Shaeffer (2002) divided the impacts into three main areas: (1) loss of social and
family support; (2) decreased access to services, and (3) stigma and discrimination. This next section explores these areas in detail.

Loss of Social and Family Support

Children may lose parental support and care in a number of ways – through
illness and death, abandonment, or emotional distancing. The loss of one
or both parents puts psychological and social pressure on children. The
relatives and neighbors or institutions that assume the care of orphaned
children may not provide the same level of love and compassion that parents would. Decline in parental health places children under increased
stress as they worry about their ill parent(s). Then as household income
falls, additional demands are placed on the children, and normally supportive communities and schools react negatively to the parent's illness
(Brown and Sittitrai 1995).

In a study in India (Verma et al. 2002), children experienced additional
stress after a parent's death due to the increased need to help support the
family, separation from siblings, placement in new family environments,
and difficulties in finding marital partners. Community safety nets for psychological support of children are usually nonexistent, and it is not practical for children to access either discussion and support groups targeted at
adults or informal counseling through religious institutions.

In the early 1990s a study at a major hospital in Thailand (Janjaroen
and Khamman 2004) found that HIV-positive women were five times as

likely to abandon their children at hospitals as uninfected women, a trend also observed in another study in Chiangmai (Brown and Sittitrai 1995) during the same period. Mothers' concerns about their ability to care for the child properly, coupled with more traditional concerns (family break-down, illegitimate births, single motherhood, and poverty, for example) all contributed to abandonment (Mielke 1994: 308). Many abandoned children ended up in institutional care, again with little psychosocial support.

Only a handful of studies have documented the psychosocial stresses on children orphaned or affected by HIV. Devine (quoted in Wijngaar-den and Shaeffer 2002) found that Thai parents sometimes physically dis-tanced themselves from their children, fearful of giving them HIV. He also reported that stigma and discrimination forced children to cut short the normal grieving process, creating problems later in life. Im-Em (reported in Wijngaarden and Shaeffer 2002) found separation and divorce sometimes followed marital problems resulting from HIV, creating further stress for children. In a participatory appraisal of needs of children affected by AIDS in Cambodia (KHANA 2000), children reported the difficulties of caring for ill parents, relocation, separation from siblings, concerns about being infected themselves, pressure not to discuss their parents' situation, and not having anybody to explain to them what was happening. All these fac-tors have a strong impact on a child's psychological, social, and physical well-being.

In addition, families affected by HIV often suffer financial difficulties. Once one or both parents become ill, the household faces a spiral of decreas-ing income and increasing expenditures. As income earners fall ill, other family members are forced to stay home to care for them while medical care costs rise. Families who have been living in rented homes or on rented land may lose their housing. In Asia, as in Africa, most often it is the father who falls ill and dies first, because he was the first in the family to con-tract HIV. After his death, funeral costs sap family savings and household income may fall substantially, threatening food security. In a study of AIDS-affected households in Northern Thailand in 1993, Pitayanon, Kongsin, and Janjareon (1997) found that the income of households experiencing an AIDS death was half the income of those with no death. In about 10 percent of cases, grandparents who lose sons and daughters to AIDS are raising their grandchildren (Knodel and Im-em 2003), and because in Asia grandparents traditionally depend on their children for financial support, these house-holds sometimes have economic problems. Substantial economic problems have also been reported in India within families with an AIDS death. Gen-der inequities in employment mean that widows who take over their hus-band's work often make half the income, pushing the family into poverty. The work demands on the widow create a need for the girls in the fam-ily to take over domestic chores and for boys to work, sometimes forc-ing them to forgo education (Association François-Xavier Bagnoud n.d.).

Decreased Access to Services

Children orphaned and affected by HIV in the region have decreased access to education, health care, and social services. Loss of educational opportunity in AIDS-affected families is a recurring theme in each of the countries studied, disproportionately affecting poorer families. In Yunnan, China, school expenses for a single child are almost one-fifth of the average annual income, and in a sample of thirty-one HIV-affected households, fourteen children from seven households had dropped out of school (China HIV/AIDS Socio-Economic Impact Study Team 2002). In Sangli district, India, 4.3 percent of children in families with an AIDS death were withdrawn from school compared with 2.6 percent in families with no death (Verma et al. 2002). In Thailand, 7 percent of AIDS-affected households reported children that were forced to leave school as a result of social discrimination (Pitayanon et al. 1997). The loss of services also extends to health care and other social services. For example, in Sangli, one-quarter of households with an AIDS death reported that children were unable to visit the health care center when needed, compared with only 8.7 percent in the households with no death (Verma et al. 2002). When children cannot read or write, they have limited access to information and difficulty accessing some social services. If they have little or no education, they will have few opportunities for good employment in the future. Both Janjaroen and Khamman (2004) and Gordon et al. (1999) point to a strong need for better targeting of social and educational support services to reach those children in greatest need.

Theft of the inheritance or property of children orphaned by AIDS has been reported in Cambodia, and asset stripping has been seen in India (Association François-Xavier Bagnoud n.d.; KHANA 2000). These children have no access to legal advice, and no support from the legal system to protect their inheritance and property rights. These losses – coupled with savings lost to medical and funeral expenses and income lost when primary wage earners die – worsen the already difficult situation of children affected by HIV.

Stigma and Discrimination

Stigma and discrimination create major problems for children affected by HIV and their families in the region. Many of the problems could be readily managed if communities were supportive, but experience has shown that this is not always so in Asian-Pacific societies. Busza (1999) describes stigma and discrimination around the region, varying from rejection of families by communities in Indonesia, to dismissal from work in a number of countries, to refusal to provide traditional burials for people with HIV and AIDS in Cambodia. The impacts on children often take the form of social ostracism, including being rejected as playmates or at social gatherings, and denial of entry to schools (Pitayanon et al. 1997; Verma et al. 2002). One should not underestimate the level of psychological stress that constant verbal and physical manifestations of stigma and discrimination create for affected children and their families. A survey in a district in Maharashtra, India (Verma et al. 2002) found that one-fifth of the children in households with an AIDS death had experienced some form of discrimination directly against them. In a Northern Thailand study (Pitayanon et al. 1997) a similar percentage of children experienced discrimination.

The effects of stigma and discrimination may be economic as well as social, affecting child welfare. In Maharashtra, discrimination against adults with HIV was even more extensive and pervasive than that against children, and it directly affected their ability to support their families and provide for their children (Verma et al. 2002). In Northern Thailand, half of the families studied reported social discrimination against adults with AIDS (Pitayanon et al. 1997). Some experienced serious economic impacts on the household, including loss of employment and refusal to use the services of the family business. For people raising their orphaned grandchildren, the refusal of day-care centers to care for children whose parents have died of HIV has limited the grandparents' ability to work (Safman 2002). If prolonged, the economic difficulties resulting from stigma and discrimination will have numerous negative impacts on children, including poor nutrition, forced withdrawal from school, and an inability to obtain health care. Unfortunately, it is hard to assess the exact magnitude of stigma and discrimination because few systematic studies are available in the region. As the epidemic evolves to affect more people, social responses in some places are becoming more tolerant, but continued discrimination is clearly an issue that requires close attention in programmatic efforts.

AT HEIGHTENED RISK: VULNERABLE CHILDREN AND YOUTH IN ASIA AND THE PACIFIC

Large numbers of children in the region are in especially difficult circumstances. In addition to children orphaned by and affected by AIDS, there are those without protective family care (street children, child laborers, migrant children, and children in institutional care, for example), children who have been drawn into sex work, children affected by armed conflict, and children of extremely poor families. The number of these children is hard to estimate, and no census has ever been taken. There is clear evidence, however, that they exist in almost every country in the region. Factors such as economic need, unstable social and living environments, coercion from adults, lack of family and community support, and discrimination, among others, increase the vulnerability of these children to HIV infection. Information is largely anecdotal or the product of smaller studies, but a picture emerges of children in serious need of help and support.

Trafficking in children for sexual exploitation is a major problem throughout the Asia-Pacific region. The risk of HIV to children in commercial sex is often even greater than the already high risk of their adult clients. Being much younger, they are physiologically more vulnerable to vaginal or anal trauma, which increases the odds of infection. In negotiating condom use with clients they lack bargaining power, are physically weaker, and are perceived as more likely to be HIV-free. Lacking a legal status, they are often unable to access health services, including essential treatment for sexually transmitted infections (STIs). They also cannot escape the psychological and physical trauma of involvement in commercial sex.

UNICEF, the University of Cambridge, and Childwatch International conducted a review of children and prostitution in the mid-1990s (Ennew et al. 1996). The researchers concluded that while it was difficult to estimate the number of children involved in sex work, the practice was a growing problem requiring more attention and concrete action, especially when such trafficking occurred in locations with high prevalence of HIV and STIs. Research by the United Nations Economic and Social Commission for Asia and the Pacific (1999) on sexually abused and exploited children in six Mekong area countries reached the same conclusion, finding that one-third of the surveyed sex workers in Cambodia were between twelve and seventeen years of age. The International Labor Organization, the United Nations Development Programme, UNICEF, and UNAIDS (the Joint United Nations Programme on HIV/AIDS) are addressing the problem of child trafficking, but progress is slow.

Increased vulnerability to HIV infection results from a multitude of factors, such as street culture, economic need, limited power in relationships, physical weakness as compared with adults, and lack of protection by – or even being targeted for arrest by – authorities. Among street children in Jakarta, for example, it was reported that older boys practiced a rite of initiation through anal sex with younger boys who wanted their protection (Black and Farrington 1997). Many street children in Thailand use sex to help them establish a sense of closeness with other youngsters, while also obtaining protection and sexual release.

Condom use remains uncommon. Many children, especially girls, are forced to sell sex to survive. In one study half of the young girls on the street in Delhi (Rajkumar 2000) reported selling sex, most often to drunken men. Sexual activity (both male-male and male-female) almost always occurred without a condom. In studies of orphans in India, boys were often sent off as migrant laborers to Mumbai, a high-HIV-prevalence area, to help the family make ends meet, even though most HIV in the home area was attributed to returning migrants (Association François-Xavier Bagnoud n.d.). Many of the two hundred thousand children in the slum areas of Kolkata were sexually active by age twelve, newly arrived young girls were often raped, and many looked to "sugar daddies" to protect themselves

(Association François-Xavier Bagnoud n.d.). Young girls did not remain on the street long because they were quickly pulled into prostitution or conscripted into domestic work or sweatshop labor. Children in all of these varied difficult circumstances clearly have special protection, prevention, and care needs that must be addressed by programs tailored to their specific circumstances.

EVOLVING PATTERNS OF SEXUAL RISK AMONG YOUTH IN THE REGION

UNAIDS (2002) estimates an HIV prevalence rate of only 0.1 percent in East Asian and Pacific youth between fifteen and twenty-four years of age, and a rate of roughly 0.3 percent in South and Southeast Asia. However, this low prevalence may be misleading, masking high levels of underlying and evolving risk as the epidemic in the region grows. Because age at first intercourse is higher in many parts of Asia and the Pacific than in other heavily HIV-affected regions, these figures include many sexually inactive youth in the younger age ranges. Once these youth become sexually active, the risk can become quite high. Half of new HIV infections occur among youth (UNAIDS 2002).

Sex workers and clients are predominantly youth, that is, between the ages of fifteen and twenty-four. Many of those who inject drugs start young, and the majority of young men who have sex with men in the region receive no information about their risk or how to protect themselves. Nor can current prevalence figures fully reflect the dynamic changes occurring in the sexual and drug-using behaviors among young people that are rapidly expanding their risk of HIV exposure.

As the age at marriage increases, the number and proportion of single youth and the rate of premarital sex are growing. The proportion of single male youth is growing from 83 percent in 1990 to an expected 96 percent in 2025. The corresponding change for females is even higher: 62 percent to 93 percent (Westley and Choe 2002). In many countries, as the number of single youth increase, premarital sex rates will also grow, exposing increasing numbers of young people to HIV risk. Traditional patterns of sexuality in Asia have given young men considerable sexual latitude while severely constraining the behavior of young women. Comparisons of premarital sexual activity from the six countries studied in the Asian Young Adult Reproductive Risk Project (Choe et al. 2004) illustrate this disparity (see Figure 7.1). In most Asian countries, young men are at least three times as likely as young women to be sexually active, with anywhere from a few percent to almost 60 percent of young men aged twenty to twenty-four reporting premarital sex before age twenty (Xenos et al. 2002). In most countries the majority of premaritally sexually active young men have partners other than their future wives. For example, surveys in the

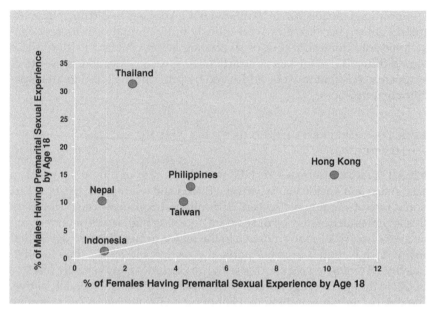

FIGURE 7.1. Percentage of males by percentage of females with premarital experience by age 18. *Source:* Choe et al. 2004; data from Taiwan and Hong Kong from
unpublished Asian Young Adult Reproductive Risk Project (AYARR) Tables.

Philippines, Taiwan, and Thailand found that almost 90 percent of the sexually active young men (ages fifteen to twenty-four) had first sex before
marriage, almost always with someone to whom they would not be married later. By contrast, less than 30 percent of sexually active young women
in Thailand and the Philippines had sex before marriage and two-thirds of
the time it was with their future spouse (Choe et al. 2001).

A large proportion of premarital sex is commercial, with a high potential for current and future HIV transmission. The imbalance in male-female
premarital sexual activity creates a high demand from young men for sex,
but limits the supply of females. As a consequence, much of the sexual
activity occurs through commercial sex. Their limited bargaining power
and the large number of clients makes sex workers particularly vulnerable
to HIV and other STIs. STIs in turn increase the HIV risk for both sex workers and clients. In addition to the more traditional brothel- and bar-based
services, new forms of sex work have been evolving, including services
in restaurants and barbershops as well as services ordered by telephone
or the Internet; in many countries, increasing numbers of teenage girls are
trading sexual services for goods or fashion accessories. HIV transmission
does not occur only in sex work, though. Virtually all the single male clients
will later marry, potentially exposing their future wives to HIV. Sexual risk

is cumulative – summing together the past and present risk of all past and present sexual partners. Thus, while most women living with HIV in Asia and the Pacific have little or no history of risky behavior (beyond sex with their husbands), they have contracted HIV as a consequence of their husbands' past or present behaviors.

Changes in the sexual behavior of women in the region are exposing more young women to risk of HIV infection. However, male-female behavioral patterns are in flux across the region, changing more rapidly in some countries than in others. In contrast to findings in the Philippines and Thailand, almost 70 percent of sexually active women in Taiwan reported having sex prior to marriage, most commonly not with their future husband (Choe et al. 2001). Increasing female risk activity has also been observed in surveys of other more industrialized countries, including Japan, where 31 percent of eighteen-to-twenty-four-year-old males and 24 percent of same-aged females reported nonregular partners in the past year (Kamakura, Kihara, and Komatsu 2001; Ono-Kihara, Kihara, and Yamazaki 2002). Similar patterns of more equal levels of sexual behavior among males and females are often seen in the Pacific. However, while rates of female sexual activity are increasing, traditional male behavioral patterns linger. In the same survey in Japan, 16 percent of eighteen-to-twenty-four-year-old males had visited a sex worker in the past year. This behavior creates a situation in which increasing numbers of young women are at much higher risk for HIV infection by virtue of their own sexual activity in relationships that they often view as "exclusive" but their partners do not. Patterns of sexuality are evolving in this direction around the region, albeit at different rates in different countries. Most often sex in the context of a relationship occurs without contraception, potentially putting both partners at risk of HIV infection.

EVOLVING PATTERNS OF RISK THROUGH DRUG USE

Injection-drug use remains a serious problem for youth and carries significant risk for HIV. Needle sharing in injection-drug use is one of the most efficient means of transmitting HIV, and prevalence among injection-drug users around the Asia-Pacific region is extremely high: 40 percent in Thailand, 80 percent in Manipur, 60 percent in Myanmar, and 50 percent in Indonesia. (US Bureau of the Census 2004). Although the size of the injecting population is not well documented in most places, drug use continues to be a significant issue among youth in Asia and the Pacific. In a nationwide youth survey in the Philippines, 2.5 percent of males and 1.8 percent of females reported having injected drugs at some time (Balk, Cruz, and Brown 1997). Studies of young military conscripts in Thailand found the proportion with a history of injection-drug use growing from 1 percent in 1991 to 4.2 percent in 1997 (Nelson et al. 2002). In some high drug use areas in China and Vietnam, anecdotal reports suggest that 5 percent or more of young males have injected. While these numbers may seem low, recall that they apply to a large population of youth in the region, that they are very likely to be underreported, and that HIV is highly prevalent among injection-drug users. Studies (such as Pisani and Winitthama 2001) of injection-drug users around the region find that many are clients of sex workers and often have other sexual partners, usually without using condoms. This practice creates serious potential for HIV to enter sexually active youth populations.

Users of other psychoactive substances are also at risk and the number of young drug users is growing. While injection-drug use represents the most immediate and serious risk in terms of HIV infection, use of psychoactive substances (alcohol and other noninjected drugs) creates intoxication that increases sexual risk among youth (Podhisita, Xenos, and Varangrat 2001; Sattah et al. 2002). Despite the higher risk associated with injecting, prevalence is often high among noninjection-drug users as well. For example, in Haiphong, Vietnam, HIV prevalence among young (under thirty) noninjection-drug users was 46 percent, compared with 74 percent among injectors (Nguyen et al. 2001).

In revisiting its 1997 review of drug use in Southeast Asia, the Centre for Harm Reduction noted two significant trends (Reid and Costigan 2002). First, regionally, the age of initiation among drug users has been decreasing, and a small but increasing number of Asian women are using drugs. Second, methamphetamine use by both injection and noninjection routes has been rising rapidly, especially among youth, to become the drug of choice in a number of Southeast Asian countries (see "Methamphetamine use is heightening risks" 2002). For example, among people under twenty-one years of age in Hong Kong who come into contact with various government drug agencies for treatment and control, heroin use had dropped threefold, from 72.5 percent in 1995 to 26.1 percent in 2000, while amphetamine use had increased from 1.8 percent to 58.1 percent over the same period (Laidler 2000). In a study of fifteen-to-twenty-one-year-old students in Northern Thailand, 41 percent of males and 19 percent of females reported having used methamphetamines at some time, primarily through noninjection routes (Sattah et al. 2002). In that study, and in several others (Gleghorn et al. 1998; "Methamphetamine use is heightening risks ..." 2002; Nemoto, Operario, and Soma 2002; Rawson, Washton, Domier, and Reiber 2002), those who use methamphetamines are much more sexually active than those who do not. The intoxication associated with use of such drugs also reduces the ability to make sound decisions, negotiate for safer sex, and make proper use of condoms. Thus, drug use and associated sexual behavior represent a growing HIV risk for youth in the region.

PROTECTING CHILDREN FROM HIV AND ITS IMPACTS:
THE WAY IS KNOWN

Programs to protect children in the region from HIV and its impacts have two major approaches, both of which are absolutely essential to addressing children's current and future needs: Prevention through preemption, and the provision of care and support. Prevention through preemption includes:

- programs to protect present and future parents from HIV, and
- programs to protect newborns and babies from HIV infection.

The provision of care and support for orphaned, infected, and affected children includes:

- programs to reduce the psychological, economic, social, and educational consequences of HIV for children orphaned and affected by HIV and their families,
- programs to provide care and support for children living with HIV and their families, and
- programs to reduce stigma and discrimination.

A discussion of strategies currently being used in the region to accomplish these goals and concrete examples of activities that have proven successful follows.

Preemption: Protecting Parents from HIV and Children from Orphaning

The primary means of preventing future pediatric infection, the impacts of HIV on children, and orphaning is to prevent HIV infection in parents. Most of the individuals engaging in risky behaviors are male. If prevention programs reach them, HIV epidemics will slow radically and levels of HIV infection can be kept low. This is the first line of defense, and if prevention resources are mobilized and targeted appropriately, they are remarkably effective in Asian settings (Brown 2003; Phoolcharocn et al. 1998).

The future parents of Asia are the youth of today. An essential part of averting future parental infection and reducing the number of AIDS-affected families and children is to work with youth to adopt safer behaviors and build AIDS-resistant societies. At least five components are essential to this strategy.

PROVIDE YOUNG PEOPLE WITH KNOWLEDGE AND INFORMATION. While knowledge alone is not enough to change behaviors, it is an essential prerequisite if young people are to take the steps needed to protect themselves and their peers from HIV. Knowledge about HIV/AIDS and the options for protecting oneself from HIV infection (including condoms and delaying onset of sexual activity) varies widely across the region but is generally insufficient. While youth in some countries (Thailand and Cambodia, for example) know a lot (see "Measure DHS+ Indicators Database"; Sittitrai et al. 1994), knowledge elsewhere is extremely low. For example, while 85 percent of fifteen-to-nineteen-year-old girls in Vietnam had heard of AIDS, only 27 percent knew the three primary means of avoiding infection (UNICEF, UNAIDS, and WHO 2002). In much of South Asia knowledge among young women is even lower. In the Nepal DHS survey in 2001, only half of the young women in the fifteen-to-nineteen age category had heard of AIDS; in India in 1998–99 this number was a low 29 percent (Measure DHS+ Indicators Database). National programs on AIDS in schools and life-skills training for both in-school and out-of-school youth are urgently needed to educate Asian-Pacific youth, especially young women, to live in a world with HIV.

DEVELOP THE LIFE SKILLS YOUNG PEOPLE NEED TO PROTECT THEMSELVES. Once armed with knowledge, young people must develop the skills to make appropriate decisions, negotiate safer behavior, resist peer pressure, and locate the necessary supplies and services for prevention, care, and support regarding reproductive health, HIV/AIDS, and STIs. Life skills training programs in Asia were pioneered early at the Thai Red Cross Society AIDS Research Center and have been adopted as a strategy for youth by several large-scale regional collaborations, including the Mekong Project for Southeast Asia, the Asian Red Cross/Red Crescent AIDS Task Force, and UNICEF for the entire region.

Asian-Pacific school systems tend to be conservative, however, and full adoption of life skills with strong HIV/AIDS components has been slow in the region. Furthermore, not all youths can be reached through the schools because large numbers of students in Asia do not complete the primary grades. Thus, there is a strong demand for sustained programs for out-of-school youth who are often mobile and at higher risk for HIV. Life-skills approaches have been incorporated into prevention efforts throughout the region by organizations such as the Cambodian Red Cross for young military and police, Mith Samlanh for street children in Cambodia, Center for Development and Population Activities for out-of-school young women in India, and the Breaking Through the Clouds project for migrant children and youth in China, Myanmar, and Thailand.

REDUCE SOCIAL, ECONOMIC, AND LEGAL FACTORS THAT CREATE VULNERA-BILITY. Vulnerability results from societal factors that affect adversely the ability to exert control over one's own health (UNAIDS 1998). A combination of personal, service-related, and societal factors can influence the vulnerability of young people to HIV infection. For example, adults often cite "cultural norms" as a reason for denying sex and HIV/AIDS information and access to contraception and condoms to youth, even as many become sexually active. Poverty and fear of authorities leave many youth vulnerable to sexual exploitation through selling sex or forced sex. Gender inequalities in educational opportunity (with the resulting lack of earning opportunities) and cultural practices of young women supporting their parents make it difficult for young girls in some societies to resist pressure to enter sex work. Programs to reduce HIV risk are necessary but not sufficient to protect young people; effective programs must also address the social, legal, economic, and cultural factors in the environment that keep young people from making the choices needed to protect their health.

Interventions and structural changes to reduce vulnerability can take many forms: literacy programs; expansion of educational and employment opportunities; legal protection of property rights; protection against physical violence; food security; and elimination of social stigmatization. Programs may need to be aimed at changing cultural norms, gender inequality, or service-provider attitudes that create barriers to youth protecting themselves from HIV. Programs might expand educational and appropriate employment opportunities for young people, and also reduce legal barriers to youth accessing reproductive health service.

Numerous programs seek to reduce vulnerability among young people. For example, UNICEF's "25 by 2005" initiative seeks to identify girls in six countries in South Asia who are not in school and help them enroll. Thailand's comprehensive program to prevent child prostitution, especially among rural girls, supports continuing education, expanded employment opportunities, and orientation of parents on the risks of sex work (UNAIDS 1999). The World Food Programme provides food aid to encourage school children to attend class, and it also supplies food to take home to their families to ensure sustained attendance. In some cases rations are specifically provided to families that send girls to school to help compensate parents for the loss of their daughters' labor.

GUARANTEE ACCESS TO YOUTH-FRIENDLY HEALTH SERVICES AND SUPPLIES. Asian societies tend to be conservative when it comes to matters of sexual behavior and drugs and particularly sensitive when these matters involve youth. Parents, teachers, and societies in general have a difficult time discussing these matters with youth or in public forums and operate from a false assumption that youth are not sexually active. Thus the public and policymakers are often opposed to establishing and funding youth-friendly reproductive health services, effectively denying condoms, STI services, and confidential counseling to youth.

In addition, many young people are embarrassed to buy condoms because of social stigma. In some places this problem has been addressed by strategic placement of vending machines or ready availability of condoms in marketing outlets, but elsewhere it remains a major barrier to prevention.

Possible strategies to remove these barriers to obtaining a means of prevention include expanding availability of condoms in places where risky behavior occurs, implementing peer education and distribution mechanisms (condom cafes in Vietnam, for example), or creating youth-friendly health services that acknowledge young people's sexual nature without being judgmental. These efforts should be supported by national campaigns to give the public a realistic understanding of current patterns in youth sexuality, so that the need for condom availability and youth-friendly services can be understood as protecting the lives of the next generation.

PROMOTE AND FACILITATE THE PARTICIPATION OF CHILDREN AND YOUTH. No one knows the needs of young people better than young people themselves. This recognition on a global scale has led to the realization that children and youth themselves can and should be the leaders, designers, and implementers of extremely effective and relevant HIV/AIDS efforts. However, the tendency of Asian-Pacific societies to have very hierarchical educational and social systems with children at the bottom has slowed the adoption of youth-centered approaches in the region (China HIV/AIDS Socio-Economic Impact Study Team 2002).

Attention needs to be given to building capacity among young people to participate effectively in these efforts in a sustained way. Additional capacity building is needed to enable adults and organizations to accept and facilitate young people's participation. Projects around the region have demonstrated that youth in Asia and the Pacific are as prepared to take the lead in prevention and care as their peers anywhere in the world. For example, in Hong Kong, TeenAIDS has been a major force in supplying HIV peer education programs in the schools. The Life Skills Training Youth Peer Education Program on Reproductive Health, STIs, and HIV/AIDS of the Asian Red Cross/Red Crescent AIDS Task Force is operating in twelve countries, working with locally appropriate youth populations. In Vietnam, youth have been taking an expanding role through the youth unions and condom cafes and in a Save the Children UK/People's Committee peer education project, largely managed and staffed by young people. Many more excellent examples exist around the region; nonetheless, such efforts remain too limited and existing programs are not doing enough.

Preemption: Protecting Children from Perinatal Infections and Loss of Their Mothers

Many HIV-positive husbands were infected as clients of sex workers or as drug injectors when they were younger. In many cases the men have not yet infected their wives, which provides a major opportunity to protect children from HIV and double orphaning by protecting their mothers from infection. Expanding confidential or anonymous voluntary counseling and testing (VCT) services for at-risk individuals and couples through either vertical or integrated reproductive health services would allow these couples to take steps to prevent husband-to-wife transmission. Should that effort fail, the accessibility of VCT services as part of family planning or antenatal care services can help couples make reproductive health decisions that reduce their probability of having an infected baby – through contraception, antiretroviral therapy to prevent mother-to-child transmission, or avoidance of breastfeeding.

Short-course antiretroviral therapy should be provided to newborns and infants to prevent perinatal infection. On a regional basis, over sixty thousand newborns are infected perinatally each year. With modern methods of preventing mother-to-child-transmission (PMTCT) – including administering antiretroviral drugs before birth, during labor, and after delivery – most new infections would be preventable if mechanisms can be created to deliver these services in developing countries (Newell 2001). In a review of mother-to-child transmission prevention in Asia, Preble and Piwoz (2002) point out that most Asian governments facing high HIV prevalence have in fact implemented transmission prevention policies, but few have moved beyond the pilot stage.

Pilot programs in Cambodia, India, and Thailand provide important lessons for other countries regarding VCT services, addressing stigma and discrimination, and organizing PMTCT services. They have also highlighted major issues that will need to be addressed in many Asian-Pacific settings, including low rates of antenatal care, high levels of stigma and discrimination, and weak health care infrastructures. Thailand (where some of the earliest testing of short-course PMTCT approaches was conducted) has demonstrated that national implementation of PMTCT is feasible in Asian settings (Shaffer et al. 1999). Efforts on a large scale began in the private sector in 1996 when, using donated funds, the Thai Red Cross Society, in partnership with many public and private hospitals, began providing the full 076 protocol – the standard treatment of AZT in the United States – to many HIV-positive pregnant women (Pancharoen, Ananworanich, and Thisyakorn, n.d., Thisyakorn et al. 2000). Once the efficacy of short-course antiretroviral treatment was established, increasing pressure to act quickly came from the local level, with some Thai CDC regional offices implementing broad coverage PMTCT programs as early as 1997. Regional operational tests were undertaken in 1997 and 1998 and short-course antiretroviral drugs became national policy by 2000. Early results found that 93 percent of women were tested, and 69 percent of those who tested positive received drugs for PMTCT through the national program (Kanshana and Simonds 2002).

The best approach to providing a supportive environment is to keep children with HIV with their families. One of the early arguments advanced against PMTCT programs was that they created orphans (some of whom would be living with HIV themselves) who would have a short, harsh life after their parents died. The major progress in reducing antiretroviral costs, along with growing recognition of the right to treatment for HIV, has spawned new programs known as MTCT-Plus or MTCT+ (Mitka 2002). Recognizing that the child's needs are best served by providing a supportive and enduring family environment, these programs are providing antiretroviral drugs to the mother on a lifelong basis, not just during pregnancy.

In Asia, the Thai Red Cross Society is currently piloting MTCT-Plus in three sites in Bangkok. Its program will also include antiretroviral drugs for the father, helping to ensure the sustainability of the family unit. As Thailand expands programs to support antiretroviral care for all, these initiatives will reduce the number of children born with HIV, provide a family environment for children born to HIV-infected mothers, and reduce the burden on society of children affected by HIV. But these actions will not yield their full benefits unless they are coupled with national campaigns to reduce stigma and discrimination.

Care and Support: Reducing HIV's Consequences for Children

No matter how effective prevention efforts are, children affected and orphaned by HIV will be with us for decades to come. Their psychosocial, economic, health, and educational needs are real, and those needs are best met by building on the strongest traditional support mechanisms in the region: family and community.

The strong, multigenerational extended family structure in Asia and the Pacific can handle much of the burden of children affected by HIV. A detailed review of the response to the Asian financial crisis in Indonesia, the Philippines, and Thailand (Gordon et al. 1999) found that these societies had been remarkably effective in protecting children from its negative impacts. The primary coping mechanism was families, which drew on extended family resources and internally reallocated family resources to protect their children. With support from the social safety nets provided by communities and by governmental, NGO, and international NGO (INGO) support schemes, families sustained children's health while simultaneously protecting their educational opportunities. While the largely anecdotal evidence presented in this chapter tends to focus almost exclusively on the problems HIV creates for children, limited systematic studies have shown that the majority of families affected by HIV have managed to deal with illness and death without suffering lasting economic damage. For example, in Thailand most extended families have successfully reallocated resources to support parents who have lost a child to AIDS (Knodel and Im-em 2003). Similar responses should prove effective in protecting children from the effects of AIDS.

In Thailand, grandparents have often stepped in to care for grandchildren when both of their parents have died. Most grandparents still receive support from one or two other children as well, so the family network provides resilience (Knodel et al. 2002). In other cases, aunts or uncles take on children orphaned by HIV. Despite early fears to the contrary, most Asian families have rallied around their members with HIV and AIDS, providing them with care and support. If countries successfully mount the prevention programs needed to keep HIV prevalence low, Asian-Pacific families should remain a strong foundation for the society to handle much of the burden.

Should prevalence grow substantially, however, the capacity of family networks may be stretched thin, as it has been in parts of Africa. External forces, such as the economic crisis that hit the region in the late 1990s and a persistently weak global economy, have also contributed to a continuing trend of land loss, indebtedness, and migration, weakening family structures and ties. These negative effects can be reversed, however, if governments, NGOs, and INGOs implement strategic programs to revitalize traditional family and community safety nets rather than building dependence on vertical programs or institutional efforts.

Under any circumstances, some families will need support, especially in more heavily affected or impoverished areas. Poverty can be a major constraint, especially when medical care costs rise, formula is needed for newborns, or the major source of income is lost. The studies on economic impact in Thailand and India have clearly shown that poor families have a harder time meeting the needs of their members when AIDS strikes (Janjaroen and Khamman 2004; Knodel and Im-em 2003; Pitayanon et al. 1997). Stigma and discrimination also may prevent some families from providing care and support for affected members, as has been reported in parts of India (Verma et al. 2002). Therefore, a need will remain for targeted subsidy programs to support medical and education costs, programs to provide free baby formula to those who cannot afford it, and income generation projects to help families cope, including microcredit and skills training efforts. This is the role of the social welfare branches of government, NGOs, INGOs, and the communities themselves. Some programs exist around the region: baby formula support for HIV-positive mothers from the Thai government; efforts around the region to identify families in need and direct financial assistance to them; and scholarship programs in a number of countries for children orphaned by AIDS to keep them in school. But one of the major challenges faced by these programs is identifying the families and children most in need of support while being sensitive to the potential for stigmatization in the community from disclosure of their identity.

Communities have a key role to play in supporting families and orphans and creating an environment free from stigma and discrimination. They must also do more. AIDS is not unique – it is one of many major problems that affect communities, and community coping mechanisms already exist to deal with them. The same response that is enlisted when a flood or drought hits can be used to deal with AIDS. Government, NGOs, business and community leaders, and international funders should work collaboratively to help the community revive or establish community safety nets for the elderly, orphans, and the poor and adapt these to the HIV/AIDS situation.

Successful examples exist of community responses. Northern Thailand has been particularly successful in building community-wide programs for prevention and care that address the needs of their members. A good example is the Support the Orphans project in Sanpatong district (Devine 2001). A district coordinating committee was set up and worked with educators, social welfare workers, NGOs, community-based organizations (CBOs), and organizations of people living with HIV and AIDS to identify those in greatest need. These families were then targeted for education subsidies or income generation funds. District hospitals worked with others to provide home-based care for people with AIDS. Schools, CBOs, and individuals worked to provide psychosocial support for children seriously affected by HIV/AIDS. These types of partnerships, where communities and agencies work collaboratively to identify those in need and fill those needs based on local knowledge, are more likely to be sustainable. However, community management and coordination skills must be developed and community capacity built to provide the necessary services to make them a reality. These efforts can benefit tremendously from the concrete support of multilateral and bilateral partners in the forms of funding, best-practice strategies, and sharing of experiences from other countries.

Keeping children integrated in communities is essential. It is widely recognized that institutional approaches for orphans and vulnerable children are a last resort in Asia and the Pacific. Again, use of existing community resources to provide care and support for orphans has been a widely used coping strategy. For example, the Nyemo II project in Cambodia seeks to strengthen the ties of HIV-positive women to their extended family networks to ensure reintegration of the children after the mother's death. Temples, pagodas, and schools have been used in some places to encourage supportive community attitudes; in some cases they have taken male orphans to keep them integrated in the community.

Efforts to build community day-care centers for children affected by HIV have expanded the ability of orphans' primary caregivers to maintain their income and keep caring for the children. Local NGOs and schools have also taken a role in providing support for orphaned and affected children. For example, the Child Friendly Schools initiative of the Life Skills Development Foundation (n.d.) provided self-esteem and bereavement-support training to teachers, administrators, parents, and community leaders. That program also organized camps for affected children and their caregivers and organized Friends Help Friends groups for children to assist other children affected by HIV or parental separation.

These efforts at community-based care and support offer the best hope for long-term sustainable responses. By using existing and strategically placed social and cultural institutions, they keep children tightly integrated with their communities, reducing the social problems they could face in the future.

Care and Support: Reducing Stigma and Discrimination

Stigma and discrimination are major barriers to an effective response to protect children. In Asia and the Pacific, as in other regions, early fear-based prevention campaigns and public emphasis on stigmatized populations left a residue of negative attitudes toward those with HIV and AIDS. Stigma and discrimination interfere with reducing HIV transmission and providing appropriate care for children and families affected by HIV. A pilot study of the impacts of stigma and discrimination on mother-to-child transmission in India (Chase and Aggleton 2001) found numerous stigma-related barriers to protecting children. In health care settings, delivery services were denied to some HIV-positive pregnant women and doctors sometimes told parents of ill children with HIV that no treatment was possible. Affected families were sometimes ostracized; their children were denied entry to some schools; and their employment was sometimes terminated, all of which had a direct impact on the ability to prevent transmission to children, provide appropriate care, and maintain a stable family environment. Nor are these isolated incidents: Problems have been seen in a variety of forms throughout the region (Busza 1999).

Keeping people with HIV healthy and working is an effective strategy for caring for children affected by HIV. Stigma and discrimination in employment, housing, and access to health, social, and legal services are often the major barriers to providing effective care for children in families affected by HIV. If a family member with HIV loses work, or the family business loses customers, family welfare suffers and the children along with it (Pitayanon et al. 1997). Although antiretroviral drugs are increasingly available at lower cost around the region, loss of income may make them unaffordable, with lethal consequences that further impoverish the family. Yet if workplaces, communities, and society in general become more supportive of them, people living with HIV can continue providing for their families and their children. How then can these supportive environments be built?

In a review of programs to reduce stigma and discrimination in communities, workplaces, health settings, and the media, Busza (2001) found that the most effective approaches mainstreamed compassion and support into ongoing community development projects or institutions. For example, the projects of the Population and Community Development Association in Northern Thailand required people living with HIV and those without HIV to apply jointly for income-generation loans. Factory-based programs involving participatory outreach (such as the Friends Tell Friends program of the Thai Red Cross and Thailand Business Coalition on AIDS) built supportive attitudes in the workplaces. It is particularly important to engender nondiscriminatory attitudes among children, who often have not yet formed negative attitudes.

Schools can also play a major role both with children and the surrounding communities. In a Save the Children UK project in Chiangmai, primary school headmasters and teachers were used as a catalyst for outreach activities in the local community (Hennessey 2001). Using the schools as a central resource to promote compassionate responses and caring attitudes proved extremely successful. Experience has shown that successful efforts to reduce stigma and discrimination must be serious, continuous, and large-scale. Therefore, as these innovative programs are implemented, the societal environment must be changed by altering attitudes and practices at a national level toward those affected by HIV. One critical component of these efforts is to design and implement national information and education campaigns for the public and service providers with the full participation of people living with HIV/AIDS and their families.

Care and Support: Caring for Children Living with HIV and Their Families

Even if comprehensive coverage with antenatal PMTCT programs is achieved, many children in the region still will be born with HIV. The therapies currently available on a large scale in developing countries do not prevent a third to half of perinatal infections (Newell 2001). Not all mothers choose to accept PMTCT even when it is offered (Temmerman et al. 2003). Some children may still become infected through breastfeeding if the mother cannot afford high-quality formula – and a number of factors including strong social stigma in this region may make this difficult. Finally, not all mothers in Asia and the Pacific receive antenatal care, limiting their opportunities to determine their HIV status and receive antiretroviral therapies. Children living with HIV require supportive community and family environments, appropriate medical care, education, and support for their emotional, social, and economic needs in dealing with their HIV status and its associated problems.

Children with HIV tend to be symptomatic and live longer than many think, requiring ongoing medical management. Many policymakers mistakenly assume that the majority of children born with HIV infection die within their first year or two. This assumption has not been borne out by cohorts of perinatally infected children in Western countries, where only one-quarter to one-third of children living with HIV had died by age five (Barnhart, Caldwell, and Thomas 1996; Blanche et al. 1997; Langston et al. 2001). Children in the United States, for example, commonly live to adolescence and beyond.

In a report on the impact of HIV on children in Thailand, Brown and Sittitrai (1995) estimated the number of children currently living with HIV if a median survival time of six years was used instead of the conventional two years. This longer survival time more than doubled the estimated number of children living with HIV and requiring ongoing medical care. Using similar survival numbers, the Thai Working Group on HIV/AIDS Projection (2001) estimated that the number of children living with HIV will rise steadily through the next decade – from 44,000 to 65,000 by 2013. This projection does not include the potential effect of antiretroviral therapies on survival, which may drive these numbers up substantially over the next several years. Recent studies of pediatric survival with HIV in Thailand (Chearskul et al. 2002) found a median survival of roughly five years, comparable to the number used by the Working Group.

Furthermore, studies of children born with HIV have shown that few go beyond six months without developing some HIV-related symptoms (Bamji et al. 1996; Chearskul et al. 2002; Diaz et al. 1998; Galli et al. 1995). This finding means that Thailand must prepare for a minimum of fifty thousand children requiring ongoing medical management for HIV for the foreseeable future. Medical infrastructures throughout Asia and the Pacific need to prepare care projections of this type to anticipate and budget for the future medical care needs of children with HIV. These include not only strengthening the formal health system, but also building sufficient capacity and allocating resources for family and community care and support.

FOREWARNED, BUT UP TO THE CHALLENGE?

Many of the countries in Asia and the Pacific have a rare opportunity to learn from their more heavily affected counterparts in the region about coping with the devastating impacts of HIV. Thailand and Cambodia have shown that aggressive and appropriately focused prevention efforts can reverse the increase of HIV prevalence on a national level (Phalla et al. 1998; Phoolcharoen et al. 1998). Numerous regional efforts have proven that young people can serve as a major prevention resource by changing their behaviors to protect themselves from HIV and providing support for their HIV-affected peers. Northern Thailand's experience demonstrates that even in a severe epidemic, families and communities can rise to the task of protecting and caring for their children (Devine 2001).

The damage HIV does to children can be anticipated, reduced, and perhaps even eliminated, but this question remains: Are Asia and the Pacific up to the challenge? Unfortunately, the answer to date is no. Other than Thailand and Cambodia, most Asian countries have made little or no progress in setting up the comprehensive coverage of at-risk populations needed to prevent HIV from becoming a serious epidemic. In most countries, programs for sex workers and clients, drug users, men who have sex with men, and sexually active youth have remained mostly at the pilot stage rather than going to scale. Political commitment remains weak.

During the UN General Assembly Special Session on HIV/AIDS in New York in 2001, not a single head of government or state attended from the Asia-Pacific region. Most Asian-Pacific leaders still have not dedicated the resources needed to prevent HIV, much less to address its long-term consequences for children and their families. Most have not allocated a substantial national budget for the AIDS response, nor have they sought to raise public awareness and support for the programs needed or for people living with HIV. Major challenges remain to sustain intensified prevention efforts and make progress in access to care and support, even in "successful" countries such as Thailand and Cambodia.

It may take a decade or more, but in the absence of effective programs, HIV in most Asian countries will reach prevalence levels previously seen only in Africa. This spread of HIV will translate to millions of children orphaned and affected by AIDS. But too many Asian-Pacific voices ignore the evidence and stand firmly opposed to educating young people about protecting themselves. Concerned that teaching young people about condoms and contraception will encourage increased sexual behavior, leaders fall back on a single approach of "social evils" or abstinence that denies the realities of adolescence and the right of young people to protect themselves.

Despite vigorous efforts, many of the HIV-affected children most in need of psychosocial, economic, and educational support remain isolated from sources of that support. In many parts of the region, frightening levels of stigma and discrimination still hold sway – interfering with the ability to provide appropriate support and care for children living with HIV and their families. In this atmosphere of complacency, inaction, and inability to make tough political decisions, HIV spreads – inexorably and inevitably – and the number of affected children grows.

What must be done? In the UN General Assembly Special Session on HIV/AIDS in 2001, all member states signed the Declaration of Commitment on HIV/AIDS, which includes commitments to orphaned and vulnerable children. In 2005, the world will see whether they are keeping their promises. If the right choices are made, HIV can be contained and children in Asia and the Pacific can be protected. At the same time, families and communities must be strengthened to provide care and support for children affected by HIV and AIDS and their parents. Both of these require sustained commitment and action from all levels of civil society in the following interrelated areas:

RAISE AWARENESS AND MOTIVATE A RESPONSE. The complacency must end. Policymakers, opinion leaders, and the general public must learn that substantial risk for HIV exists in every country in the region, that HIV epidemics evolve on time scales of decades in this part of the world, and that today's children and young people urgently need to learn to live in a world with HIV. Every person must be convinced of HIV's real and devastating impacts on children. HIV must be kept high on global, regional, and national agendas, and public awareness must be raised to support the right political decisions and large-scale efforts to address the problem.

BUILD AND SUSTAIN COMMITMENT TO CREATE POLICIES AND INCREASE RESOURCES. Heads of government and state must lead the response – with more than just an occasional speech. They must make a sustained commitment to containing HIV and caring for orphaned and affected children. They must build that same commitment in the institutions under their control and reflect that commitment in budgets, policies, and programs that adequately address local prevention and care needs. They must demonstrate and encourage a commitment to youth that the next generation is prepared to sustain. They must mobilize other leaders from all sectors and levels of society to lead and contribute to responses – to prevent HIV, to care for children living with and affected by HIV, and to ensure that locally relevant, sustainable responses are developed. Limited progress has been made in the region in this respect. At the end of 2001, the ASEAN Heads of Government Summit held a special session on HIV/AIDS. A report on the progress of the AIDS response has become a standing item on the summit agenda. In addition, Thailand demonstrated its political commitment by hosting the 15th International AIDS Conference in July 2004, the first time this major conference was organized in a developing country in the region. But much, much more is needed.

FORM PARTNERSHIPS THAT INVOLVE YOUNG PEOPLE IN AN INTEGRAL WAY. The government alone cannot handle HIV; programs require partnerships that include the private sector, NGOs, families, affected communities, and international partners, who contribute funding and technical expertise to build local capacity. Partnerships among government ministries through multiministerial AIDS plans and the integration of the AIDS response into the national development agenda are important, as are partnerships in the private sector in the form of "business coalitions on AIDS." Horizontal or "South-to-South cooperation" to share experiences among developing countries is also a crucial form of partnership. Involving affected communities has been the hallmark of successful HIV programs globally, and this remains true of programs for children and youth. Programs have often treated communities, children, and youth paternalistically, not contributing necessary resources, not building their capacity, not involving them in the design, content, and implementation of programs. This paternalism must end; communities, children, and youth must be accepted as full partners, as the only ones who truly understand their situation, their needs, and what will be effective in reducing risk and building support for affected peers. They must also be provided with resources and support for local capacity building.

EXPAND THE KNOWLEDGE BASE. Support the development, dissemination, and utilization of strategic information on children and HIV in the region. As we know, knowledge to date about the impacts of HIV on children and how to address them is largely anecdotal, based on a few heavily affected parts of the region and a limited number of aggressive though primarily small-scale efforts. Asia and the Pacific is a diverse region, though, and health, education, and social infrastructures vary. Some economies are strong, others are weak. Thus, approaches to prevent HIV and protect children from its impacts must be adapted and tailored to local needs, economic circumstances, and infrastructure capacity. Heads of government and state, other political leaders, and program managers must have access to certain key information for making strategic decisions on policy, resource allocation, and programs. Country-specific and regional information will be needed both by donors – to make decisions on funding – and by the media – to influence the public in favor of effective policies and to engender supportive attitudes. Governmental offices, NGOs and INGOs, CBOs, and communities will need locally relevant information to design, plan, implement, and evaluate their programs. These groups must cooperate, coordinate, and contribute to ensure that appropriate strategic information is identified, collected, summarized, disseminated, and utilized.

GO TO SCALE. Finally, efforts must move beyond the demonstration project phase. Without large-scale or national coverage, the course of the epidemic cannot be altered and achievements to date can be lost. Without sustained large-scale efforts, young people will not adopt safer sexual practices. Without large-scale programs to build the coping capacity of families and communities, their safety nets may ultimately fail. To date, too few countries have taken effective and successful programs to the scale where they can have a serious impact on the epidemic. Five conditions must be met in order to effectively bring a program to scale: (1) national leaders must declare their intention and commitment to scaling up effective programs; (2) supportive policies must be issued; (3) capacity must be built at both national and local levels; (4) communities, including children affected by HIV, people living with HIV, young people, and others, must have ownership; and (5) sufficient human and financial resources must be allocated. Communities in the most heavily affected parts of Asia and Africa have shown the way to build effective responses to protect their children from the grassroots up – they have embraced HIV as a problem for their communities, mobilized resources and commitment, and dealt with it. The challenge now is for Asian-Pacific leaders to take these lessons to scale.

The choices are difficult because effective programs require increased commitment, resources, and actions. They require a new way of working together, and they require politicians and religious leaders to make tough political decisions on fundamental issues that have not been addressed before. Only by making these difficult choices can Asian-Pacific societies hope to provide their children all the protection they deserve from HIV/AIDS and its impacts.

ACKNOWLEDGMENTS

The authors wish to acknowledge the dedicated assistance of Chutima Chaitachawong and Supreeya Aksornpan in gathering resources used in the preparation of this chapter. We wish to acknowledge the kind support of the UNICEF East Asia Program Regional Office in providing access to and assistance in locating relevant documents. We would like to thank our former Thai Red Cross colleagues, Nonthathorn Chaiphech and Greg Carl, for their feedback on the chapter and their hard work on behalf of the children of Asia over the years. And finally, we would like to thank our colleagues at East-West Center and the UNAIDS Secretariat, including Mahesh Mahalingam and Neff Walker, who have helped in formulating our thinking, provided much of the background we have used, and provided constructive comments.

Disclaimer: The material presented herein and the views expressed are those of the authors and do not necessarily represent the policies or views of their respective organizations.

References

Association François-Xavier Bagnoud. n.d. *Orphan alert 2: Children of the HIV/AIDS pandemic; The challenge for India.* http://www.albinasactionfororphans.org/learn/ORPHANALERT2.pdf
Balk, D., G. Cruz, and T. Brown. 1997. *HIV/AIDS risk in the Philippines: Focus on adolescents and young adults.* Working Papers, Population series no. 93. Honolulu: East-West Center.
Bamji, M., D. M. Thea, J. Weedon, K. Krasinski, P. B. Matheson, P. Thomas, G. Lambert, E. J. Abrams, R. Steketee, and M. Heagarty. 1996. Prospective study of human immunodeficiency virus 1-related disease among 512 infants born to

infected women in New York City. The New York City Perinatal HIV Transmission Collaborative Study Group. *Pediatrics Infectious Disease Journal* 15 (10): 891–8.

Barnett, T., and P. Blaikie. 1992. *AIDS in Africa: Its present and future impact*. London: Belhaven Press.

Barnhart, H. X., M. B. Caldwell, and P. Thomas. 1996. Natural history of human immunodeficiency virus disease in perinatally infected children: An analysis from the Pediatric Spectrum of Disease Project. *Pediatrics* 97 (5): 710–16.

Black, B., and A. R. Farrington. 1997. Preventing HIV/AIDS by promoting life for Indonesian street children. *AIDScaptions* 4(1) June.

Blanche, S., M. L. Newell, M. J. Mayaux, D. T. Dunn, J. P. Teglas, C. Rouzioux, and C. S. Peckham. 1997. Morbidity and mortality in European children vertically infected by HIV-1: The French Pediatric HIV Infection Study Group and European collaborative study. *Journal of Acquired Immune Deficiency Syndromes* 14 (5): 442–50.

Brown, T. 2003. *HIV/AIDS in Asia*. Asia-Pacific Issues no. 68. Honolulu: East-West Center.

Brown, T., and W. Peerapatanapokin. 2004. The Asian Epidemic Model: A process model for exploring HIV policy and programme alternatives in Asia. *Sexually Transmitted Infections* 80 (suppl.): i19.

Brown, T., and W. Sittitrai. 1995. *The impact of HIV on children in Thailand*. Bangkok: Thai Red Cross Society.

Busza, J. 1999. *Literature review: Challenging HIV-related stigma and discrimination in Southeast Asia; Past successes and future priorities*. New York: Population Council/Horizons. http://www.popcouncil.org/pdfs/HORIZONS_paper.pdf

———. 2001. Promoting the positive: Responses to stigma and discrimination in Southeast Asia. *AIDS Care* 13 (4): 441–56.

Chase, E., and P. Aggleton. 2001. *Stigma, HIV/AIDS, and prevention of mother-to-child transmission: A pilot study in Zambia, India, Ukraine, and Burkina Faso*. London: UNICEF and the Panos Institute.

Chearskul, S., T. Chotpitayasunondh, R. J. Simonds, N. Wanprapar, N. Waranawat, W. Punpanich, K. Chokephaibulkit, et al. 2002. Survival, disease manifestations, and early predictors of disease progression among children with perinatal human immunodeficiency virus infection in Thailand. *Pediatrics* 110 (2, pt. 1): e25.

China HIV/AIDS Socio-Economic Impact Study Team. 2002. Limiting the future impact of HIV/AIDS on children in Yunnan (China). Chapter 9 of *AIDS, public policy, and child well-being*, ed. G. Cornia. Florence: UNICEF. http://www.unicef-icdc.org/research/ESP/aids/aids_index.html

Choe, M. K. n.d. Risk-taking among Asian youth: Findings from the AYARR Project, Asian Young Adult Reproductive Risk. PowerPoint presentation. Available at http://www.worldbank.org

Choe, M., H.-S. Lin, C. Podhisita, and C. Raymundo. 2001. Sex and marriage: How closely are they related in the Philippines, Taiwan, and Thailand? Research brief 12 presented at AYARR International Conference, Taipei, November 26–29. http://pisun2.ewc.hawaii.edu/ayarr/

Choe, M. K., S. H. Hatmadji, C. Podhisita, C. Raymundo, and S. Thapa. 2004. Substance use and premarital sex among adolescents in Indonesia, Nepal, the Philippines, and Thailand. *Asia-Pacific Population Journal* 19(1): 5–26.

Devine, S. 2001. *A multi-sectoral approach to planning services for AIDS orphans: San-patong district, Chiangmai.* Bangkok: UNICEF Office for Thailand.

Diaz, C., C. Hanson, E. R. Cooper, J. S. Read, J. Watson, H. A. Mendez, J. Pitt, K. Rich, V. Smeriglio, and J. F. Lew. 1998. Disease progression in a cohort of infants with vertically acquired HIV infection observed from birth: The Women and Infants Transmission Study (WITS). *Journal of Acquired Immune Deficiency Syndromes* 18 (3): 221–28.

Ennew, J., K. Gopal, J. Heeran, and H. Montgomery. 1996. *Children and prostitution: How can we measure and monitor the commercial sexual exploitation of children? Literature review and annotated bibliography.*, Cambridge: Centre for Family Research; Oslo, Norway: Childwatch International.

Galli, L., M. de Martino, P. A. Tovo, C. Gabiano, M. Zappa, C. Giaquinto, S. Tulisso, et al. 1995. Onset of clinical signs in children with HIV-1 perinatal infection: Italian Register for HIV Infection in Children. *AIDS* 9 (5): 455–61.

Gleghorn, A. A., R. Marx, E. Vittinghoff, and M. H. Katz. 1998. Association between drug use patterns and HIV risks among homeless, runaway, and street youth in northern California. *Drug and Alcohol Dependency* 51 (3): 219–27.

Gordon, J., S. Bessell, B. Borrell, G. Coombs, T. Jones, K. Horton-Stephens, R. Mauldon, S. Ranck, and B. Warner 1999. *Impact of the Asia crisis on children: Issues for social safety nets.* Canberra: Centre for International Economics. http://www.ausaids.gov.au/publications/pdf/impact-asiacrisis-children1999.pdf

Hennessey, C. 2001. *Research on available and potential support systems for children infected/affected by HIV/AIDS in Thailand.* Bangkok: Save the Children UK.

Janjaroen, W., and S. Khamman. 2004. Perinatal AIDS mortality and orphanhood in the aftermath of the successful control of the HIV epidemics: The case of Thailand. Chap. 7 of *AIDS, public policy, and child well-being,* ed. G. Cornia. Florence: UNICEF. http://www.unicef-icdc.org/research/ESP/aids/aids_index.html

Kamakura, M., M. Kihara, and R. Komatsu. 2001. The current status, trends, and determinants of the HIV epidemics in Japan. Paper presented at Mapping the AIDS Pandemic Network meeting, Melbourne, October.

Kanshana, S., and R. J. Simonds. 2002. National program for preventing mother-child HIV transmission in Thailand: Successful implementation and lessons learned. *AIDS* 16 (7): 953–9.

KHANA (Khmer HIV/AIDS NGO Alliance). 2000. *KHANA appraisal of needs and resources for children affected by HIV/AIDS in Cambodia.* http://www.aidsmap.com/about/intl_HIV_AIDS/Intl_AIDS_HIV_children.asp

Knodel, J., and W. Im-em. 2003. The economic consequences for parents of losing an adult child to AIDS: Evidence from Thailand (revised). PSC Research report no. 02-504. Population Studies Center at the Institute for Social Research, University of Michigan, October. http://www.psc.isr.umich.edu/pubs/papers/rr02-504.pdf

Knodel, J., W. Im-em, C. Saengtienchai, M. VanLandingham, and J. Kespichayawat-tana. 2002. The impact of an adult child's death due to AIDS on older-aged parents: Results from a direct interview survey. PSC Research report no. 02-498. Population Studies Center at the Institute for Social Research, University of Michigan, April. http://www.psc.isr.umich.edu/pubs/papers/rr02-498.pdf

Laidler, K. A. J. (with D. Hodson and H. Traver). 2000. *The Hong Kong drug market: A report for UNICRI on the UNDCP Global Study in Illicit Drug Markets.* Hong

Kong: Centre for Criminology, University of Hong Kong. http://www.unodc.un. or.th/material/document/Kong.PDF

Langston, C., E. R. Cooper, J. Goldfarb, K. A. Easley, S. Husak, S. Sunkle, T. J. Starc, and A. A. Colin. 2001. Human immunodeficiency virus-related mortality in infants and children: Data from the pediatric pulmonary and cardiovascular complications of vertically transmitted HIV (P(2)C(2)) Study. *Pediatrics* 107 (2): 328–38.

Life Skills Development Foundation, Chiangmai, Thailand. n.d. 'Child-friendly' community schools approach for promoting health, psychosocial development, and resilience in children and youth affected by AIDS. Report from the Child Friendly Schools project for AIDS affected children in three provinces of northern Thailand. www.unicef.org/lifeskills/cfs_caba.doc

Mason, C. J., L. E. Markowitz, S. Kitsiripornchai, A. Jugsudee, N. Sirisopana, K. Torugsa, J. K. Carr, R. A. Michael, S. Nitayaphan, and J. G. McNeil. 1995. Declining prevalence of HIV-1 infection in young Thai men. *AIDS* 9 (9): 1061–5.

Measure DHS+ Indicators Database. http://www.measuredhs.com/hivdata/ Accessed Sept. 8, 2003.

Methamphetamine use is heightening risks among gay youth: 'Club drugs' dull safe-sex sensibilities. 2002. *AIDS Alert* 17 (10): 121.

Mielke, J. C. 1994. Child abandonment and HIV/AIDS in Northern Thailand: Implications for relocation of abandoned children into family and community networks. Ph.D. diss., University of Hawaii.

Mitka, M. 2002. MTCT-Plus program has two goals: End maternal HIV transmission and treat mothers. *Journal of the American Medical Association* 288 (2): 153–4.

Nelson, K. E., S. Eiumtrakul, D. D. Celentano, C. Beyrer, N. Galai, S. Kawichai, and C. Khamboonruang. 2002. HIV infection in young men in northern Thailand, 1991–1998: Increasing role of injection drug use. *Journal of Acquired Immune Deficiency Syndromes* 29 (1): 62–8.

Nemoto, T., D. Operario, and T. Soma. 2002. Risk behaviors of Filipino methamphetamine users in San Francisco: Implications for prevention and treatment of drug use and HIV. *Public Health Reports* 117 (suppl. 1): S30–8.

Newell, M. L. 2001. Prevention of mother-to-child transmission of HIV: Challenges for the current decade. *Bulletin of the World Health Organization* 79 (12): 1138–44.

Nguyen, T. A., L. T. Hoang, V. Q. Pham, and R. Detels. 2001. Risk factors for HIV-1 seropositivity in drug users under 30 years old in Haiphong, Vietnam. *Addiction* 96 (3): 405–13.

Ono-Kihara, M., M. Kihara, and H. Yamazaki. 2002. Sexual practices and the risk for HIV/STDs infection of youth in Japan. *Japan Medical Association Journal* 45 (12): 520–5.

Pancharoen, C., J. Ananworanich, and U. Thisyakorn. n.d. Preventing Parent to Child Transmission & HIV: The Thai Experience. http://www.idthai.org/ Download/HIV/PMTCT.pdf.

Phalla, T., H. B. Leng, S. Mills, A. Bennett, P. Wienrawee, P. Gorbach, and J. Chin. 1998. HIV and STD epidemiology, risk behaviors, and prevention and care response in Cambodia. *AIDS* 12 (suppl. B): S11–18.

Phoolcharoen, W., K. Ungchusak, W. Sittitrai, and T. Brown. 1998. Thailand: Lessons from a strong national response to HIV/AIDS. *AIDS* 12 (suppl. B): S123–35.

Pisani, E., and B. Winitthama. 2001. *What drives HIV in Asia? A summary of trends in sexual and drug-taking behaviors.* Bangkok: Family Health International.

Pitayanon, S., S. Kongsin, and W. Janjareon. 1997. The economic impact of HIV/AIDS mortality on households in Thailand. In *The Economics of HIV and AIDS: The Case of South and South East Asia,* ed. D. E. Bloom and P. Godwin, New Delhi: Oxford University Press.

Podhisita, C., P. Xenos, and A. Varangrat. 2001. *The risk of premarital sex among Thai youth: Individual and family influences.* Honolulu: East-West Center.

Preble, E. A., and E. G. Piwoz. 2002. *Prevention of mother-to-child transmission in Asia: Practical guidance for programs.* Washington, DC: Linkages Project.

Rajkumar, V. 2000. *Vulnerability and impact of HIV/AIDS on children in selected areas of Delhi, Rajasthan, Tamil Nadu, and Maharashtra.* New Delhi: Save the Children UK.

Rawson, R. A., A. Washton, C. P. Domier, and C. Reiber. 2002. Drugs and sexual effects: Role of drug type and gender. *Journal of Substance Abuse Treatment* 22 (2): 103–8.

Reid, G., and G. Costigan. 2002. *Revisiting "the hidden epidemic": A situation assessment of drug use in Asia in the context of HIV/AIDS.* Fairfield, Victoria: The Centre for Harm Reduction.

Safman, R. 2002. *Unto the thousandth generation? The reproduction of risk among Thai youth affected by HIV/AIDS.* http://www.iussp.org/Bangkok2002/S06Safman.pdf

Sattah, M. V., S. Supawitkul, T. J. Dondero, P. H. Kilmarx, N. L. Young, T. D. Mastro, S. Chaikummao, C. Manopaiboon, and F. Griensven. 2002. Prevalence of and risk factors for methamphetamine use in northern Thai youth: Results of an audio-computer-assisted self-interviewing survey with urine testing. *Addiction* 97 (7): 801–8.

Shaffer, N., R. Chuachoowong, P. A. Mock, C. Bhadrakom, W. Siriwasin, N. L. Young, T. Chotpitayasunondh, et al. 1999. Short-course zidovudine for perinatal HIV-1 transmission in Bangkok, Thailand: A randomised controlled trial. Bangkok Collaborative Perinatal HIV Transmission Study Group. *Lancet* 353 (9155): 773–80.

Sittitrai, W., P. Phanuphak, J. Barry, and T. Brown. 1994. A survey of Thai sexual behaviour and risk of HIV infection [letter]. *International Journal of STD and AIDS* 5 (5): 377–8.

Temmerman, M., A. Quaghebeur, F. Mwanyumba, and K. Mandaliya. 2003. Mother-to-child HIV transmission in resource poor settings: How to improve coverage? *AIDS* 17(8): 1239–42.

Thai Working Group on HIV/AIDS Projection. 2001. *Projections for HIV/AIDS in Thailand: 2000–2020.* Bangkok: Dept. of Communicable Disease Control, Ministry of Public Health.

Thisyakorn, U., M. Khongphatthanayothin, S. Sirivichayakul, C. Rongkavilit, W. Poolcharoen, C. Kunanusont, D. D. Bien, and P. Phanuphak. 2000. Thai Red Cross zidovudine donation program to prevent vertical transmission of HIV: The effect of the modified ACTG 076 regimen. *AIDS* 14 (18): 2921–7.

UNAIDS (Joint United Nations Programme on HIV/AIDS). 1998. *Expanding the global response to HIV/AIDS through focused action: Reducing risk and vulnerability; Definition, rationale, and pathways.* Geneva: UNAIDS.

_____. 1999. *Reducing girls' vulnerability to HIV/AIDS: The Thai approach.* Geneva: UNAIDS.

_____. 2002. *Report on the global HIV/AIDS epidemic.* Geneva: UNAIDS.

UNICEF, UNAIDS, and WHO (World Health Organization). 2002. *Young people and HIV/AIDS: Opportunity in crisis.* New York: UNICEF.

United Nations Economic and Social Commission for Asia and the Pacific. 1999. *Background document on the Mekong Project on Sexual Abuse and Sexual Exploitation of Children and Youth: Research and intervention phases.* UNESCAP HRD course on psychosocial and medical services for sexually abused and sexually exploited children and youth. Bangkok: UNESCAP.

United Nations Population Division. 2001. *World population prospects: The 2000 revision.* New York: United Nations.

USAID (United States Agency for International Development), UNICEF, and UNAIDS. 2002. *Children on the brink 2002: A joint report on orphan estimates and program strategies.* Washington: TvT Associates/The Synergy Project, USAID. http://www.unicef.org/publications/pub_children_on_the_brink_en.pdf

_____. 2004. *Children on the brink 2004: A joint report of new orphan estimates and a framework for action.* New York: USAID. Available at http://www.unicef.org

U.S. Bureau of the Census, International Program Center, Population Division. 2004. HIV/AIDS Surveillance Database. 2004 edition. Washington, DC.

Verma, R. K., S. Salil, V. Mendonca, S. K. Singh, R. Prasad, and R. B. Upadhyaya. 2002. HIV/AIDS and children in the Sangli district of Maharashtra (India). Chap. 8 of *AIDS, public policy, and child well-being,* ed. G. Cornia. Florence: UNICEF. http://www.unicef-icdc.org/research/ESP/aids/aids_index.html

Westley, S., and M. Choe. 2002. Asia's changing youth population. In *The future of population in Asia,* by East-West Center, 57–67. Honolulu: East-West Center.

Wijngaarden, J., and S. Shaeffer. 2002. The impact of HIV/AIDS on children and young people: Reviewing research conducted and distilling implications for the education sector in Asia. Paper prepared for the workshop Anticipating the Impact of AIDS on the Education Sector in Asia, Bangkok, Thailand, December 12–14.

Xenos, P., S. Achmad, H.-S. Lin, P.-K. Luis, C. Podhisita, C. Raymundo, and S. Thapa. 2002. *Marriage and sexual experience indicators for Asian youth: A graphical presentation.* AYARR CD. Honolulu: East-West Center.

8

Troubled Tapestries

Children, Families, and the HIV/AIDS Epidemic in the United States

Barbara H. Draimin and Warren A. Reich

The HIV/AIDS epidemic in the United States humbles those who try to ameliorate its impact on children and families. Certainly, more resources are available than in Africa or Asia and the scale of the epidemic is much less daunting, but the problems of affected families and communities are so entrenched and unyielding that efforts to address the problems directly related to the disease reach only the most visible aspect of troubled families' lives. Despite the differences in culture, resources, and experience with disease between the United States and other areas affected by the global epidemic, at the most basic human level there are also strong similarities. Parents grieve the deaths of children; grandmothers take on the care of their grandchildren; children's lives are irrevocably altered by a parent's death. There is much in common and much to learn from each other, even as we pursue different strategies to treat the wounds.

In this chapter we present a brief review of the HIV/AIDS epidemic in the United States and New York City and the response of The Family Center to the epidemic. We focus on some of the issues relating to children and families that have been the hardest to address and resolve, and conclude by suggesting some practices that reflect what The Family Center has learned over the past ten years.

THE FAMILY CENTER: A TEAM APPROACH

In 1988, Barbara Draimin began working directly with families with HIV/AIDS in New York City, first through the Department of AIDS Services of the New York City Human Resources Administration, and then from 1992 on as the founder and director of The Family Center, a nonprofit agency devoted to serving parents with life-threatening illnesses and their children. The agency assists families in making plans for the future care and custody of children, counsels parents, children, and other family members about living with illness and bereavement, and offers children recreational and mentoring opportunities. Staff also serve new caregivers who take responsibility for the children after a parent's death. Although most of the families are dealing with HIV/AIDS, some parents have cancer or other diseases. After the World Trade Center attacks of September 11, 2001, services were provided to low-income, mostly minority, families of people who were killed, injured, or otherwise directly affected by the sudden loss of a loved one.

The Family Center is supported primarily by federal, state, and New York City government grants, and to a lesser extent by foundation grants and corporate and individual donations. Starting with a staff of five, the agency has grown to include forty-five social workers, attorneys, and counselors. There are two locations: the original site in lower Manhattan and a more recent one in the Bedford-Stuyvesant section of Brooklyn, where HIV/AIDS is endemic. Through the years parents, children, and family members have told us about their pain, vulnerability, and despair, but they have also demonstrated adaptability, resilience, and faith.

It is difficult to discuss some HIV/AIDS-related issues openly without offending both the people whose lives have been enmeshed in poverty and discrimination and their advocates. HIV/AIDS began with and still evokes blame. Nevertheless, the interrelated problems must be faced forthrightly if there is to be any hope of reducing the impact of this still lethal virus. HIV/AIDS in the United States demonstrates both the strengths and weaknesses of our society.

THE EVOLUTION OF HIV/AIDS IN THE UNITED STATES

To understand the particular challenges facing families and children affected by HIV/AIDS in the United States, it is important to sketch the broader context. The HIV/AIDS epidemic in the United States has evolved in very different patterns from the HIV epidemic in Africa, although the link to injection-drug use has similarities to the epidemics in Asia and may presage the impact of the disease in Eastern Europe. It has now been more than twenty years since the first cases of death from a previously unknown immune deficiency were reported to the federal Centers for Disease Control and Prevention (CDC).

There have been major successes: Notably, the advent of highly active antiretroviral treatment (HAART) in the early 1990s has prolonged lives, although the drugs have significant and often debilitating side effects. Perinatal transmission has been reduced dramatically – from 35 percent in 1995 to 3 percent in 2003 – through aggressive programs of voluntary HIV testing and treatment of pregnant women. Transmission through contaminated blood and blood products (the early source of infection for large numbers of hemophiliacs and transfusion recipients) has been virtually eliminated. In the 1980s children with HIV rarely lived into their teens; now there are many eighteen-to-twenty-year-olds who were infected perinatally. While many are living relatively normal lives, others are having problems adjusting to adolescence, integrating HIV prevention into their developing sexual lives, and planning for a future where none existed before.

While HIV/AIDS has become a treatable disease, it is still a leading cause of death in adults in their thirties and forties. Primary and secondary prevention have proven to be elusive, although research has identified many of the psychosocial, cultural, and contextual barriers to consistent, long-term behavior change. Stigma and discrimination persist. Despite the progress that has been made on HIV/AIDS as a medical problem, it resists solution as a social problem.

In the United States the earliest and most publicly affected group was gay men – in epidemiological terminology, "men who have sex with men." The gay male community was both devastated and empowered by the epidemic. Mostly white, urban, and middle-class, gay men had only in the previous decade begun to assert their rights and freedoms. As the death toll mounted in previously healthy men, they founded their own service organizations, created care networks, captured media attention, and successfully advocated for governmental and private sector funds for treatment, prevention, and care. This remarkable example of community mobilization is all the more impressive given the widespread stigma associated with homosexuality and the reluctance of many in power to address the crisis.

The second group to be identified with HIV/AIDS had no comparable social capital or material resources. These were male and female injection-drug users (IDUs), who transmitted HIV primarily through sharing contaminated needles and secondarily through sex. Initially concentrated in the East and West Coast cities where illegal drugs entered the country, HIV has since moved to other parts of the country.

Drug use often brings involvement with the criminal justice system as well as HIV/AIDS. Many families are struggling with all three problems (Barreras, Drucker, and Rosenthal 2005). IDUs who are HIV-infected are disproportionately black or Hispanic, poor, and stigmatized not only by the wider society but also by their own communities. There were, to be sure, overlapping risky behaviors; some men who had sex with men were also injection-drug users, and some drug users had sex with men and also with women. Women and men traded sex for drugs. The links of transmission involved complex social networks.

Although AIDS in women was first reported in 1981, the disease was largely considered a male disease; the only women considered at risk were IDUs who shared needles. The risk of heterosexual transmission to women was at first dismissed and then exaggerated. Because the symptoms of the disease in women are often different from those in men, women with AIDS and their advocates in 1994 successfully pressed the CDC to change the case definition, thereby more accurately representing the toll of the disease on women and bringing more women into care. Everything about HIV/AIDS in the United States has taken on a political dimension, even something as apparently objective as a disease definition (Levine and Stein 1994).

When it became clear that pregnant women could transmit the virus to their fetuses, public and professional attention focused on "AIDS babies." Emotional accounts of the plight of these infants, many left in hospitals as "boarder babies," created both waves of sympathy for them and anger toward their mothers. Babies were labeled "innocent victims"; by implication their mothers and the gay men who, it was believed, had "started" the epidemic were "guilty." It took years for pediatricians and obstetrician-gynecologists to regard the mother and child as a family unit. Uninfected children who lived in families where the mother and newborn or other family member had HIV/AIDS were largely ignored. These children became visible only when the parent died and a decision had to be made – sometimes at the deathbed or at the funeral – about who would take them in.

The following is a snapshot of some of the most salient features of the epidemic in the United States (CDC 2004):

- Through the end of 2002, 886,575 people had been diagnosed with AIDS: 718,275 men, 159,271 women, and approximately 9,300 children under age thirteen.
- Over half of the total adult cases (501,669) have died; over 5,000 children under age fifteen have died.
- Although men continue to account for the largest number of AIDS diagnoses and reported HIV infections, the proportion among women has been steadily growing. In 1986, only 7 percent of AIDS cases were among women, but by 1999 that percentage had increased to 18 percent. As of mid-2003, almost a third (32 percent) of newly reported HIV infections were among women. Approximately 180,000 women are estimated to be living with HIV infection (Lee and Fleming 2003). This phenomenon has been called the "feminization" of the HIV epidemic in the United States (Wingood 2003).
- By 1995, more women were becoming infected through heterosexual transmission than through drug use.
- Younger women are disproportionately at risk; an estimated quarter to one-half of all persons who acquire HIV heterosexually do so when they are teenagers or in their early twenties.
- African Americans (12.3 percent of the population) account for 39 percent of the AIDS cases. More than half of new HIV infections are reported among African Americans.
- Hispanics, who now outnumber African Americans in the United States, account for 19 percent of the new infections.

- Approximately 100,000 children and adolescents have lost their mothers to the disease (Lee and Fleming 2003). An estimated double or triple that number have an HIV-infected mother.
- While the number of people with HIV or AIDS is rising faster in the rural South than in other regions of the United States (Scavnicky and Williams 2004), New York is the hardest-hit city in the country. Fourteen percent of people in the United States living with AIDS are in New York City; seventeen percent of all AIDS deaths have occurred there. As of December 31, 2003, there were 83,249 people living with HIV/AIDS, including 1,486 children aged newborn to twelve, 1,125 adolescents thirteen to nineteen, and, 23,255 women twenty years and older (New York City Department of Health and Mental Hygiene 2004).

In sum, HIV/AIDS in the United States has become a disease largely (although not exclusively) of ethnic minorities, younger people, and, increasingly, women.

PUBLIC AND PRIVATE RESPONSES TO HIV/AIDS IN THE UNITED STATES

Over the past twenty years, enormous efforts have been made to address some of the family problems created or exacerbated by HIV/AIDS. Unlike the response in Africa and Asia, programs in the United States have largely focused on the ill parent, not the orphaned child. Even programs specifically geared toward children have been targeted at HIV-infected children and sometimes their siblings. In the early years, and to a large degree even now, services are provided by newly created HIV/AIDS service organizations, not established governmental or private child welfare agencies.

Where older organizations have added HIV/AIDS to their mission, it has not generally become a major focus. These efforts are even less visible because of more reliable treatment for parents and HIV-infected children and teens, and especially because of the decrease in HIV-infected infants. While the emphasis on the parent is certainly essential for children's well-being, there is a serious lack of services, especially housing and mental health services, after the parent's death.

Most governmental funding for HIV/AIDS services comes through the federal Ryan White Comprehensive AIDS Resources Emergency (CARE) Act of 1990, which Congress has renewed periodically. Funds are allocated to highly affected cities, statewide programs and prescription drug reimbursement, early intervention at federally funded clinics, women and children's programs, and programs for health provider education. Local and state planning councils decide how to spend the allocated funds, with many advocates competing for their particular subgroup. Families and children (particularly uninfected children) do not have the most powerful voices in these discussions. The CARE Act is targeted to people with HIV; consequently, these services end when they die or leave the home. There is no effective follow-up plan for children in families where the parent has HIV/AIDS.

Housing Opportunities for People with AIDS (HOPWA), another federal program, began in 1992 to serve HIV-infected people with limited financial resources. These funds can be used for a broad range of housing sites, as well as for supportive services such as health care, drug treatment, mental health services, nutrition, and others. There are provisions to fund larger housing units for families. However, when the person with HIV or AIDS dies, the family is no longer eligible for housing under HOPWA, leaving some children homeless.

Other services may be available for HIV-infected people through home- and community-based waivers under Medicaid, the federal–state program that provides health insurance for very-low-income people. Under the waivers, states can use their federal Medicaid allotment for home care and other services rather than institutional care. The services usually available include case management, homemakers, personal care, and respite care for caregivers. Again, eligibility depends on the HIV-infected beneficiary, not the family.

The official child welfare system responded to the HIV/AIDS epidemic primarily through the foster care system. In New York City, for example, the city agency now known as the Administration for Children's Services (ACS) gave foster parents who cared for children with HIV an enhanced living allowance in order to alleviate the problem of boarder babies. The agency also became flexible in their requirements for becoming a foster parent, allowing many gay and lesbian couples and other nontraditional families to foster, and often adopt, these children.

Most children, however, stayed within the family, whether in an informal arrangement with a grandmother or aunt or the more formal kinship foster care, in which a relative is certified to be a foster parent and receives financial support comparable to a nonfamily caregiver. Kinship foster care had already been established in the 1980s at the height of the crack cocaine epidemic. Even though many parents were unable to care for their children, it was recognized that remaining in the extended family was in the children's best interests. Many families affected by HIV/AIDS have long and complex relationships with various governmental bureaucracies – housing, justice, family court, child welfare, public assistance, Medicaid, and more. They may be followed by staff from different agencies who have separate reporting and monitoring practices.

African American and Latino churches are typically the most powerful voices in their communities, but church leaders were reluctant to acknowledge HIV/AIDS in their midst, adding yet another source of sorrow and despair to an already heavy burden. The stigma attached to homosexuality and drug use is still a barrier to more extensive involvement. Many religious leaders have begun to address HIV/AIDS in positive ways and several organizations, such as the Black Leadership Coalition on AIDS, the Latino Commission on AIDS, and Balm in Gilead, have taken on this mission. Nevertheless, in terms of direct services to children and families, religious bodies have not been prominent organizational players. Some families prefer to use services with no church connections because they do not want to disclose family member's HIV status, fearing rejection and isolation.

ONE CLIENT'S STORY

Statistics and formal programs, of course, tell only part of the story. Each person who is counted (and all those who are not) is an individual with a unique life history and experiences. The following description of the life and death of "Deborah," a Family Center client, includes many of the factors that make serving families with HIV/AIDS so challenging.

Case Study
Deborah, a thirty-nine-year-old African American mother with AIDS, was referred to The Family Center by the New York City Department of Social Services. The service goals were to stabilize her living arrangements, offer custody planning for her two sons, Mark, aged sixteen, and Elvin, aged five, and support all of them through her illness. Deborah was not married to either of the boys' fathers. She said that Mark's father had died of AIDS and she did not know whether Elvin's father was alive. The boys were growing up without any significant men in their lives. The only males other than peers that they met were the occasional teacher and the occasional boyfriend.

Deborah did not want to talk about her childhood. She had little education, having dropped out after sixth grade to join her friends on the street. She had her first child in her mid-teens. She never held a job (she frequently said that staying on welfare was her full-time job). Deborah could be friendly one minute and abusive the next. At her best at parties, she loved to dance and socialize. She was frequently not in her "party" mode, however, and then she was depressed and angry. Although she was suspected of using drugs, she did not admit substance abuse to any of the six staff who worked with her for more than five years. She kept her inner turmoil private because she wanted the outside world to think of her as strong.

Deborah dismissed the efforts of doctors, lawyers, case managers, and social workers to help her. Her multicultural workers were often frustrated with their inability to build a trusting relationship. She had access to HAART drug therapy but did not like the side effects. Often she failed to return to the doctor to adjust the dosages and would simply stop taking the drugs.

Deborah could not or refused to accept attempts to influence her behavior and attitude. On one occasion she joined a group of clients who were learning and practicing job-interviewing skills. Deborah was being videotaped in a mock job interview. When the other clients critiqued her tight skirt and flashy jewelry as inappropriate in a business setting, she became very defensive. "If I have to take off just one of my nineteen gold bangles, it's not worth the job," she said.

Mark, her older son, deeply resented his mother's erratic behavior. He floated between his two grandmothers' homes, often staying away from school. He felt guilty about leaving Elvin behind but did not know how to set and accomplish his own goals. Elvin tried to be perfect in order to please his mother, his teachers, and his relatives. But he did not want to leave his mother home alone and often missed school to make sure she took her medication or went to the clinic. Deborah loved her sons, but she could not be consistently supportive of them. At home her anger and depression were always present, and her sons were her first target.

Deborah did not lack involved social service providers, but their interventions with her, the children, and the family as a whole took place under the cloud of unacknowledged and untreated drug use. Deborah died in 2001, alone, in pain, and angry. Many people wanted to help, but no one was able to build rapport with her that would make a difference. She was an example of a parent with AIDS for whom all the available resources could not overcome her drug use, psychological problems, and lack of coping skills.

There was much greater success in working with other members of Deborah's family. After Deborah's death, the agency continued to serve her sisters and children. The sister who is Elvin's guardian received legal and counseling services. Elvin has a buddy (an adult mentor matched to him by The Family Center), consistently attends activity/therapy groups, and goes to sleep-away camp for four weeks every summer.

Deborah's example illustrates how difficult and frustrating it can be to serve some families with HIV/AIDS. Certainly a number of factors may have contributed to her substance abuse, inconsistent behavior, and lack of trust (including generations of oppression, diminished social capital, and a racially divisive culture, among countless others). Nonetheless, acknowledging limitations on all levels in serving families like hers encourages professionals to share responsibility in creating new and more effective ways to help.

THE SOCIAL CONTEXT OF FAMILIES AFFECTED BY HIV/AIDS

Several key issues emerge from Deborah's story. Separately or in combination, these issues affect a large majority of families with HIV/AIDS: health care, mental health, substance use, fathers, poverty (in terms of income and housing), and secrecy and stigma.

Health Care

In the United States, where over forty-three million people, including nine million children and adolescents, lack health insurance and therefore access to health care except in emergencies, medical services are erratic and often inadequate. This is especially true in the poor and minority communities where HIV/AIDS is most prevalent. Access to therapeutic drugs that the rest of the world seeks is by no means guaranteed in the United States. Many IDUs and others are diagnosed very late in the disease, when they do not respond as well to therapies. When effective drug therapies became available, some physicians did not want to give them to parents suspected of illegal drug use – though empirical studies (for example, Gange et al. 2002) have debunked the myth that adults whose lives revolve around drugs are incapable of using prescription drugs appropriately.

Even for families with HIV/AIDS who do have health care coverage through Medicaid, health care is not provided in an environment that supports a doctor-patient relationship of trust and respect. The distrust of the African American community, particularly in the area of health care, has been well documented. Assessment, treatment, and follow-up depend on trust in the system and in individual doctors, nurses, or therapists who represent the system. Long waits, short visits, and meeting with a different provider each visit are not conducive to building this kind of relationship.

A mother with HIV/AIDS may fail to keep a medical appointment because she is too overwhelmed by daily crises, has no one to stay with her children, does not have money to take a taxi and is too weak to take the subway, or for many other reasons. By the time she desperately needs care, it is late in the episode and often late in the night. She is often seen by an emergency department doctor whose primary responsibility is to stabilize her condition. The doctor either admits the patient to the hospital or sends her home with a clinic referral. She will likely never see that doctor again, and her conviction that the health care system does not work for her will be reinforced.

Mental Health

High rates of undiagnosed and untreated mental illness further weaken the physical health and family stability of women with HIV/AIDS. A survey conducted as part of a study funded by the National Institute of Mental Health found that 55 percent of mothers with AIDS had scores on a mental health screening measure (the psychiatric Symptom Index) strongly indicating major depressive disorder (Silver et al. 2003). One in six clients reported a history of psychiatric illness. These women report that they rarely receive consistent, high-quality mental health services – a finding that clearly signifies a serious unmet need for ongoing treatment and support. Clients who miss more than two or three appointments are sometimes discharged from care. For the reasons cited above, too many clients fall through the cracks in this system. Clearly, there needs to be longer engagement, home-based work, and a tolerance of the approach-avoidance conflict many of these clients manifest.

High rates of domestic violence, depression, and untreated drug and alcohol abuse further complicate care delivery. Domestic violence is often the root cause of homelessness for single women and women with children. Together these factors compound the already formidable challenge facing service providers. It was never clear whether Deborah's history included violence, but it seemed likely given her angry outbursts and her inability to trust others.

Substance Use and Abuse

Casual and chronic substance abusers are more likely to engage in high-risk behaviors, especially unprotected sex (Leigh and Stall 1993). Parents take drugs for many reasons. Many mothers have been brought up in families where drug use was common; many others self-medicate to relieve the trauma of childhood sexual abuse and family violence. Drugs and alcohol grip these mothers with a powerful force that often overrides their ability to care for their children. They may alternate between lavishing their children with presents and punishing them harshly for trivial acts. They may disappear for days or weeks and then reappear as though nothing has happened. Children, not unexpectedly, are confused and terrified by this unpredictable behavior.

Drug treatment appropriate for women is hard to find, and even when it is available, parents may not take advantage of it. Removal of the child by child welfare agencies seems to be one of the few stimuli to motivate a parent to enter treatment. Child welfare agencies alternate between a strong belief in family preservation (doing everything possible to keep a family intact) and child protection (acting quickly to remove children from an environment suspected to be dangerous). The latter approach is especially prominent when serious cases of abuse and neglect are reported.

Fathers

About 10 to 15 percent of families with HIV/AIDS are headed by a father. In most of these cases the mother has died. These fathers are often not given the attention and credit they deserve and do not have the support system available to other fathers.

A second group of fathers have irregular or little contact with their children. Most often they have other women and other children, which leaves little time, affection, and resources for the children left behind. They make a few telephone calls and make promises they do not keep. The relationship between the fathers and mothers is often filled with conflict, hostility, and unresolved issues. There may have been drug use, incarceration, sexual abuse, abandonment, another woman, or another man. There is almost always the issue of child support. While the father withholds or has no money, the mother uses the only power she has: access to her household and his children. Still, the father has legal rights. He must consent to any custody plan unless he is determined by a court to have abrogated his rights.

Deborah, for example, was very angry with her younger son's father. She told some workers she was afraid of him. She told other workers that he was probably not the biological father because she had been unclear at the time about who the father really was. Deborah's highly ambivalent relationship with the fathers of her sons made helping her and her children complex.

The father is often blamed for bringing HIV/AIDS into the family. Many fathers identify as being heterosexual but have sex with men as well as women. They contribute to the spread of HIV/AIDS and they either do not know it or cannot admit it to themselves or anyone else. Living on the "down low," they secretly have sex with men while maintaining sexual relationships with women (Denizet-Lewis 2003; King 2004). These men do not relate to the terms "homosexual" or "bisexual" and thus are often not reached by prevention or treatment messages coming from minority HIV organizations and other groups.

Poverty of Income and Housing

Families with no formal work history and little housing space are among the hardest to help. AIDS has been especially prevalent in women of color who bore children when they did not have the opportunity to stay in or return to school. Early motherhood too often means early public assistance, which in turn means low income and substandard housing, even in New York where rent assistance for people with HIV is substantially higher than standard rent assistance for low-income people. The demand for housing far exceeds the need, creating situations in which seven people might be living in a one-bedroom apartment. This lack of privacy within a chaotic family with too little structure can lead to severe boundary issues and, in the worst situations, to sexual experimentation and abuse, often by siblings, boyfriends, or other relatives living in the same home. It also leads to moving from apartment to apartment. Some clients move as often as three times a year to find better housing, to preempt eviction, or to avoid bill collectors.

Many studies have found a direct relationship between higher HIV incidence and lower income (for example, Diaz et al. 1994). Possibly the most intractable poverty, however, is poverty of hope and opportunity. The poverty of spirit that Michael Harrington (1962) writes about in *The Other America* too often characterizes families affected by HIV/AIDS.

Many parents with HIV/AIDS have no formal work history. Their untaxed, unreported income comes from work outside the traditional system. Poverty, drug use, and illness have prevented them from getting a basic education and steady taxable employment. They cannot help their children with homework or create a household culture that values work. Children who do not see adults working become nocturnal; their lives revolve around sleeping late, hopelessness, the building stoop, and the corner store. They attend school irregularly. They are not shown opportunity or the way to exploit it should it appear. In a vibrant, competitive city filled with creativity and innovation, these young people are more isolated and unconnected than the recent immigrants who throng the streets.

Secrecy and Stigma

Although the issue of HIV is more open now than it was in 1995 when The Family Center was established, there is still great reluctance to discuss private issues such as sexual behavior and drug use. How much does a child know about his or her parents' drug use (one kind of illness) or HIV status (another kind of illness)? Parents hiding many secrets pass enormous burdens onto their children. Interviews with parents and new guardians reveal significant difficulties with disclosure, both within and outside the family unit (Bauman and Silver 2001). Some of the parents interviewed and many of those who had died had chosen not to inform all or some of their children of their HIV status. In a study of the mental health needs of adolescents in families with AIDS, 39 percent of youth interviewed did not know about the HIV status of their living or deceased parent (Draimin, Hudis, and Segura 1992).

Many parents said that their decision not to inform was based on a desire to protect the child. Often they felt that a child, even an adolescent, was too young or immature to understand or deal with the information. Many said they simply did not wish to burden the children with the knowledge that their parents were very sick and probably going to die. Others said that they feared youngsters would inadvertently reveal the parent's HIV status to others, potentially resulting in discrimination toward the entire family.

Informing their children about their HIV diagnosis was one of the most difficult tasks these parents faced during the course of their illness. In cases where the parent had not informed the child, the new guardian was left to wrestle with this issue after the parent's death. In some cases, parents felt that disclosing their HIV diagnosis to their children had been a huge mistake. One mother who had disclosed to her eighteen-, fifteen-, and seven-year-old children on the advice of her hospital social worker compared the experience to "dropping a bomb with no plan for the clean-up." In this family and others, the adolescent children most frequently coped with a parent's illness by refusing to discuss matters such as future custody arrangements. These young people's experiences were also characterized by social isolation: Of the 61 percent of youth interviewed by Draimin, Hudis, and Segura (1992) who knew about their parents' HIV status, none had shared that information with his or her best friend. Similarly, few families had chosen to reveal their HIV status outside the family. In cases where neighbors and others in the community suspected that a family member might have HIV, these families were often subjected to harassment, threats of violence, and the need to relocate to neighborhoods where their anonymity could be better protected.

CUSTODY PLANNING

Custody planning represents an important step in parents' acceptance of their illness and in the ability to plan for their children's future. Many parents assume that a family member will take care of their children and that there is no need to make a plan. Among the strengths of black families are strong kinship bonds and adaptability of family roles (Hines and Boyd-Franklin 1982). Latino families often make informal adoptions with *compadres* and *comadres* – godparents who accept responsibility for the care of children should their parents be unable to do so (Garcia-Preto 1982).

For these and other reasons, in 53 percent of the families we studied where the parent with AIDS was alive, there was no viable custody plan for the adolescent children (Draimin 1995). Custody planning for older adolescents was particularly problematic, because their growing independence and acting out behavior made relatives reluctant to accept guardianship responsibility. It was not unusual for a relative to agree to be the guardian for the younger children but refuse responsibility for the adolescent. In several of the families interviewed, older adolescents went to great lengths to try to keep all of their siblings together in one household. In some cases, this goal pitted older adolescents against adult family members who might have wished to take custody of the younger children but who had no interest in accepting the older adolescent into their home.

While many families shy away from involvement with lawyers and courts and do not have assets to distribute in a traditional will, in fact the legal system has been modified in some states to provide more flexibility. Under standby guardian laws, parents can declare their choices for a future guardian for their children, and these guardians can establish a legal status that gives them priority over other individuals (Figure 8.1). Convincing parents to use this option and then following them through the vicissitudes of their own or the standby guardians' lives remains difficult, as the case of Maria illustrates.

In the United States, guardianship of children is covered by state, rather than federal, law. Laws in effect at the early stages of the HIV epidemic had significant limitations. Parents could use a standard will to express a preference for a guardian, but after death a probate court might not approve the choice. Parents could also transfer guardianship while alive but this would limit their rights as a parent. Standby guardianship laws were developed to provide parents with HIV or any life-threatening conditions another option, and have been enacted in 22 states and the District of Columbia.

While specific provisions vary by state, in general the laws permit a parent to designate a specific person to be guardian in case of death or incapacity. The parent's choice is approved by a court, which investigates the proposed guardian and the family situation. The guardianship can go into effect during the parent's lifetime (for example, while a mother is hospitalized), or it can be activated after death. The parent retains considerable control, determining when the guardianship should begin (except in cases of mental incapacity or other limiting condition), and can withdraw the authority and change guardians. The parent and guardian share decision-making responsibility, with the guardian deferring to the parent while he or she is alive. A legally approved standby guardianship is the most effective way to ensure that a parent's choice is not overridden in court by another family member.

Source: National Adoption Information Clearinghouse 2003.

FIGURE 8.1. Standby Guardianship Laws

Case Study

Maria is a sixty-one-year-old Puerto Rican grandmother who is separated from her third husband. She has already raised five daughters and is currently caring for five of her grandchildren, four girls – Casey, eleven; Sophia, nine; Jasmine, eight; and Monique, seven – and a boy, José, eight. Three of the girls are from her daughter Irma. José and Monique are from her daughter Luz. Maria lives in a two-bedroom apartment in subsidized housing.

Maria became the caregiver for Irma's children as the result of a neglect case filed by police against Irma three years ago. At that time the three girls were found steps away from the scene of a drug transaction that involved Irma and her partner, Roberto. On short notice, Maria was called from Puerto Rico to come to a Long Island police precinct to pick up her grandchildren, who were in the custody of ACS. After establishing herself in an apartment and on the recommendation of the ACS worker, Maria was granted kinship care of her grandchildren.

After three years Irma died of AIDS. Maria was told that she had to petition the family court to obtain guardianship of the children or they might eventually be removed from her care. When she went to court, Roberto, the girls' father, was brought from jail to attend the hearing. When he requested visitation rights, Maria's lawyer objected, stating that Roberto had not established paternity and had never expressed interest in the children before. Maria was also very upset by the possibility of Roberto's being in her life, because she believed that he had infected her daughter with HIV. Ideally, Maria wanted to adopt the girls but she was told that if she did so she might lose the subsidies from the foster care agency that she needed to support them.

Maria assumed the care of Luz's children, José and Monique, when Luz was accused of neglect and ACS removed the children from her care. Maria went to court and petitioned to have the children placed with her. Maria wanted to keep the children in the family, even though accepting guardianship meant that she would be able to receive only public assistance for the children, not the generally higher foster-care subsidies.

Maria had difficulty talking about Irma's death with the children. All three of Irma's girls attend special education programs and receive counseling at a local mental-health clinic. Although Maria has attended several grief workshops in the community, she does not see the value of "remembering such a bad time with children who already have problems" (adapted from McKelvy and Draimin 2002: 154–5).

In discussing this case, McKelvy and Draimin (2002) conclude that Maria's case is typical in a number of ways, including her conviction that even though she could barely afford their care, her grandchildren were better off with her than with strangers. She was also caring for two sets of children with different visitation and guardianship requirements. Finally, all members of the family were affected by multiple losses, which were made more complicated by Maria's reluctance to talk about her daughter. Her reasons are not uncommon. She felt that it would make life harder for the children, and because the family had suffered enough already, there was no sense talking about pain from the past.

PRACTICES THAT SUPPORT FAMILIES AND CHILDREN

Based on The Family Center's decade of experience working with families and children affected by HIV/AIDS and conducting research that informs this work, we have developed a set of practice guidelines that seem to us to offer the best possibilities for overcoming the many challenges these families face. Nevertheless, perhaps the most sobering lesson is that new situations and dilemmas frequently make us reexamine policies and procedures. This constant process of reappraisal is essential, but these principles and practices have served us well.

1. *The family is our client; the child's future is our focus.* In complex families, there are mothers, fathers, grandparents, and unrelated kin who often do not have goals and priorities in common. To serve only one member of the family is often to participate in the blaming and disintegration already present. Family-centered care begins with creating a genogram (a schematic representation of the family relationships), which reinforces the family's belief that we care about and will serve the whole family. An example of a genogram is shown in Figure 8.2; it represents Deborah – the woman whose story was presented earlier in the chapter – and her sons

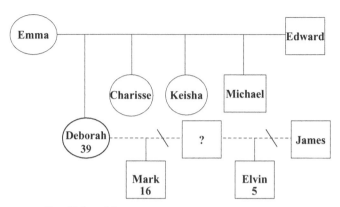

<small>FIGURE 8.2.</small> Deborah's genogram

and siblings. Deborah's genogram is relatively simple – two children from two fathers, no grandparents. Others are much more complicated.

Focusing on children's needs acknowledges everyone's love for children and helps adults have a common goal. Adults learn that reasonable people may have different viewpoints about the best ways to address children's needs, and that challenging another person's love for the children is the least effective way to resolve these differences.

2. *We deliver services where it is convenient for the client, usually at home.* For an ill parent with (on average) three children, coming to meet professionals at the office can be a daunting task. Initiating services at clients' homes gives them the opportunity to show the professionals their space and possessions. It also demonstrates the kind of willingness to be accommodating that is necessary to engage the hardest-to-serve clients.

3. *We always honor the parent's decision-making responsibility for the child.* This standard applies to a decision about whether to disclose the nature and extent of the illness, to the selection of a future caregiver, and to other decisions related to family functioning. Parents sometimes make decisions different from the ones other family members or professionals might prefer. Professionals must acknowledge the parent's role and responsibilities while helping them appraise the positive and negative consequences of each decision. At times, this principle troubles some staff members, particularly when a parent's decision seems risky or problematic. Supervisors work closely with staff to help them respect the parent's decision-making autonomy and to work toward forming the best possible plan under the circumstances. Staff are trained to assist parents in carefully assessing the strengths and weaknesses and likely success of their plans, but they do not attempt to dissuade a parent from a decision or particular course of action.

There is one exception, however. Social workers are legally and ethically required to report suspected cases of child abuse or neglect, and clients are apprised of this responsibility. The decision to file a report is not always clear-cut, because the facts may be ambiguous and because it is not always clear that being removed from the home will lead to a more secure environment for the child. Often these situations do not involve the parent as the abuser but another person in the home, either a relative or a boyfriend. When a case is reported to ACS, the parent is almost always informed ahead of time so that trust and communication are not disrupted.

4. *Following the death of the parent, we continue to support the children and their new families.* Governmental and private funding sources tend to be disease-focused and stop funding services within a month after an ill parent dies. It is critical to forge varied funding streams so that services to the new family can continue for a year or two after the death. A family needs help during the transition and after. Usually there are children in the new family who now have more crowded housing and less time with their caregiver. Helping the caregiver with the loss, helping the orphaned children enter the new family setting, and assisting children with their new and bigger family is very crucial work. Especially when services to the parent have been challenging to provide, there is much work to be done to help children in their new households.

5. *We offer services to the family when clients first learn about their illness or anytime before or after their death.* Transitions are difficult and unpredictable. It is always a good time to plan, though we never know when is the best time to start. The family is best served by a coordinated interdisciplinary team, including a lawyer, social worker, psychotherapist, substance use counselor, and entitlement specialist. Sometimes many different approaches do not seem to work and the best we can do is stay with a family. Some of the most challenging clients get the most services but do not really get what they need. Deborah was a case in point.

6. *We emphasize staff recruitment, training, and support.* Working with ill and dying parents is hard. Staff need many supports to grow, learn, and feel fulfilled. Limited success is also hard for staff to accept, especially after a huge expenditure of time and effort. Attention to staff needs reduces turnover and provides leadership opportunities. Celebrating successes is very important. So is acknowledging the power of loss. It is helpful to look at the impact on staff as multiple clients die. We provide opportunities for staff to express their feelings and to remember and honor clients who have died.

7. *We evaluate and reflect.* Consumer satisfaction ratings and periodic consumer input on issues related to design and delivery of services are important, but they tell little about effectiveness in creating more secure futures for children. A strong commitment to rigorously assessing the strengths and weaknesses of service content and delivery is essential. At The Family Center, program evaluation includes quarterly case review, detailed data base compilation of all services delivered, and longitudinal,

randomized-control group outcome evaluation studies on child mental health and adjustment. In addition, needs assessments are a critical first step in designing new programs that truly meet the needs of ill parents and their children. These kinds of data are also instrumental in obtaining funding, though we should recognize that rigorous collection and analysis of "soft" data on the effectiveness of social programs presents a special challenge not usually faced by medical providers.

Each worker and each family has to determine whether our efforts and time were invested wisely. Although we try to measure that, and often can, we are also never quite sure. Living with the commitment to helping others but wondering how we might have done more or done it differently is the professional's ultimate marathon. Did we help Deborah and her children, and can we be satisfied with modest accomplishments? Elvin, her younger son, has been receiving services for almost ten years, is rarely depressed, and has learned new ways to express his feelings. We will never be absolutely sure how much of a difference we made, but we kept trying. With very complicated families, that is often the most important message we give. By inviting professionals into their lives, our clients have demonstrated the courage to try to address their problems. The tapestry is woven from the risk they take and the understanding and respect we provide.

References

Barreras, R. E., E. M. Drucker, and D. Rosenthal. 2005. The concentration of substance use, criminal justice involvement, and HIV/AIDS in the families of drug offenders. Journal of Urban Health: Bulletin of the New York Academy of Medicine 82(1): 162–70.

Bauman, L., and E. Silver. 2001. Disclosure of maternal HIV/AIDS to children. Poster presented at the annual meeting of the Pediatric Academic Societies, Baltimore, May.

CDC. 2004. National Center for HIV, STD, and TB Prevention: Basic statistics. http://www.cdc.gov./hiv/stats.htm

Denizet-Lewis, B. 2003. Double lives on the down low. *New York Times Magazine*, August 3.

Diaz, T., S. Y. Chu, J. W. Buehler, D. Boyd, P. J. Checko, L. Conti, A. J. Davidson. 1994. Socioeconomic difference among people with AIDS: Results from a multi-state surveillance project. *American Journal of Preventive Medicine* 10:217–22.

Draimin, B. H. 1993. Adolescents in families with AIDS: Growing up with loss. In *A death in the family: Orphans of the HIV epidemic*, ed. C. Levine, 13–23. New York: United Hospital Fund.

———. 1995. A second family? Placement and custody decisions. In *Forgotten children of the AIDS epidemic*, ed. S. Geballe, J. Gruendel, and W. Andiman, 125–39. New Haven: Yale University Press.

Draimin, B. H., J. Hudis, and J. Segura. 1992. The mental health needs of well adolescents in families with AIDS. New York: New York City Human Resources Administration, Division of AIDS Services. March.

Gange, S. J., Y. Barrón, R. M. Greenblatt, K. Anastos, H. Minkoff, M. Young, A. Kovacs, M. Cohen, W. A. Meyer III, and A. Muñoz. 2002. Effectiveness of highly active antiretroviral therapy among HIV-1 infected women. *Journal of Epidemiology and Community Health* 56:153–9.

Garcia-Preto, N. 1982. Puerto Rican families. In *Ethnicity and family therapy*, ed. M. Goldrick, J. K. Pearce, and J. Giordano, 164–86. New York: Guilford Press.

Harrington, M. 1962. *The other America*. New York: Macmillan.

Hines, P. M., and N. Boyd-Franklin. 1982. Black families. In *Ethnicity and family therapy*, ed. M. Goldrick, J. K. Pearce, and J. Giordano, 84–107. New York: Guilford Press.

King, J. L. 2004. *On the down low: A Journey into the lives of "straight" black men who sleep with men*. New York: Broadway Books.

Lee, L. M., and P. L. Fleming. 2003. Estimated number of children left motherless by AIDS in the United States, 1978–1998. *Journal of Acquired Immune Deficiency Syndromes* 34 (2): 231–6.

Leigh, B., and R. Stall. 1993. Substance use and risky sexual behavior for exposure to HIV. *American Psychologist* 48:1035–45.

Levine, C., and G. Stein. 1994. *Orphans of the HIV epidemic: Unmet needs in six U.S. cities*. New York: Orphan Project.

McKelvy, L., and B. Draimin. 2002. Their second chance: Grandparents caring for their grandchildren. In *Invisible caregivers: Older adults raising children in the Wake of HIV/AIDS*, ed. D. Joslin, 151–69. New York: Columbia University Press.

National Adoption Information Clearinghouse. 2003. Statutes-at-a-glance: Standby guardianship. Available at: http://naic.acr.hhs.gov

New York City Department of Health and Mental Hygiene. 2004. *HIV Epidemiology Program: First Quarter Report* 2(1). http://www.nyc.gov/html/doh/pdf/dires/dires-2004-report-qtr1.pdf

Scavnicky, M., and K. Williams. 2004. Epidemiology of HIV/AIDS in the south. Paper presented at the National HIV/AIDS Update Conference, Miami, March 28.

Silver, E. J., L. J. Bauman, S. Camacho, and J. Hudis. 2003. Factors associated with psychological distress in urban mothers with late stage HIV/AIDS. *AIDS and Behavior* 7:421–31.

Wingood, G. M. 2003. Feminization of the HIV epidemic in the United States: Major research findings and future research needs. *Journal of Urban Health* 80:67–76.

9

Interventions to Support Children Affected by HIV/AIDS

Priority Areas for Future Research

Douglas Webb

In a field of study and practice as diverse and dynamic as HIV/AIDS care and impact mitigation, it is imperative to continuously reappraise both the evolving situation and the assumptions underlying current actions. The priority remains the implementing of effective and scaled-up responses to the pandemic. To keep asking the right questions, researchers and practitioners must understand the range of operational possibilities. The impetus for reappraisal comes from many sources: situation and needs analyses on the ground, empirical field and clinical research, changes in nongovernmental organization (NGO) and government priorities, scenario planning, and the availability of resources that can be directed toward further research.

Most crucially, political pressure is now increasingly being exerted on governments to fulfill obligations outlined in the United Nations (2001) Declaration of Commitment on HIV/AIDS, an outcome of the United Nations General Assembly Special Session on AIDS (UNGASS). Rather than research for its own sake, studies must be linked to the development of operational assistance to guide and scale up action. At the same time, inaction due to lack of knowledge is itself not acceptable. Governments and other key stakeholders must "act on data which is already available. . . . It is not necessary to wait for data before starting work" (Loudon 2003).

The immediate information needs are overwhelmingly practical and geared toward practitioners and policymakers. More difficult to ascertain, but still vitally important, are the theoretical bases for both the research and the reconsideration of research directions. Development models based on macroeconomic theory are being turned on their heads by the unprecedented demographic shift created by the decimation of the productive generation of adults lost to HIV/AIDS.

While arguably there is no dominant paradigm in terms of understanding societal responses to HIV/AIDS, conceptual differences do dominate many policy discussions, notably the emergence of "rights-based" approaches, which often sit uncomfortably with more traditional notions of child welfare and needs-driven responses. The paucity of critical analyses of the impacts of HIV/AIDS on children is reflected in the fact that only ninety-four of the thousands of abstracts presented at the 15th International AIDS Conference in Bangkok in July 2004 referred to orphans or vulnerable children (though this was substantially higher than the sixty-nine abstracts presented at the previous international conference in Barcelona two years earlier). While large scientific conferences arguably do not represent the overall state of knowledge on the pandemic, the construction of a research agenda focused on the impacts of HIV/AIDS on children is clearly driven not by academic interest or competing sociodevelopment models, but by the urgency of responding practically, at scale, to an unfolding humanitarian crisis.

Three of the leading international agencies concerned with HIV/AIDS and children have agreed on five key strategies to guide action (USAID, UNICEF, and UNAIDS 2002, 2004). These five priorities relate to family support, community-based responses, direct service support to children and young people, governmental responsibilities, and the wider mobilization of civil society. These areas provide a framework for highlighting some of the knowledge gaps and debates arising in discussions of the socioeconomic impacts of AIDS on children. The focus in this chapter is on intrafamily and community-wide impacts and their mitigation, and while the lessons learned come from sub-Saharan Africa, they have validity across all contexts.

WHICH AIDS-AFFECTED CHILDREN NEED SUPPORT?

The disparity of operational definitions used in interventions to assist children affected by HIV/AIDS reflects the host of different program approaches, underlying philosophies, and an incomplete knowledge base about who is most vulnerable. Community-based programs often target children in "especially difficult circumstances," a broad category that can include both maternal and paternal orphans under eighteen. While acknowledging international epidemiological definitions, practitioners must also investigate local definitions of orphanhood and vulnerability more generally, which may include abandoned children (as in Romania), children living in destitute households, or those whose parents are sick or unemployed or whose caregivers are elderly (Harber 1998). Defining a child as an orphan may itself reinforce the youngster's feelings of being different, which could impede integration into a foster family. Similarly, the concept of "vulnerable children" can be interpreted as disempowering, undermining approaches that emphasize resilience within children and their communities (Tolfree 2003).

In resource-poor, high-HIV-prevalence countries, the impulse to target orphans for welfare assistance on the grounds that, a priori, they are more vulnerable than non-orphans is misguided. Its persistence is linked to the concept of orphan care and support as represented in (mainly British) Western-centric models of social welfare inherited from colonial administrations. Despite being evident in the earliest orphan enumeration studies in Uganda in the late 1980s, the fundamentally alien conceptual basis of this approach is too often overlooked. Imposed definitions of orphanhood overlooked preexisting concepts of clan ownership of children that incorporate flexible notions of parenthood and parental roles taken by adults within the extended family (Dunn 1992; Hunter 1990).

Needs assessments of orphans in Zimbabwe and Zambia point out that, in terms of the key indicators of nutritional status, access to health care, and access to education, the situation of orphans is often not dramatically different from that of non-orphans at a local level (Foster et al. 1998; Manda, Kelly, and Loudon 1999; McKerrow 1996). At national levels, however, distinctions can be made between orphans and non-orphans, for example in relation to school enrollment levels (Monasch and Boerma 2004; World Bank 1997). But the fallacious assumption that this remains true at all local levels can lead to accusations of favoritism and reverse discrimination, in direct violation of the principles of the United Nations Convention on the Rights of the Child.

The impacts of the epidemic are rarely homogeneous, and simple categorizations of children into donor- or program-friendly groupings are misguided. Community definitions of vulnerability are often very different from and contradict the macroindicators used by policymakers. Neglecting this principle could ultimately lead to counterproductive interventions that result in further discrimination against children affected by HIV/AIDS.

Because many practitioners now prefer to rely on local definitions of vulnerability rather than externally defined categories, however, the operational research agendas linked to each program will be less amenable to cross-cultural comparisons. Local definitions introduce a subjective aspect to meta-analyses that may hamper the ability to define generic best practices, which in any case are often difficult to define.

Inappropriate targeting of children or their families has also led to bizarre situations where to be labeled as AIDS-affected is seen locally as desirable because it is likely to bring outside benefits. A young South African woman reportedly commented that "I love this HIV. Yes, I like this HIV/AIDS because we have grants to support us" ("Families tipped into destitution" 2002). Evolving patterns of discrimination and stigma now reflect not only perceptions of the disease itself but also the welfare responses provided to those affected.

FAMILY RESPONSES

Families are the first line of response, and family capacity to care for children is the primary determinant of child welfare. A truism perhaps, but there are still large knowledge gaps regarding intrafamily dynamics and the ways in which families respond to the morbidity and mortality associated with HIV/AIDS.

First, little is understood about how the ages at which the children in the household are orphaned determine their own and the family's ability to cope in different social and economic environments. Such data, if available, could feed into models that themselves generate predictive estimates at local levels, giving greater impetus to policy planners to be proactive rather than reactive. The most recent edition of *Children on the Brink* (USAID et al. 2004) extends the estimates of orphans from age fifteen to eighteen, and stresses a developmental perspective for considering children's needs. Age at orphanhood is crucial because it partly determines the nature and severity of children's psychological morbidity, developmental impacts, and practical problems. For example, age determines whether children drop out of school, whether they engage in paid or unpaid labor, or whether they are capable of self-support in child-headed households, either as a provider or as a dependent. Malnutrition among younger children, for example, can have severe, long-term impacts on brain and other physical development. In addition, parental or guardian loss in early childhood, in school-age years, and in early or late adolescence affects children in different ways, psychologically and in terms of developmental disruption.

End-outcomes of orphanhood are often a starting point in understanding the impacts of parental loss. Studies consistently indicate that orphans are disproportionately represented in marginal groups of young people, whether in groups of sex workers and street children in Zambia or in child domestic workers in Ethiopia (Connolly and Monasch 2002). To understand these factors and to monitor labor-related migration patterns, incidence studies of orphans within a longitudinal framework are required. To date, most such studies have been demographic and concentrated in Eastern Africa, with relatively little research in Southern Africa, the region with highest HIV prevalence and rates of urbanization.

The impacts of HIV/AIDS on families relate directly to increased vulnerability to infection. While this concept is generally accepted, describing the causal pathways and options for intervention is far more complicated. Special attention must be paid to orphaned girls, who are particularly vulnerable when they lack parental protection. Working with young children and adolescents in Zambia, Shah and Nkhama (1996) found that a girl was more likely to get pregnant if she lived with a grandparent rather than her biological parents. A Ugandan study found that orphaned girls were more than twice as likely as other girls to be sexually active (Bagarukayo et al. 1993). Evidence from New Zealand and the United States shows that teenage girls whose fathers were absent from the home when they were young were more likely to become sexually active earlier and more likely to get pregnant than girls whose fathers were present (Nowak 2003). Psychology and poverty may combine to increase girls' vulnerability to sexual exploitation or likelihood of entry into commercial sex work.

Girl orphans may be (informally) fostered because of their value in obtaining bride price and because they can provide unpaid domestic labor and coerced sexual services. There have been few studies to date of sexual activity, psychological profiles of orphans, and tracking through biological markers such as early conception, sexually transmitted diseases, and HIV prevalence rates compared with other children that would quantify such assumptions of risk or clarify specific points of vulnerability. It should be possible to adapt studies conducted in Western contexts to sub-Saharan Africa, which would provide important insights into the relationship between HIV/AIDS in the family and children's consequent vulnerability to HIV infection, as well as cross-cultural comparisons (Barber 2000).

Only when sexual behavior has been understood can intervention measures be adequately developed. HIV prevalence studies of prepubescent children and adolescents can be carried out ethically and with little inconvenience to subjects, especially with the advent of saliva- and urine-testing techniques, as studies in Zimbabwe (for example, Cowan et al. 2002) have successfully demonstrated. Following a cohort of orphans over a short period could provide data that will draw attention to this highly vulnerable yet relatively invisible population. Few serosurveys have been conducted among children, let alone orphans. A notable exception is a study (Shisana 2002) in South Africa among children aged two to fourteen that estimates the prevalence among girls and boys to be 5.2 percent and 5.9 percent, respectively.

THE PSYCHOSOCIAL CONSEQUENCES OF AIDS FOR CHILDREN

The essential differences between orphans and other children may be material and financial in most contexts, but they are undoubtedly psychological everywhere. Children living in families affected by HIV/AIDS often find themselves in unpredictable, uncertain, and crisis-prone situations. Because of their still-maturing cognitive and emotional development, sometimes these children are unable to understand the complexities of the disease, let alone their own fears, anxieties, stigma, and evolving responsibilities. The need to understand the psychosocial dimensions of orphanhood in developing countries has never been more pertinent, despite the recent plethora of work in this area in the developed world (Regional Psychosocial Support Initiative 2003).

Patterns of psychological morbidity in children are being documented, however. In a study (Poulter 1997) of sixty-six households with chronically ill patients and seventy-five control households in Lusaka, Zambia, children of sick adults were significantly more likely than other children to show signs of psychological disturbance, that is, to be unhappy, worried, lonely, or fearful of new situations. In addition, when the parent was ill, many of the children changed their behavior and become worried, internalizing the possibility of death. In Brazzaville, Congo, studies (such as Makaya et al. 2002) indicate that double orphans have a more severe psychological profile than single orphans. Children of sick parents are significantly more likely to show depressive than antisocial behavior, which may be linked to a greater tendency to feel fatalistic and powerless over their situation. The parent's death exacerbates this behavior. In Uganda, one study found that non-orphans also tend to be more positive and optimistic about the future than bereaved children (Sengendo and Nambi 1997). Orphans' higher rates of depression are manifested in more physical complaints (both as a child and later as an adult), lower self-esteem, increased likelihood of being involved in fights, playing truant, and appearing miserable, unhappy, tearful, or distressed. In Zimbabwe, research on commercial farms has highlighted the tendency of orphans to reject extended family support, play truant, place a high priority on the search for wages, and be more likely to migrate, even at a young age, in search of work (Ledward 1997). For teenage girls, the quest for economic security is hampered by the stigma attached to orphans, which restricts their desirability as marital partners but not necessarily as sexual partners (Saoke and Mutemi 1994).

While not discounting the importance of the adverse material conditions linked to orphan status, it is imperative to examine the programmatic implications and mitigation practices on addressing the psychosocial needs of children in affected communities. Pediatric and youth counseling is an area requiring urgent operational research, as is the sociomedical and social welfare structures that are responsible for facilitating such work. Western counseling practices will need to be adapted in order to develop wide-scale and realistic means of addressing the psychological welfare of AIDS-affected children. Needs assessments have led to the development of training manuals for outreach health and community workers in Malawi (for example, Cook 1998; Cook, Ali, and Munthali 1998) and Uganda (Save the Children UK 2003). Without consistency within program approaches, however, impact assessment and intervention evaluation will remain very difficult.

While home care services have tended to focus on the adult patient, there is a need to operationalize home care that considers the needs of child caregivers as well as other children within the affected family. Such a structure, founded on and adapting existing principles of home care, would develop the skills of home visitors on relating to the children, while identifying and referring cases of child illness and behavioral and emotional problems.

A more sophisticated support system would incorporate elements of intrafamily HIV disclosure and the longer-term stages of succession and inheritance planning. These are often termed "memory" approaches. While evidence suggests that inheritance planning may be more crucial in urban areas (Magalla et al. 2002), the determinants of vulnerability regarding succession and inheritance are poorly understood in virtually all contexts, beyond general differentiations along the lines of matrilineal or patrilineal descent. Practitioners typically do not know about appropriate accountability mechanisms, the relative merits of formal versus customary inheritance practices, and who the right arbitrators are in inheritance cases, beyond the catch-all subgroup of "community leaders." Inheritance of property by children, and the associated emergence of child-headed households, may well be resisted in contexts where unsupervised children are considered to be socially disruptive and counter to cultural and traditional norms, as is reportedly true in Uganda (Bennell, Hyde, and Swainson 2002). The development of good practices is urgently needed in this area and is underway through community-based groups such as the Salima AIDS Service Organisation in Malawi and the National Community of Women Living with AIDS in Uganda (Lindsay Smith and O'Brine 2000).

Practitioners need case definitions with minimum care standards for affected children, as well as some type of surveillance to act as an early warning system of unsustainable levels of community stress. This stress will manifest itself differently depending on the site. In the Democratic Republic of Congo, for example, stress, stigma, and poverty have combined to increase accusations of sorcery toward (mostly orphaned) children, resulting in ever-growing levels of child abandonment ("Congo casts out its 'child witches'" 2003), and in Northern Tanzania against elderly grandmothers, many of whom care for orphans ("Raising the issue of rights in Africa" 2003). The potential roles of community health workers, social workers, and, in particular, teachers need to be articulated regarding initial case notification, referral, and indeed intervention with affected families. Undertaking such studies is programmatically complicated because the most vulnerable children are often hidden, abandoned, or simply missing.

Measures of orphan welfare that look at health, education status, and other more immediate indicators often fail to identify more subtle forms of difference between orphans and other children. Two-thirds of a sample of orphans in Namibia reported increases in levels of emotional problems and "stress" (Social Impact Assessment and Policy Analysis Corporation 2002). Similarly a study of orphans of adults who died of AIDS found that 73 percent were above the cut-off point for the post-traumatic stress symptoms. These children were also significantly more likely to have concentration problems, report having no good friends, show somatic symptoms and report constant nightmares, compared to non-orphans (Cluver et al. 2005) Adapting and incorporating into rapid assessment procedures such psychometric screening tools as the Child Behaviour Checklist and the Social Response Questionnaire (SRQ20) – which measure manifestations of stress in children, young people, and caregivers – may well help to identify those with greatest need (Poulter 1997).

The longer-term social sequelae of an increased incidence of adult depressive illness linked to maladaptive childhood grieving are currently difficult to imagine, but with over a quarter of all children and young people now growing up in these circumstances in many sub-Saharan countries, this question is worth taking seriously. The challenge for those concerned with social policy and social welfare is the translation of findings from Western contexts (Geballe, Gruendel, and Andiman 1995), where psychological and social support is relatively accessible, to contexts where the extent of the problems is greater and social welfare structures are nascent or even absent. Regional programs, such as the Zimbabwe-based Regional Psychosocial Support Initiative, are at the forefront of understanding and defining interventions for orphans and affected children.

Immediate operational research can focus on methods of child participation in intervention design and implementation – as a psychosocial intervention in and of itself. The danger of exclusion (the separation of affected children from family structures, or at best considering them a distinct social group, which remains the dominant program design approach), could lead to mass social dependency in the most affected areas. The reality of childhood is changing far more quickly than are welfare responses (Germann 2003).

CHILDREN AS CAREGIVERS

Children are often cast in caregiving roles for their sick parents, elderly relatives, or younger siblings. These children experience multiple losses. In South Africa, for example, in 7 percent of a sample of AIDS-affected households, a child was the primary caregiver for a sick adult ("Families tipped into destitution" 2002). Childhood itself is truncated as normal activities such as play often give way to basic needs of survival. Children who are required to care for younger siblings or to engage in extra domestic chores complain of lack of time to play or to interact socially with peers. Thus they are unable to develop the relationships and social circles that could prove crucial when the household experiences periods of extra stress and depends on outside assistance. In Malawi, orphans' tendency to form friendships with other orphans potentially could result in social stratification rooted in patterns of stigma and discrimination (Cook 1998; Save the Children UK 2001). In urban Zambia, orphans are expected to finish school quickly in order to find paid work and contribute financially to the household (Nampanya-Serpell 1998). For girls and young women acting as caregivers, this shift from dependence to income production can lead to potentially exploitative sexual relationships with older men. The quest for stability and security often results in unwanted pregnancy, single motherhood, and a continuation of the spiral of poverty as well as the risks of HIV infection.

Beyond the role of children as caregivers of adults, it is important to explore and enhance the awareness and understanding of service agency personnel about the productive roles children aged six to fourteen can play in the health care, emotional support, and informal education of younger siblings. The incorporation of children as constructive resources within the network of care provided for especially vulnerable children is now a necessity as intrafamily support is stretched. The research focus should be on finding the correct balance between protecting children from exploitation and recognizing their relative value in the domestic economy and as a contribution to overall social capital.

A case in point is education. The opportunity costs of education increase for many households as the priority shifts toward utilizing the child's productive capacity in domestic, agricultural, or waged work. Research is needed to examine the changing value of child productivity, and the potentially damaging consequences for the child's own (especially educational) development. Where the educational status of a child is prioritized in a household experiencing an adult death, the relative value of maintaining the child in school needs to be assessed against other household welfare indicators, especially nutritional status. External agencies also seem most concerned about enrollment rates without also addressing the equally important aspects of retention and attainment while in school.

Evidence from Burundi and Zimbabwe (Connolly and Monasch 2002) shows that mothers keep children in school following the death of the father, despite increasing poverty within the household. In Manicaland, Zimbabwe, paternal death has increased orphan girls' chances of completing primary education, in contrast to the opposite outcome with maternal death (Nyamukapa, Foster, and Gregson 2003). Other research (Bennell et al. 2002) on causes of absenteeism from schools in Botswana, Uganda, and Malawi paints a complex and inconsistent picture where the degree of attendance is dependent on the sex of the child, parental status, length of previous schooling, and perhaps most important, the socioeconomic status of the household. More understanding of household economies in communities affected by HIV/AIDS and gender dimensions of decision making is needed to ensure that decisions made by adults and parents are in the best interests of the child (Save the Children UK 2001).

Not all families affected by HIV/AIDS manage to cope. Households that disintegrate are lost to researchers and surveillance as its members are either absorbed by other households or enter a life outside any household unit. Where adults die and a child becomes the household head, the continuation of the household structure indicates at least minimum viability as a caring model. Despite the undesirability of the child-headed household as a care option, its prevalence is on the increase and must be taken into account by those wishing to understand and support community coping mechanisms. In Zimbabwe, estimates suggest that twenty-five thousand children currently live in such households, with this figure projected to rise to one hundred thousand by 2020 (Germann 2003). In genocide-wracked Rwanda, not only is the occurrence of fostering far above average for an African country (Monasch 2003), but the number of children living in child-headed households is also extremely high – between two and three hundred thousand children in 2003 (Jose Bergua, UNICEF Rwanda, personal communication (November 2000). The child-headed household may indeed be viable if appropriate monitoring and support connections within the community are established. Semiformal visitor programs do exist; but beyond a handful of case studies (for example, Lee 2000), good practices are again lacking. Child rights analyses could consider children heading households as manifestations of child empowerment, but this view should not obscure the need to ensure minimum standards of welfare and prevention of exploitation through the establishment of locally based monitoring mechanisms. In fact such standards of protection are not in place. Some child-headed households, for when supported by an external agency, can experience exploitation from within the community, as reported in southwest Uganda (Luzze 2002).

EXTENDED FAMILY SUPPORT

Because of its sexual mode of transmission, HIV/AIDS generally causes the death of both parents within a relatively short period, creating a critical need for alternative caregiving arrangements for surviving children. The extended family, especially in sub-Saharan Africa, generally constitutes the major resource for addressing this need. Family systems vary dramatically, however. In particular, the degree of active participation and responsibility expected of aunts and uncles, grandparents, and older siblings in the care and socialization of children under the age of fourteen varies significantly from one society or culture to another. The debate over whether the extended family system is coping or not distracts attention from the far more important task of assessing how extended families react, what assistance is needed, and when.

Studies in the important area of caregiving experiences are very limited despite the urgent need to understand the nature and extent of caregiver "burnout," the degree of financial and material assistance to caregivers, and motivation for working with and caring for HIV/AIDS-affected children. The resilience of the extended family as the support unit continually surprises researchers and commentators, who possibly overlook the crucial role that informal or spontaneous fostering and household recomposition has traditionally played in times of household crisis. Research is still needed to identify the differences between functional and dysfunctional HIV/AIDS-affected families, the strength of family support systems, communication networks, patterns of closeness and partnerships, and the role of religion and culture in influencing caring patterns. These determinants themselves will most likely differ by ethnicity, culture, and socioeconomic status. Informal or spontaneous fostering, for example, can occur for many reasons, especially the fulfillment of cultural obligations or economic necessity. Trade-offs between domestic labor and reciprocity predominate. The degree to which outcomes of child welfare differ according to these varying causal mechanisms is largely unexplored, and policy makers are still unaware of which informal fostering processes should be supported. Timing of the fostering, for example, may be critical. Evidence from Namibia (Social Impact Assessment and Policy Analysis Corporation 2002) suggests that children who move to live with a caregiver well before – years before, in many cases – the death of their parent(s) cope better with the transition than children who are moved in the most traumatic period following death.

Intervention designers should be aware also that fostering could be appropriate even in cultures where it is deemed untraditional. Conversely, fostering in situations where it is the norm does not necessarily mean that the arrangement is in the child's best interests (Tolfree 1995, 2003). The appropriateness of informal fostering hinges on questions of parental motivation and the likelihood of permanency for the placement. There are no tools to assist program designers and project workers arbitrating in such crucial decisions, potentially allowing continued abuses and exploitation to flourish in areas of high adult mortality.

The potential role – indeed the promotion – of children as agents in the decision-making process regarding their fostering options is also poorly understood, despite its centrality within rights-based approaches. Evidence does suggest, for example in Malawi, that adults do not consult children in arranging the foster placement and use different criteria than children in making this decision. While children emphasize their desire to be in a household with loving and caring adults, the current process of fostering is based largely on economic criteria, identifying households that can afford to take on another child (Mann 2003). Similarly in Zambia, only 11 percent of orphans who had been moved into another household had been consulted in the decision (Volle et al. 2002). While we would expect the outcomes for children to be improved where they are involved in the decision-making process, the various cultural contexts of child–adult relationships defy the definition of the ideal "toolkit" for community project workers. In the case of Malawi especially, the dominant tradition militates against child consultation, but until evidence is forthcoming from other contexts, programmatic engagement in this area will be restricted. Where models of facilitating community dialogue have proved successful regarding HIV prevention – most notably in the example of the "Stepping Stones" package (Shaw 2002) – the key lesson is that such engagement is time-intensive and requires great facilitator skill. Application of successful models to issues concerning the impacts of HIV/AIDS on child welfare at the community level is emerging but still in its pilot stages.

The dispersal of siblings is a key outcome that is considered harmful in HIV/AIDS-affected households. In many African societies, the traditional response to parental death is to divide the caregiving responsibilities for the surviving children among adult relatives. Studies (for instance, Mutangadura and Webb 1998) have shown that the dispersion of orphaned siblings often occurs after considerable internal family dispute. In Zambia, as many as two-thirds of orphans were separated from their siblings following parental death, an outcome that may be more likely in rural settings (McKerrow 1996). Despite the stated intention of communities to keep siblings together when they become orphaned, very often the children are separated. In contrast, in Namibia sibling dispersal is much less common, leading to a situation where the vast majority of caregivers are looking after more than one orphan child (Social Impact Assessment and Policy Analysis Corporation 2002).

Consequences of sibling separation have been described but again are poorly understood when the aggregation of family separation is considered. Orphans who are separated and taken care of in different households within the extended family have more reported emotional problems than those who are kept together as one unit in the same household (Nampanya-Serpell 1998). The impact of the deprivation of sibling contact on family bonding and future ties can only be imagined. Typically, children from about the age of six, participate actively in the care and nurturing of younger siblings, much more so than in the Western families for which many of the institutionalized practices of adoption, fostering, early education, and health care were originally developed.

The emotional problems of separated siblings may be related to discriminatory treatment in the new household in terms of domestic chores or meal rations, poor relations with stepparents or guardians, or the loss of connection with family ancestry. Initial studies suggest that children employ various adaptive strategies upon relocation, including becoming withdrawn and absorbed in solitary activities, entering a negotiation role with foster parents over work roles and well-being, or even remigrating to a new social environment (Ansell and Young 2002). In Namibia, most relocated orphans go through an initial period of crying and fighting with other children in the household before adapting to the new situation (Social Impact Assessment and Policy Analysis Corporation 2002). Research in Uganda and Lesotho also describes how children who had lived in urban areas but were transferred to rural areas after the death of their parents tended to be depressed and poorly adjusted to rural conditions (Ali 1998; Sengendo and Nambi 1997).

The combined trauma of losing parents and losing contact with siblings no doubt is considerable, especially when the reasons for separation or parental death are not explained to the child. The nature of this suffering, in both the short and the long term, is an urgent area for study. That research is needed must be emphasized so that practitioners and policymakers do not overlook the impact of sibling dispersal. Intervention assistance should focus on ensuring that orphans in an adopted household do not experience or perceive discrimination. This issue is very complex and requires careful and sensitive attention.

MISSING THE MOST VULNERABLE?

Counting orphans accurately and defining their vulnerabilities compared with other children is problematic. The current orphan macrodefinitions and estimates mask vulnerabilities apart from parental death. First, an unknown number of children are living with parents who are suffering from HIV-related illnesses, while many more are living with asymptomatic HIV-positive parents. Many children in sub-Saharan Africa live in households other than those with one or both biological parents, and between 10 and 15 percent of all children are fostered by relatives (Monasch and Boerma 2004). The loss of a foster parent can be as traumatic to such children as the loss of a parent, and many foster parents also are dying because of AIDS. Their children can go unreported in models and enumerations.

Second, defining the cut-off point for childhood at the fifteenth birthday (which has been the norm for demographic measures) detracts attention from the material and psychological needs of older adolescents and the increasingly important phenomenon of "orphans of orphans," when an orphan girl's vulnerability to sexual exploitation leads to HIV infection and AIDS, an early death, and her children becoming orphaned. This as yet poorly described sociodemographic shift is already beginning and is likely to characterize at least 10 percent of children in severely affected countries in the future.

To complicate matters, under-enumeration, especially of young children, is also common. At the time of the counting, young children may be away from the household with a caregiver or may not be described as orphans due to stigma or because they have been adopted by foster parents. Disabled children are also hidden at the time of surveys, enumeration, or census. Over-enumeration can also occur because respondents may hope to gain any benefits attendant to orphan status. Children in single-mother households may be over-enumerated if they are counted as paternal orphans or under-enumerated if the paternal status is unknown.

The few actual enumeration studies (which were based on empirical household surveys rather than on estimated positive HIV serostatus rates) measured orphan prevalence, not incidence. That is, the number of orphans in a given location was recorded, rather than the rate at which children were expected to be orphaned. In Zambia it has been estimated that anywhere from 15 to 50 percent of children below the age of eighteen have lost either one or both parents (McKerrow 1996). These wildly varying estimates point to limitations in the surveillance methodology and sampling techniques. Differential mortality rates in adults and the propensity of chronically ill patients to migrate have led to a process of orphan clustering (UNICEF 2003). In Zimbabwe this process may well mean a concentration in rural areas or periurban areas, hidden away from the urban-based surveyors. The numbers of chronically ill patients are proportionately greater in rural areas, indicating that the going-home-to-die phenomenon continues, along with the possibility of "child dumping" in rural areas. In a study of AIDS-affected households in South Africa, one in ten had sent a child to live in another household, usually with an aged relative ("Families tipped into destitution" 2002). The simplest two scenarios here are: An ill mother returns to her parents' village, taking her children with her, but dies soon after; or a widower in an urban area sends children to live with maternal relatives in rural areas or another town. Numerous case studies (for example, Guest 2001; Social Impact Assessment and Policy Analysis Corporation 2002) demonstrate both the complexities of illness and death-related migration, and the dangers of overgeneralization (Ansell and Young 2003).

Clusters of orphan households may also occur in poorer urban areas as households affected by HIV/AIDS experience greater levels of poverty and are forced to move in an intraurban pattern, which often involves moving to a new house with a lower rent (Mutangadura and Webb 1998). In other words, the areas of highest incidence of orphans (urban areas with highest HIV prevalence rates) may not be the areas with highest relative

orphan prevalence because of urban-to-rural and urban-to-urban relocation. Further surveillance is required to fully establish the relative clustering of orphans in either (or both) periurban or rural areas rather than
central urban–upper income zones. Research also needs to unravel the relevant causal pathways: Are there more orphans in poor households, or
does having an orphan push the family (further) into poverty? In 1999 the
Zambia Participatory Assessment Group (cited in Subbarao, Mattimore,
and Plangemann 2001: 9) estimated that over 70 percent of households
keeping orphans were in the "very poor" category, whereas only 10 percent of households were in the "rich" category.

CLOSING THE INFORMATION GAP: WHAT IS BEING EVALUATED
AND FOR WHOM?

The effectiveness of interventions and the potential to sustain them also
need to be explored, yet many monitoring and evaluation techniques
and structures are either inadequate or inconsistent in design. For example, where community-based initiatives such as income generation are
assessed, their impacts on children are usually forgotten or discussed anec-
dotally. If the welfare of children in impacted communities is integrally
linked to the welfare of adults, these indirect outcomes of initiatives must
be explored more systematically (see Chapter 2). Evaluations can overlook
the indirect and noneconomic costs altogether in evaluation frameworks
that focus on short-term results and tangible outputs.

Similarly, the institutional roles of different organizations need an honest
appraisal. The approaches and methods of faith-based organizations, government institutions, school bodies, and NGOs can conflict with each other.
The potentially adverse implications of local ideological and direct competition, especially for resources in assisting affected children, are rarely
considered. The competition for resources and ideological dominance in
support structures is manifest in many different contexts – for example,
in Eastern Europe, in terms of the institutionalized care of orphans, and in
many African countries where foreign financial support often encourages
the development of discreet, visible outputs such as orphanages, in direct
contradiction to expressed government policy (Dunn, Jareg, and Webb
2003). Media coverage of such developments may give a false impression
of the availability of external financial support, which would discourage
communities from being proactive and from using local resources to meet
child-support needs.

The integration of rights-based approaches into program design and
evaluation provides a context for these developments. Rights-based
approaches are struggling to move beyond the level of rhetoric into a practitioner framework. Many involved in project design and development still

need specific tools for rights-based programming. The Convention on the Rights of the Child is a powerful advocacy tool and potentially extremely useful in guiding program design and evaluation (Tarantola and Gruskin 1998; Chapter 5 in this volume). Advocates of rights-based programming must anticipate conflict, however, when differing views of what constitutes a rights violation emerge. As the use of child labor grows in importance for severely affected (particularly rural, agriculture-based) communities, and the opportunity cost of education increases, how will a rights-based perspective be received in these contexts? Researchers and practitioners alike are obliged to share their findings in this new and vital area of impact-alleviation research.

Understanding who needs research-generated information and why is vital. The agenda alluded to here is being defined by international agencies keen to "take to scale" interventions that have proved effective, in a collaborative effort that relates to the fulfillment of key articles within the United Nations (2001) Declaration of Commitment on HIV/AIDS. Research questions necessarily relate to the links between intervention practices and policies, rather than an overarching conceptual paradigm or competing hypotheses. Equally important, the agenda is not being defined with the participation of those who are most affected – mothers, families, their locally based community representatives, and, of course, the children themselves. Affected communities sadly remain the subject, not the object, of this operational research, and the voices of the affected remain marginalized. This is a key challenge for those seeking to improve the lives of those most affected by the pandemic.

There must be more effective partnerships between academic institutions, affected communities, and international development agencies. These partnerships should emphasize participatory research methods to complement the macroassessments that have little direct relevance to context-specific, locally designed and owned interventions. Where information is generated, do affected communities receive it in a way that is practical and applicable to their immediate needs? Rarely – and this can only stifle a shared ownership of the emerging knowledge, or at the very least create a polarization of the real meaning, or hermeneutics, of the impacts of HIV/AIDS. In terms of subject matter, the complexity of the situation too often defies generalization, and its unquantifiable human nature is lost once the frame of attention goes beyond the local scale, beyond the methods favored by anthropology.

CONCLUSION

Identifying the priorities for research is a subjective exercise, because advocating for more and better research is relevant in most aspects of HIV/AIDS

248 *Douglas Webb*

prevention and care. In relation to HIV/AIDS and children, however, several areas do stand out (USAID and Family Health International 2001):

- A consensus on definitions is urgently needed and must be the responsibility of leading organizations, such UNAIDS and UNICEF. Consensus would facilitate better learning between projects, allow uniformity in policy design, and ease the establishment of systematic surveillance.
- Psychosocial impacts of HIV/AIDS on children are a vital area for research, particularly in resource-poor contexts. The family context of coping is often mentioned but inadequately studied; we are only beginning to understand community coping in the form of household recomposition, child migration, the changing domestic roles of children, and the emergence of new demographic features such as abandoned children, child-headed households, grandparent-headed households, unprecedented numbers of widows, and single-parent families.
- A major area of concern is how the extended family and traditional mechanisms of caring for orphans are changing and being undermined by the epidemic.

Why are these important and very challenging questions (also summarized in Figure 9.1) not being studied extensively and supported with the same fervor as, say, vaccine initiatives, sexual behavior studies, and demographic modeling? In no way belittling other vital research agendas, we must collectively recognize and reverse the marginalization of children and AIDS as an area of urgent inquiry. The responsibility for children affected by HIV/AIDS within governments most often falls to the weakest ministries, those on the margins themselves of donor attention and financial influence. Externally dominated research agendas prioritize the means of achieving coverage or performance targets and generally avoid areas that are complex and difficult to define at any scale, such as the impacts of AIDS on child rights.

Through the active articulation of current research requirements, we can focus attention on information gaps, keep children on the HIV/AIDS research agenda, and further involve those closest to the epidemic. These research priorities will change as our levels of knowledge, as well as the epidemic itself, changes. The danger remains that unless good information is produced and disseminated we will only slip further behind in our attempts to respond effectively to this unprecedented crisis, with its extremely serious implications for children and the subsequent development of societies.

Defining differences in concepts surrounding AIDS, vulnerability, and children
  Child and community vulnerability
  Orphanhood

Direct impacts on children
  Age at orphanhood and nature of outcomes
  Sexual risk behaviors and variation by orphan/parental status, especially in
    girls, using both qualitative and biological markers
  Serosurveys among children
  Emotional responses to repeated bereavement and how this varies by age
    and nature of child-care responses
  Consequences of sibling dispersal

Family and community responses
  Nature and extent of exploitative fostering of children, especially girls
  Needs of children as caregivers
  Determinants of vulnerability regarding succession planning and inheritance
    rights
  Potential roles of children and young people as a resource in family and
    community care
  Opportunity costs of education for AIDS-affected children
  Viability and robustness of child-headed households, and the necessary
    conditions for their support
  Informal fostering and its social rules; how these vary and can be externally
    supported
  Nature and degree of child consultation in fostering decisions
  Decisionmaking related to sibling dispersal after adult death
  Factors involved in mortality-related child migration
  Orphan clustering in rural and urban contexts – determinants and variations
    between countries
  Nature and extent of growth of institutional and residential forms of child
    care

Programs and interventions
  Development of targeting methods that are inclusive, rights-based and not
    discriminatory
  Good-practice definition in supporting and counseling bereaved children
  Development of child-focused home-care structures, with appropriate
    screening and referral systems
  Defining good practices and core processes in succession planning in
    different contexts
  Evaluating AIDS impact mitigation efforts from a child perspective
  Noneconomic costs in community involvement in an externally facilitated
    response designed to benefit orphans and vulnerable children
  How to operationalize a research agenda with inclusion of those most affected
  Means of measuring child, family, and community levels of stress and
    maladaptation

FIGURE 9.1. Priority Research Issues

ACKNOWLEDGMENTS

This chapter is based on an earlier report written by Douglas Webb, Geoff Foster, Hugo Kamya, and Namposya Nampanya-Serpell for G. Foster and C. Levine, *The White Oak Report: Building International Support for Children Affected by AIDS* (New York: Orphan Project, 2000). Additional thanks to Naomi Honingsbaum and Roeland Monasch.

References

Ali, S. 1998. Community perceptions of orphan care in Malawi. Paper presented at "Raising the Orphan Generation" conference, Pietermaritzburg, June.

Ansell, N., and L. Young. 2002. Young AIDS migrants in southern Africa. Project report, Department for International Development, Brunel University. http://www.brunel.ac.uk/depts/geo/dfidreport3.pdf

——— 2003. Fluid households, complex families: The impacts of children's migration as a response to HIV/AIDS in Southern Africa. *The Professional Geographer* 55(4): 464–79.

Bagarukayo, H., D. Shuey, B. Babishangire, and J. Karin. 1993. An operational study relating to sexuality and AIDS prevention among primary school students in Kabale district of Uganda. African Medical and Research Foundation, Entebbe.

Barber, B. 2000. Connection, regulation, and psychological autonomy: Key protective factors for children and adolescents. Unpublished paper, Department of Sociology, Brigham Young University, Provo, UT.

Bennell, P., K. Hyde, and N. Swainson. 2002. The impact of the HIV/AIDS epidemic on the education sector in sub-Saharan Africa: A synthesis of the findings and recommendations of three country studies: Botswana, Malawi and Uganda. Centre for International Education, University of Sussex Institute of Education. http://www.sussex.ac.uk/usie/PDFs/cie/aidssynpublished.pdf

Cluver, L., F. Gardner, S. Seedat and L. Wild. 2005. Risk and Protective Factors in the Psychological Health of Children experiencing orphanhood by AIDS: Summary Sheets 4. Cape Town Child Welfare Society/University of Oxford.

Congo casts out its "child witches." 2003. *The Observer* (London). May 11.

Connolly, M., and R. Monasch. 2002. Global perspectives. Paper presented at the 2002 Eastern and Southern Africa Regional Workshop on Children Affected by HIV/AIDS, Windhoek, Namibia, November 25–29.

Cook, M. 1998. *Starting from strengths: Community care for orphaned children; A training manual supporting the community care of vulnerable orphans; Facilitator's guide.* Victoria: Unit for Research and Education on the Convention on the Rights of the Child, School of Child and Youth Care, University of Victoria; and Zomba: Department of Psychology, Chancellor College, University of Malawi. http://web.uvic.ca/iicrd/pub_train_manual.html

Cook, P. H., S. Ali, and A. Munthali. 1998. Starting from strengths: Community care for orphaned children in Malawi: Final report. Prepared for the International Development Research Centre (IDRC), Centre for Social Research, Ottawa.

Cowan, F. M., L. F. Langhaug, G. P. Mashungupa, T. Nyamurera, J. Hargrove, S. Jaffar, R. W. Peeling, 2002. School-based HIV prevention in Zimbabwe:

Feasibility and acceptability of evaluation trials using biological outcomes. *AIDS* 16:1673–8.

Dunn, A. 1992. The social consequences of HIV/AIDS in Uganda. Working paper no. 2, Save the Children UK.

Dunn, A., E. Jareg, and D. Webb. 2003. *A last resort: The growing concern of children in residential care: Save the Children's position on residential care.* London: Save the Children UK, under the auspices of the HIV/AIDS Coordinating Group of the International Save the Children Alliance. Available at http://www.savethechildren.net

Families tipped into destitution. 2002. *Mail and Guardian* (Johannesburg). September 27.

Foster, G., R. Shakespeare, F. Chinemana, H. Jackson, S. Gregson, C. Marange, and S. Mashumba. 1998. Orphan prevalence and extended family care in a peri-urban community in Zimbabwe. In *The family and HIV today: Recent research and practice*, ed. R. Bor and J. Elford, 203–20. London: Cassell.

Geballe, S., J. Gruendel, and W. Andiman. 1995. *Forgotten children of the AIDS epidemic*. New Haven: Yale University Press.

Germann, S. 2003. Psychosocial needs and resilience of children affected by AIDS: Long-term consequences related to human security and stability. Paper presented to the World Bank Workshop on Orphans and Vulnerable Children, Washington, DC, May.

Guest, E. 2001. *Children of AIDS: Africa's orphan crisis*. London: Pluto Press.

Harber, M. 1998. Developing a community-based AIDS orphans project: A South African case study. Paper presented at "Raising the Orphan Generation" conference, Pietermaritzburg, June.

Hunter, S. 1990. Orphans as a window on the AIDS epidemic in sub-Saharan Africa: Initial results and implications of a study in Uganda. *Social Science & Medicine* 31 (6): 681–90.

Ledward, A. 1997. Age, gender, and sexual coercion: Their role in creating pathways of vulnerability to HIV infection. Master's thesis, University College, London.

Lee, T. 2000. Evaluating community-based orphan care in Zimbabwe: Monitoring and evaluation of the quality of services and programmes. Southern Africa AIDS Information Dissemination Service and Family AIDS Caring Trust, Harare.

Lindsay Smith, C., and R. O'Brine. 2000. *Memory book for Africa*. St. Albans, UK: Teaching-Aids at Low Cost. Order from: http://www.talcuk.org/index.htm

Loudon, M. 2003. 2002 Eastern and Southern Africa Regional Workshop on Children Affected by HIV/AIDS: Implementing the UNGASS goals for orphans and other children made vulnerable by HIV/AIDS (November 25–29, 2002). UNICEF, USAID, FHI, Hope for African Children Initiative, UNAIDS, Save the Children, NORAD, Sida, and the Government of Namibia, Windhoek. http://www.unicef.org/aids/aids/WINDHOEKReport.pdf

Luzze, F. 2002. Survival in child headed households: a study on the impact of World Vision support on coping strategies in child-headed households in Kakuuto County, Rakai District, Uganda. World Vision, Kampala.

Magalla, A., H. Houlihan, D. Charwe, K. Kipagasi, P. Bhatt, and A. Reeler. 2002. Urban-rural differences in programs on orphans and vulnerable children in AIDS affected areas in Tanzania. Paper presented at the 14th International Conference on AIDS, Barcelona, July.

Makaya, J., F. F. Mboussou, T. Bansimba, H. Ndinga, S. Latifou, Ambendet, and M. F. Puruehnce. 2002. Assessment of psychological repercussions of AIDS in 354 orphans in Brazzaville. Paper presented at the 14th International Conference on AIDS, Barcelona, July.

Manda, K. D., M. J. Kelly, and M. Loudon. 1999. *Orphans and vulnerable children: A situation analysis, 1999.* Joint USAID/UNICEF/SIDA/Study Fund project, Government of Zambia. Available at http:www.harare.unesco.org

Mann, G. 2003. Family matters: The care and protection of children affected by HIV/AIDS in Malawi. Report prepared for Save the Children Sweden, Stockholm.

McKerrow, N. 1996. Responses to orphaned children: A review of the current situation in the Copperbelt and Southern Provinces of Zambia. Collaborative study between UNICEF (Zambia), the Children in Need Network (CHIN) Secretariat, the Salvation Army, and Family Health Trust's Children in Distress (CINDI) Project. Also published as UNICEF Lusaka Research Brief no. 3, December 1997.

Monasch, R., and J. T. Boerma. 2004. Orphanhood and childcare patterns in sub-Saharan Africa: An analysis of national surveys from 40 countries. AIDS 18; supp. 2: S55–S65.

Mutangadura, G., and D. Webb. 1998. The socio-economic impact of adult morbidity and mortality on households in urban Zambia. *SAfAIDS News* 6 (3): 14–15.

Nampanya-Serpell, N. 1998. Children orphaned by HIV/AIDS in Zambia: Risk factors of premature parental death and policy implications. Ph.D. diss., University of Baltimore, Baltimore, MD.

Nowak, R. 2003. Absent fathers linked to teenage pregnancies. *New Scientist,* May 17.

Nyamukapa, C. A., G. Foster, and S. Gregson. 2003. Orphans' household circumstances and access to education in a maturing HIV epidemic in eastern Zimbabwe. *Journal of Social Development in Africa* 18 (2): 7–32.

Poulter, C. 1997. A psychological and physical needs profile of families living with HIV/AIDS in Lusaka. Paper prepared for Family Health Trust and UNICEF Lusaka.

Raising the issue of rights in Africa. 2003. *Ageing and Development,* July, 6–7.

Regional Psychosocial Support Initiative. 2003. Call to action: Security and stability; What happens if we neglect children affected by HIV/AIDS? Bulawayo, Zimbabwe.

Saoke, P., and R. Mutemi. 1994. Needs assessment of children orphaned by AIDS. Grantee Organisation, APMS and UNICEF Nairobi.

Save the Children UK (South Africa Programme). 2001. *The role of stigma and discrimination in increasing the vulnerability of children and youth infected with and affected by HIV/AIDS.* Pretoria: Save the Children UK.

Save the Children UK (Uganda Programme). 2003. *Care for children infected and affected by HIV/AIDS: A handbook for community health workers.* Kampala: Save the Children UK and Uganda Ministry of Health. http://www.savethechildren.org/uk/tempscuk/cache/cmsattach/1099_HIVCarehandbook.pdf

Sengendo, J., and J. Nambi. 1997. The psychological effect of orphanhood: A study of orphans in Rakai district. *Health Transition Review,* supplement to vol. 7:105–24.

Shah, M. K., and G. Nkhama. 1996. *Listening to young voices: Participatory appraisal on adolescent sexual and reproductive health in peri-urban Lusaka.* Lusaka: Care International.

Shaw, M. 2002. "Before we were sleeping but now we are awake"; The Stepping Stones Workshop Programme in the Gambia. In *Realizing rights: Transforming approaches to sexual and reproductive well-being*, ed. A. Cornwall and A. Welbourn, 128–40. London: Zed Books.

Shisana, O. 2002. Nelson Mandela and HSRC study of AIDS, household survey 2002. Human Sciences Research Council, Johannesburg.

Social Impact Assessment and Policy Analysis Corporation. 2002. A situation analysis of orphan children in Namibia. Ministry of Health and Social Services and UNICEF Namibia, Windhoek.

Subbarao, K., A. Mattimore, and K. Plangemann. 2001. Social protection of Africa's orphans and other vulnerable children, Africa region. Africa Region Human Development Working Paper. World Bank, Africa Region. Available at http://www.worldbank.org

Tarantola, D., and S. Gruskin. 1998. Children confronting HIV/AIDS: Charting the confluence of rights and health. *Health and Human Rights* 3 (1): 60–86.

Tolfree, D. 1995. *Roofs and roots: The care of separated children in the developing world.* Aldershot, Eng.: Ashgate.

———. 2003. *Whose children? Separated children's protection and participation in emergencies.* Stockholm: Save the Children Sweden.

UNICEF. 2003. *Africa's orphaned generations.* New York: UNICEF, November. http://www.unicef.org/publications/africas_orphans.pdf

United Nations. 2001. Declaration of Commitment on HIV/AIDS. Adopted by the United Nations General Assembly Special Session on AIDS, June 27. Available at http://www.unaids.org

USAID (United States Agency for International Development) and Family Health International. 2001. Orphans and other vulnerable children and adolescents in the context of AIDS. Report from the meeting on developing a research agenda, Washington, DC, February 5.

USAID, UNICEF, and UNAIDS (Joint United Nations Programme on AIDS). 2002. *Children on the brink 2002: A joint report on orphan estimates and program strategies.* Washington, DC: TvT Associates/The Synergy Project, USAID. http://www.unicef.org/publications/pub_children_on_the_brink_en.pdf

———. 2004. *Children on the brink 2004: A joint report of new orphan estimates and a framework for action.* New York: USAID. Available at http://www.unicef.org

Volle, S. J., S. Tembo, D. Boswell, S. Bowsky, D. Chiwele, R. Chiwele, K. Doll-Manda, et al. 2002. Psychosocial baseline survey of orphans and vulnerable children in Zambia. Paper presented at the 14th International Conference on AIDS, Barcelona, July.

World Bank. 1997. *Confronting AIDS: Public priorities in a global epidemic.* Washington, DC: World Bank.

10

Finding a Way Forward

Reducing the Impacts of HIV/AIDS on Vulnerable Children and Families

John Williamson

The number of children and families made vulnerable by HIV/AIDS is massive and will remain so for decades. As the previous chapters have shown, the pandemic is causing unprecedented child and family welfare problems, and the collective response in every seriously affected country falls far short of what is needed. What affected children and families require and what their own countries and the international community owe them is a combination of efforts, large and small, that collectively match the scale and duration of the impacts of AIDS. However, only a small percentage of children and families affected by HIV/AIDS are currently benefiting significantly from assistance from outside their own extended family (USAID, UNAIDS, WHO, UNICEF, and The Policy Project 2004:27). While many effective programs are in operation, there remains a huge gap between the results of these initiatives and what needs to be done. This chapter recommends strategies and interventions that, taken together, would begin to close the gap between what is being done and what must be done.

THE ELEMENTS OF AN ADEQUATE AND EFFECTIVE RESPONSE

By itself, no single intervention will make a sufficient impact on the full range of economic and psychosocial problems HIV/AIDS is causing among children and families, because the problems are too many and too varied. What is needed is a planned and coordinated set of policy, social-mobilization, and programmatic interventions by public sector and civil society actors. Achieving this goal requires a strategic response from leaders that only recently has been seen in a few countries.

If governments and other key stakeholders are to mobilize and guide strategic responses, leaders at every level of government must understand the type of collaborative responses needed and use their policy and public leadership capacities to support sustained, multisectoral commitment to the task. Uganda, Thailand, and Senegal have shown that open, committed leadership in vigorous prevention efforts can make a difference in an HIV/AIDS epidemic. UNICEF, bilateral donors such as USAID (U.S. Agency for International Development), and nongovernmental organizations (NGOs) are playing critical supportive roles, particularly in sub-Saharan Africa, in stimulating and helping to guide national policy development and planning regarding orphans and vulnerable children.

Massive, sustained action by national and international actors is essential to build an effective response to children made vulnerable by AIDS, and the primary emphasis must be to strengthen family and community capacities for protection and care. The vast majority of children orphaned by AIDS are living with a surviving parent or within their extended family, but HIV/AIDS and poverty continually erode caretakers' ability to meet even the basic needs of these children. As shown in Chapter 1, on the scale that is needed there are no viable alternatives to family and community care for orphans and vulnerable children. Unless the coping capacities of families and communities seriously affected by AIDS are reinforced, the number of children slipping through these primary social safety nets will overwhelm any feasible set of alternative-care programs.

Building family and community capacities, however, is not enough. Through school and other opportunities for learning and action, children must be prepared to meet their own needs. Governments must provide essential services and ensure protection and care for children outside family care – on the street, in child-headed households, or in residential care. Broad social mobilization is also necessary to counter stigma and discrimination and promote support for children and households in greatest need.

In 2001 the United Nations General Assembly Special Session (UNGASS) on HIV/AIDS passed the Declaration of Commitment on HIV/AIDS (United Nations 2001), which includes specific goals regarding orphans and vulnerable children (see Figure 10.1). These goals have spurred some governments to develop national policies and action plans. Their commitments and plans must be translated into adequate support to those living on the front line.

Through a series of regional workshops in Africa organized by UNICEF, USAID, and other organizations, a consensus has emerged in favor of five steps each country must take to achieve the UNGASS goals for the needs and rights of orphans and vulnerable children:

1. Carry out a collaborative national situation analysis concerning orphans and vulnerable children.
2. Develop a national plan of action.
3. Address policy issues.
4. Establish mechanisms for information exchange and collaboration.
5. Monitor and evaluate interventions.

We, the heads of state and governments, declare our commitment to . . .

65. By 2003, develop and by 2005 implement national policies and strategies to: build and strengthen governmental, family and community capacities to provide a supportive environment for orphans and girls and boys infected and affected by HIV/AIDS, including by providing appropriate counseling and psycho-social support; ensuring their enrolment in school and access to shelter, good nutrition, health and social services on an equal basis with other children; to protect orphans and vulnerable children from all forms of abuse, violence, exploitation, discrimination, trafficking and loss of inheritance;

66. Ensure non-discrimination and full and equal enjoyment of all human rights through the promotion of an active and visible policy of de-stigmatization of children orphaned and made vulnerable by HIV/AIDS;

67. Urge the international community, particularly donor countries, civil society, as well as the private sector to complement effectively national programmes to support programmes for children orphaned or made vulnerable by HIV/AIDS in affected regions, in countries at high risk and to direct special assistance to sub-Saharan Africa.

Source: United Nations 2001.

FIGURE 10.1. Goals Concerning Orphans and Vulnerable Children Included in the United Nations General Assembly Special Session on HIV/AIDS

ANALYZING THE SITUATION

Building an adequate response requires careful consideration of the factors that drive an HIV/AIDS epidemic and its social, political, and economic consequences. It is necessary to recognize the problems at the individual level – how parents, children, and orphans' guardians are affected and struggle daily to cope. But this perspective, by itself, is inadequate to guide the scaling up of responses to these problems. As stressed in the Introduction, it is also essential to take into account the magnitude and duration of the HIV/AIDS pandemic and its collective impacts. The individual and aggregate consequences of HIV/AIDS play out differently in every country. Thus, situation analysis and ongoing monitoring are essential to planning and implementing effective interventions.

Situation analysis involves gathering and analyzing quantitative and qualitative data about the social, economic, cultural, religious, historical, and demographic dimensions, as well as information on resources, capacities, and problems and the dynamic interrelationships. It also includes gathering information about a country's HIV/AIDS epidemic, including its consequences, household and community coping responses, and relevant polices and programs. Once the information has been gathered and analyzed and geographic and programmatic priorities have been identified, specific actions can be recommended. Situation analysis provides a basis for making difficult choices about how and where to direct available resources to benefit the most seriously affected children and families.

A situation analysis is also an important means of building consensus among key stakeholders. Collaboration to mitigate the impacts of HIV/AIDS becomes essential as a country's epidemic spreads. Conducting a situation analysis as a broadly inclusive, participatory process is a way to bring together key agencies and organizations – those already engaged and those who will need to be. Participants develop a shared understanding of the situation and reach consensus on the best way forward and the next steps. A participatory situation analysis should enable the organizations involved to reach consensus on priority issues and generate information on the current and future magnitude of orphaning and other impacts of HIV/AIDS on children and families. For program heads and policymakers, a situation analysis should provide clear answers to the question, Why should I care about these issues?

As has been seen in Zambia, Namibia, Uganda, and other countries, broad participation is important. Participants can include relevant government ministries or departments, international organizations, donors, NGOs and their coordinating bodies, associations of people living with HIV/AIDS, religious bodies and programs, women's associations, members of seriously affected communities, university departments, civic organizations, the business community, and other concerned groups. Actively involving stakeholders in a situation analysis increases the likelihood of their feeling ownership of the findings and being committed to implementing its recommendations. Inclusive participation means the process will take longer than one contracted out for implementation by a technical group, but the investment in time can make the difference between a report that occupies shelf space and a process that generates action.

A situation analysis should identify the geographic areas where families and communities are having the most difficulty protecting and providing for the most vulnerable children, and thus where action is most urgently needed. Identifying geographic priorities requires consideration of such information as census or survey data on orphaning and adult mortality; the pattern of spread of an epidemic; its impacts on different farming systems and other economic activities; vulnerability indicators regarding health, nutrition, education, and other factors; and the geographic reach and effectiveness of current services. Geographic priorities for action should not be based, however, only on statistical information. They also require validation through active consultation with people living and working in HIV/AIDS-affected communities.

The process should produce specific recommendations for action. Simply making a wish list will not help, though. Participants must identify what needs to be done, by whom, within a specified time frame. Considering all their recommendations, participants should organize, integrate, and present them in terms of sequence and strategic priorities. A participatory situation analysis is a springboard to generate decision making, planning, and action.

A situation analysis provides an overview of the impacts of HIV/AIDS on children, responses to the problems, and priorities for action, but because conditions will continue to evolve, ongoing monitoring is also necessary to help guide and adjust interventions over time. A system to monitor the impacts of AIDS on children and families should be one of the results of a situation analysis. The process will have identified sources of information that can be tapped periodically for ongoing monitoring of changing circumstances. One of its recommendations should identify a body to be responsible for compiling, analyzing, and disseminating relevant information to track trends (Williamson, Cox, and Johnston 2004).

A STRATEGIC FRAMEWORK

Countries with advanced epidemics have recognized that HIV/AIDS is not just a health issue but a major development issue as well. Agriculture, education, health, social welfare, community development, and business all are seriously affected, and a multisectoral, strategically linked set of responses is necessary. The beginnings of such a coordinated response are emerging in some of the worst-affected countries.

Government policy and public leadership can make a difference in the course of an HIV/AIDS epidemic. NGOs are developing effective interventions. Faith-based groups and networks are also emerging as structures with great collective potential for responding to HIV/AIDS. Their efforts are most likely to make a difference if all of these actors listen to and strengthen the capacities of families and communities who are the first line of response.

An effective response to the impacts of HIV/AIDS requires the active, ongoing collaboration of actors across all sectors. In addition to estimates and projections on orphaning, *Children on the Brink 2004* (USAID, UNICEF, and UNAIDS 2004: 22–4) presents the following five strategies to guide development of an effective national response to the impacts of HIV/AIDS on children and families. (For an earlier version of these strategies, see USAID, UNICEF, and UNAIDS 2002: 13–14).

1. Strengthen the capacity of families to protect and care for orphans and vulnerable children by prolonging the lives of parents and providing economic, psychosocial, and other support.
2. Mobilize and support community-based responses to provide both immediate and long-term support to vulnerable households.
3. Ensure access for orphans and vulnerable children to essential services, including education, health care, birth registration, and others.[1]

---

[1] *Children on the Brink 2002* (USAID, UNICEF, and UNAIDS 2002) and its two previous versions referred to building children's capacities to meet their own needs. Comments

4. Ensure that governments protect the most vulnerable children through improved policy and legislation and by channeling resources to communities.

5. Raise awareness at all levels through advocacy and social mobilization to create a supportive environment for children affected by HIV / AIDS.

These five strategies provide a framework for each country to shape its own comprehensive response. An uncoordinated collection of individual programs is inadequate: The programs must fit together into a coherent whole shaped by a national policy and plan of action. But national policies and plans will not be effective if they are simply imposed from the top. To ensure that policies and plans are grounded in reality and have legitimacy in the eyes of those expected to implement them, they must be developed with the participation of the community groups on the front line and the agencies that will be involved.

Governments have a responsibility, through laws, policies, and action, to support the coping capacities of individuals and families and provide them basic protection. Fulfilling these responsibilities requires particular attention to the situation of children and women; key elements of a framework to protect them include laws and effective structures for their implementation, such as provisions for:

- protection of children against abuse, neglect, and sexual contact with adults,
- elimination of barriers to school enrollment and completion,
- prohibition of discrimination in health care, schools, employment, or other areas based on actual or presumed HIV status,
- protection of the inheritance rights of orphans and widows,
- enactment and enforcement of laws ensuring women the right to own property,
- prohibition of harmful child labor, and
- protection and care for children without adequate family care, including children of the street, those in residential care, and child-headed households.

PROGRAMMATIC INTERVENTIONS

If the needs and rights of children made vulnerable by AIDS are to be fulfilled, a set of interventions appropriate to each country must be scaled up through increased coverage, scaled out through replication, and sustained for decades. When agencies consider possible programmatic interventions,

made during the review process of *The Framework for the Protection, Care and Support of Orphans and Vulnerable Children Living in a World with HIV and AIDS* indicated that this concept was not clear, and the current wording was substituted. This change clarifies part of the strategy, but unfortunately omits what many advocates feel is the essential element of children's active participation. The editors recommend that subsequent versions of *Children on the Brink* and *The Framework* clearly affirm the importance of children's participation.

they need to assess and compare the respective potential of alternative approaches for improving the capacities of families, communities, and vulnerable children to meet their own needs. In a country with an advanced HIV/AIDS epidemic, the most effective interventions are those that:

- fulfill children's basic needs and rights,
- are directed to the most vulnerable geographic areas, communities, and population groups,
- are targeted, in turn, by each community to its most vulnerable children and households,
- can be sustained for decades or generate ongoing improvements in coping,
- have an affordable cost per beneficiary,
- are widely replicable, and
- mesh together into an adequate collective set of responses.

Recognizing the need to provide guidance regarding programs for children affected by HIV/AIDS, UNICEF, USAID, and UNAIDS (the Joint United Nations Programme on HIV/AIDS) initiated a consultative process to forge international consensus on principles to guide programming. The process began at the 13th International AIDS Conference in Durban, South Africa, in July 2000 and incorporated feedback from subsequent regional meetings involving governments, NGOs, international organizations, the private sector, community organizations, and young people. It culminated with the formation of the Global Partners Forum in October 2003. The synthesis of this process, *The Framework for the Protection, Care and Support of Orphans and Vulnerable Children Living in a World with HIV and AIDS*, was issued in July 2004. It can be used to guide collaborative action at each level, from grassroots to national and international efforts. *The Framework* presents a version of the original five development strategies and includes program guidance on the following key points (27–30):

- Focus on the most vulnerable children and communities, not only children orphaned by AIDS.
- Define community-specific problems and vulnerabilities at the outset and pursue locally determined intervention strategies.
- Involve children and young people as active participants in the response.
- Give particular attention to the roles of boys and girls, men and women.
- Address gender discrimination.
- Strengthen partnerships and mobilize collaborative action.
- Link HIV/AIDS prevention activities, care, and support for people living with HIV/AIDS, and support for vulnerable children.

- Use external support to strengthen community initiative and motivation.

KEY INTERVENTIONS

A mix of interventions is needed to build an adequate, collective response to orphans and vulnerable children. This section gives an overview of seven categories for each country to consider as it develops its set of responses: education, community mobilization and capacity building, microeconomic strengthening at the household level, other development interventions, direct services, support grants, activities to promote the psychosocial well-being of children affected by HIV/AIDS, and a very broad set of interventions that includes HIV prevention and treatment and the care of those living with HIV/AIDS.

Education

Education is fundamental to the well-being and development of all children and is recognized as a human right by the United Nations Convention on the Rights of the Child (CRC) (United Nations 1989). Making primary education free and compulsory for all children is among the responsibilities undertaken by governments that have ratified the CRC. The reality, however, is that in developing countries there are educational costs, and typically the poorest children have difficulty attending school. The vulnerabilities caused by AIDS exacerbate attendance problems.

Paying school expenses can be a prohibitive financial burden for families affected by AIDS. Girls, on whom future family and community well-being substantially depend, are often forced to drop out before boys. From the national to the community level there have been a variety of responses to help orphans and other vulnerable children stay in school, but there are no easy answers to the resource deficits HIV/AIDS is causing (Hepburn 2001). Providing scholarships is a direct and efficient solution, but the expense makes it difficult to sustain as an escalating number of children are pushed out of school. Some ministries of education have waived school fees for orphans, which helps, but the resulting deficits in ministry and school budgets have to be made up from other sources.

Some organizations have provided supplies and equipment and constructed classrooms for schools prepared to accept orphans. Some communities have started their own basic schools to provide education for children unable to afford regular schools. The schools may be less expensive per pupil than government schools, but communities face significant challenges to support them indefinitely (Nampanya-Serpell 1999; Sikwibele, Mweetwa, and Williamson 2001). Countries such as Malawi, Uganda, and

Kenya that have eliminated all fees for primary school have seen dramatic increases in enrollment.

Some orphans are not in school simply because their guardians do not send them. Community groups concerned with orphans and vulnerable children in Zambia and Malawi have helped some students return to school by persuading guardians that these children need an education. Appeals by local religious groups, emphasis on traditional values and responsibilities, parenting skills classes, and sensitization to children's rights help motivate some care providers to send children to school.

Measures to improve household economic capacity, particularly where the participants are women, can be one of the most important and sustainable ways to address problems of educational access. Evaluations of microfinance programs involving women (for example, Adelski et al. 2001; Allen 2002; Allen, Koegler, and Rushawa 2002; Tumushabe 1999; Wright et al. 1999) have found that educational expenses are one of the primary uses of participants' income. Chapter 3 addresses these and other education issues.

Community Mobilization and Capacity Building

Community mobilization is a process through which a community (on its own or with an outside catalyst) identifies and takes action on its shared concerns. Capacity building involves strengthening or developing skills, methods, and organizational functioning. It may include linking communities with outside resources (training and information or material, financial, or technical support) or providing limited resources to the community. External resources must follow mobilization and action initiated by the community, however, not lead it. Effective mobilization is based on community ownership of a problem and a sense of responsibility to address it. Community mobilization is not a matter of persuading people to take action by giving them resources, nor to work as volunteers in an agency's program.

Communities become mobilized when residents collectively define strongly felt, shared concerns and identify how they can address these concerns themselves (Donahue and Williamson 1999). As a large number of communities have shown, people at the grassroots level are not only concerned about the growing number of orphans and vulnerable children, they are also prepared to respond to their needs using local resources. Some groups eventually secure additional funding or material support from external sources.

While many community groups have addressed the needs of orphans on their own initiative, it would be unrealistic to expect that most communities will eventually do so. Spontaneous grassroots efforts are scattered and their collective coverage is limited. The programmatic challenge is to develop ways to systematically assist communities to mobilize their responses and

The Families, Orphans, and Children under Stress (FOCUS) Program in Mutare, Zimbabwe, has mobilized volunteers to visit orphans regularly, monitor their situation, respond as appropriately as possible with community resources, distribute small amounts of externally provided material support, and refer urgent problems to government authorities. Some nine thousand needy children benefit from the program, and the cost per household visited was less than US$10 per year in 1998 and lower the next year. Its 1998 budget of US$13,800 broke down as follows: 44 percent to material assistance, 7 percent to volunteer allowances and uniforms, 5 percent to volunteer training and meetings, and 44 percent to salaries of the coordinator and assistant coordinator and administrative costs. Program efficiency was subsequently increased by integrating visiting orphans with home-based care and HIV/AIDS prevention activities. The FOCUS Program is implemented by Family AIDS Caring Trust (FACT).

FIGURE 10.2. FOCUS: A Volunteer Program in Zimbabwe

help them sustain their efforts. Programs such as those described in Figures 10.2 and 10.3 have shown that this is possible, with limited amounts of support.

Communities' strongly felt concerns for their children are the driving and potentially sustaining force behind their initiatives. Concerns are not created by the community mobilization process; rather, the coming together of mobilized communities, both rural and urban, stimulates a shift in perception from seeing the needs of orphans and, especially, vulnerable children as being the responsibility of individual households to recognizing that children's needs are a shared community responsibility that can be addressed more effectively through cooperative efforts. Because the motivation to participate comes from shared personal concerns, communities must define for themselves which children and which threats to their current and future well-being concern them most. Consequently, an outside agency cannot predetermine the specific activities or outputs that the process will generate, or even the specific issues that will be addressed. These are decisions community members must make for themselves.

Mobilizing a community or building its capacity does not necessarily mean helping it to develop a new organizational structure. It may involve enabling an existing community committee, school, religious group, women's association, or other body to broaden or strengthen its action for vulnerable children and households.

The specific kinds of capacity building needed after an initial mobilization process depend and build on a community's existing capacities, opportunities, resources, and commitment to its most vulnerable children. Capacity building may include training in writing proposals, developing and managing programs, mobilizing local resources, fundraising, or training in child development, health care, nutrition, and children's rights.

Zambia's Strengthening Community Partnerships for the Empowerment of Orphans and Vulnerable Children (SCOPE-OVC) was designed to mitigate the impact of HIV/AIDS on orphans and vulnerable children through mobilizing, strengthening, and scaling up community led responses aimed at benefiting orphans and vulnerable children. The project has organized district and community committees in twelve of the country's seventy-three districts. Collectively, these committees reached over 137,000 orphans and vulnerable children in 2002, over 26 percent of the estimated total number in these districts. In ethnically mixed urban communities and rural areas, they have helped residents to respond to children in need. Many community committees have started community schools for children too poor to attend government schools. Other community initiatives include intervening to protect abused children and organizing group income-generating projects. The district committees also provide a forum for information exchange and coordination among government, NGO, church, and business members. The SCOPE-OVC project is being implemented by CARE Zambia supported by Family Health International with funding from USAID.

Other capacity-building efforts include strengthening district and community partners to address the interrelated issues of children's psychosocial needs and household economic strengthening through training in community and resource mobilization, strategic and action planning, monitoring and evaluation, business development and microfinance services, and psychosocial support.

To supplement local mobilization efforts, the project has a small grants component aimed at helping communities and organizations scale up the support they are providing.

FIGURE 10.3. Mobilizing Communities in Zambia: SCOPE-OVC

It is an ongoing process that involves helping communities (1) identify and use their own capacities and local resources, (2) develop skills in assessment, decision making, planning, monitoring, and evaluation, and (3) link with external resources. Chapter 1 describes community action for vulnerable children (see also Phiri, Foster, and Nzima 2001).

Microeconomic Strengthening

Many of the problems of AIDS-affected children and families result from their deteriorating economic situation. HIV/AIDS-related illness and death lead directly to economic problems that undermine children's well-being in a variety of ways (see Figure I.2 in the Introduction). Consequently, improving the ability of vulnerable households to support themselves is fundamental. "Economic strengthening," however, is easier said than done. It is probably safe to say that all the major child-focused development organizations have had significant experience with failed income-generating projects. The challenge, then, is to implement approaches that work and that can be replicated with reasonable consistency. Typically, what seem most likely to fail are group income-generating projects whose profits are intended to benefit vulnerable children. They are very difficult to sustain when they are run only by volunteers, and profits, if any, are generally quite limited. What shows much more promise are microfinance services and savings mobilization approaches that enable participants to carry out their own individual income-generating activities for the benefit of their own households (Donahue 2002: 5).

Most microfinance programs do not specifically aim to benefit children, although children typically do benefit. Evaluations (Adelski et al. 2001; Barnes 2002; IFAD 2002; Tumushabe 1999; Wright et al. 1999) show that women who participate in microfinance programs spend most of their profits on household needs such as their children's school expenses, health care, and food. The Uganda Women's Effort to Save Orphans (UWESO) program, however, has shown that targeting vulnerable children is possible in a financially sustainable program (see Figure 10.4).

Microeconomic interventions are needed for the majority of vulnerable households, but children and families at the very bottom who have already slipped into destitution need immediate, direct assistance. Their community, with some outside support, is in the best position to provide such help.

The economic stability of the entire community requires attention where HIV/AIDS is widespread. If too many families are allowed to become destitute, the community safety net will be overwhelmed. Effective microeconomic interventions that help stabilize household incomes can reduce the number of people who need immediate relief as well as increase the ability of poor and less-poor households to help those more vulnerable than themselves. Sustaining the capacity of families and communities to cope with the impacts of HIV/AIDS requires ongoing interaction between community mobilization and capacity-building activities, on one hand, and interventions that build household and community economic resources, on the other. Figure 10.4 makes this point, indicating that microeconomic strengthening and community mobilization are complementary approaches, both of which are necessary. Chapter 2 describes approaches to microeconomic strengthening.

Other Development Interventions

Appropriate development interventions can be targeted to geographic areas where families and communities are having the greatest difficulty protecting and providing for their most vulnerable children. For example, one of the recommendations of an assessment conducted in Uganda (Alden, Williamson, and Salole 1991) was to upgrade roads linking villages

While evaluations have shown that microfinance programs can help households in areas affected by HIV/AIDS to better meet basic expenses, the large majority did not aim for this goal. They set out simply to provide savings and credit services (and in some cases other services, such as microinsurance) to poor people in a sustainable way without specific social goals. The Uganda Women's Effort to Save Orphans (UWESO) Savings and Credit Scheme is an exception. Founded by the First Lady of Uganda, Madame Janet Museveni, UWESO started in 1986 making charitable responses to orphans of Uganda's years of armed conflict and brutal repression. By the early 1990s, increasingly, it was responding to children orphaned by AIDS. By 1994, through grants and donations, it was paying school fees for about five thousand orphans.

Recognizing the massive and growing task it faced, UWESO began to seek a more sustainable way to respond to orphan's needs. Initially, it tried funding group income-generating activities, but as many organizations have found, the rate of economic success was very low. Then UWESO tried starting small revolving-credit schemes, but these did not prove sustainable. In 1996, UWESO took a new tack and initiated its Savings and Credit Scheme, targeting households caring for orphans and using a village banking approach complemented with health and other training. As of 2002 some one hundred thousand children were receiving ongoing benefits from the program. Evaluations have found that children of school age are in school, the quality and frequency of meals has improved, and that between 1999 and 2003 there has been substantial improvement in the well-being and economic circumstances of participating households. The loan repayment rate has been 95 percent.

Women in some of UWESO's village banking groups also benefit from information and training in health, household, and social issues. Some of the topics include business skills, improved agricultural methods, HIV/AIDS, children's rights and protection, nutrition, water and sanitation, and property rights.

Sources: IFAD 2002; Tumushabe 1999; Ntambirweki, Pelucy. "The UWESO Savings and Credit Scheme (USCS), Uganda," in White, J., Facing the *Challenge: NGO experiences of mitigating the impacts of HIV/AIDS in sub-Saharan Africa*, final draft, Natural Resources Institute, University of Greenwich, UK, November 2002; Tumushabe, J., "Quantitative Assessment of the Impact of The UWESO Development Programme," (Draft Report), Department of Population Studies, Institute of Statistics and Applied Economics, Makerere University, 2004.

FIGURE 10.4. Microfinance with a Difference: The UWESO Program in Uganda

to markets. Roads had deteriorated badly over the country's years of misrule and civil war. In a city market, the staple plantain cost ten times what it would bring in a more remote village due to transportation difficulties and the related breakdown in agricultural marketing systems.

In that situation, upgrading roads was one of the measures that offered good possibilities for improving the care of orphans in struggling communities. In other situations, supporting key agricultural inputs or tools, establishing new market linkages, and a variety of other development interventions might be effective ways of improving the economic situation of families and communities.

In most countries women bear the major burden of caring for the ill and for orphans, in addition to most household tasks and many key economic activities. Development interventions that women identify as being important deserve particular attention in mitigating the impacts of HIV/AIDS. Examples might include improving access to safe water to reduce the amount of time and effort required to carry it, supporting collaborative, community-based childcare to free women's time for economic activities, and introducing fuel-efficient stoves or planting fast-growing tree varieties to reduce the time and effort needed to gather firewood. Laws that strengthen and protect the rights of women to own land and for widows to inherit property also benefit their children.

Direct Services

Children and households who slip to the level of destitution need direct support, which is often provided by community residents or local religious groups. Formal programs that deliver direct services for orphans and vulnerable children (for example, repairing houses, paying school expenses, providing food and material assistance, and health services) are often run by NGOs or government agencies. Many service delivery programs have produced good results, but with limited geographic coverage and at a cost per beneficiary that is too high to reach more than a fraction of the vulnerable children and households.

Direct service delivery is needed in all countries, but because it is resource intensive it can be the principal type of response only in countries with a strong economic base, or in less-developed countries during the early stages of an HIV/AIDS epidemic when fewer children are affected. As the number of children made vulnerable by HIV/AIDS escalates in a poorer country, the priority must be to shore up family and community capacities to protect and care for vulnerable children. This can keep to a manageable level the number of children whose survival and well-being depend on the ongoing delivery of direct services.

Support Grants

Some developing countries with high HIV prevalence are using household-level support grants to help vulnerable households to provide more adequately for especially vulnerable children. A working paper from South Africa concluded:

[T]he most equitable, accessible and appropriate mechanism for supporting children in the context of the AIDS pandemic would be through the extension to all children of the Child Support Grant mechanism that is currently in place, and for the means test that restricts children's access to be removed. Progressive implementation of a universal Child Support Grant should be based not on providing grants in the interim to particular categories of children (such as orphans) but rather on drawing more impoverished children – irrespective of their parental circumstances – into the social security 'safety net' (Meintjes et al. 2004).

A separate study in South Africa, which included a total of 5,000 households in three provinces, found that over half of the income of these households came from current Government grant programs, old age pensions being the most significant source. Twenty-eight percent of the households were receiving child support grants (Vermaak et al. 2004).

The Progresa program in Mexico is receiving attention as a model for possible adaptation in countries with a large number of orphans. Targeting poor households with poor villages, Progresa benefits more than 20 million people through conditional cash grants. Selected households can receive a monthly cash grant for each child in grades three through nine who is in school and who attends at least 85 percent of the time. Each household is also eligible for an additional nutrition grant, conditional upon each child receiving two to four health check-ups per year, each adult having an annual check-up, and any pregnant women receiving seven pre- and post-natal checkups. The results have included increase in secondary school enrollment of more than 70 percent, a decrease of at least 20 percent in illness among children under five years of age, and a 45 percent reduction in the severity of poverty (Filmer n.d.).

Providing a large number of household support grants is beyond the means of many of the poorer countries without extensive external support, but some countries with a relatively strong economy, like South Africa and Botswana, are already using this mechanism as part of their response to the needs of orphans and other vulnerable children. Where such an approach can be sustained at scale, it is an effective way to provide support.

Activities to Promote Psychosocial Well-being

Psychosocial distress is less tangible than the material problems many AIDS-affected children suffer, but concerned organizations increasingly are addressing these issues. Enabling a family to cope more effectively with the material problems they face is a major step toward helping them deal with their psychosocial distress, but it is not enough. Effective measures to address psychosocial needs do not necessarily require separate programs; they should be incorporated into all activities for children and families affected by HIV/AIDS.

Interventions with psychosocial benefits include:

- Helping HIV-positive parents create memory books to assist them in talking with their children about important aspects of their shared past, to deal with problems related to increasing illness, and to ensure children's future care.
- Enabling children to stay in school.
- Keeping orphaned siblings together by enlisting support from families and communities.
- Encouraging religious observances or traditional ceremonies to help heal grief and promote social integration.
- Training teachers to recognize and respond supportively to children's withdrawal or disruptive behavior.
- Encouraging and supporting communities to conduct structured recreation, art, cultural, and sports activities that enable isolated orphans and other vulnerable children to integrate socially.
- Organizing regular home visiting for orphans and children whose parents are ill.
- Reducing stigma and discrimination associated with HIV/AIDS.
- Providing counseling services for children who are not responsive to other community-based interventions.

Chapter 4 addresses psychosocial issues and interventions.

HIV/AIDS Prevention, Treatment, and Care

While it is beyond the scope of this chapter to deal substantively with the wide range of approaches to prevention, treatment, and care related to HIV/AIDS, these services are directly relevant to the well-being of orphans and vulnerable children. Preventing HIV infections prevents orphaning. Treatment and care prolong the lives of HIV-positive parents, and this is one of the most important ways to help their children. What is addressed here is the need for better integration of prevention and care activities.

Among HIV/AIDS care efforts there has been increasing attention to coordination and integration of home-based care for people living with HIV/AIDS and support for orphans and vulnerable children. Programs providing care and treatment for people living with HIV/AIDS have direct opportunities to identify the needs of children in the same household. Also, linking care and prevention activities seems particularly relevant for children and adolescents. Teenagers frequently show a willingness and capacity to organize and address community problems. For example, creating a framework in which older children and adolescents meet some of the emotional or daily living needs of orphans or people living with AIDS, provides opportunities to convey and reinforce HIV-prevention messages among participants, as well as benefitting those assisted.

Because families and communities are the first line of response to HIV/AIDS, programmatic interventions must be organized in ways that make sense in terms of people's day-to-day needs and struggles. Unfortunately, the focus of HIV/AIDS programs often has more to do with the skills of the professionals planning and managing them than it does with the problems the interventions are intended to address. For example, HIV prevention programs are typically planned by public health specialists, home-based care programs by medical service providers, programs for orphans by social welfare specialists, and microeconomic interventions by relevant specialists. Often these programs are quite separate, but the people on the front line do not categorize their lives in this way. Interventions for care or prevention, if they are to be effective, must be integrated in ways that make sense in terms of the daily realities of those most affected.

SCALING UP AND SUSTAINING RESPONSES

Because the number of children orphaned by AIDS can be expected to increase and remain high for decades, responses must match the scale of these impacts and be sustained indefinitely. This is not to say that an individual program should attempt to achieve country-wide coverage. But interventions must do so collectively, and available resources must be apportioned effectively among them.

One implication of the need to identify, scale up, replicate, and sustain effective interventions is that much more attention must be given to the per capita costs of effective interventions (see Figure 10.5). It is essential to develop affordable measures that can significantly improve the survival and development of vulnerable children and that can be replicated on the same scale as the pandemic's impact.

The only realistic way to scale up is for agencies and groups to develop a collective set of responses, including grassroots initiatives, larger NGO-supported programs, action by faith communities, and national development initiatives and policies. At each level of society, from the village to the nation, concerned individuals, groups, and agencies must come together, analyze needs and capacities, and find ways to collaborate to secure the protection and care of the most vulnerable children. Each country and community must review and consider its own situation and build its own set of responses, and committed leadership is needed at every level to make this happen. There is no viable alternative to this strategy, and it is beginning to materialize.

Countries in Africa are starting to conduct national situation analyses, develop national policies and plans of action concerning orphans and vulnerable children, and develop networks through which they can

The strategic importance of basic cost-per-beneficiary analysis was highlighted during a program assessment in Malawi (Williamson and Donahue 1996). All of the program's activities were relevant to the problems of AIDS-affected children and families. They included health care needs, education, training, and psychosocial needs of children, as well as training in home-based care, support for gardening and other income-generating activities, and microfinance services. The staff of the program considered it to be community-based because many of its activities were being carried out by community volunteers. It became evident during the assessment, however, that the ongoing participation of the volunteers depended on the continuing involvement of the sizable NGO staff and the material inputs that the program provided. The NGO's plans to shift the program to another geographic area seemed likely to result in the collapse of the activities that had been started in the initial area of operation. Further, the cost per beneficiary was too high for the program to be scaled up significantly. Taking these considerations into account, the program's leadership decided to revise it radically, and they began a community mobilization approach through which less costly, sustainable, and community-owned and managed activities were initiated.

FIGURE 10.5. Considering Cost per Beneficiary

exchange information and find ways to work together on an ongoing basis. By late 2003, of the forty-six sub-Saharan countries, twenty have carried out situation analyses concerning orphans and vulnerable children, the six had developed a response policy, and seventeen had established a coordination mechanism (UNICEF 2003: 51). In addition to the obvious need for such action, a motivating force has been the goals concerning orphans and vulnerable children established by the UNGASS on HIV/AIDS in the Declaration of Commitment (United Nations 2001). Technical guidance and opportunities for information exchange are being provided through sub-regional workshops on orphans and vulnerable children organized by UNICEF, USAID, and other organizations.

Much remains to be done, however. In particular, each country needs mechanisms to channel technical, material, and financial resources as well as essential information to the community groups on the front line of response. Initially, a collaborative national response may resemble more a patchwork quilt that is continually being revised and repaired than a neat organizational structure. But the central issue will be whether the various bodies manage collectively to make a positive difference in the lives of the most vulnerable children and families.

TARGETING RESPONSES

Scaling up requires targeting responses to improve the well-being of the most vulnerable children and families and using available resources as effectively as possible. Resources may not be sufficient for even cost-effective programs to be uniformly implemented and sustained throughout a country. Targeting resources directs them where they are most needed, gathering information for subsequent targeting should be part of a situation analysis.

There are two stages of targeting. The first is to identify and direct financial and material resources to the geographic areas where families are having the greatest difficulty protecting and providing for the care of their children. This requires the use of data indicating the prevalence of problem conditions and responses, broken down to the district level or a lower administrative level, and might include rates of orphaning, adult mortality, infant mortality, malnutrition, school dropouts, income levels, and other poverty measures. Rates of children whose parents both have died can be used to identify areas where an HIV/AIDS epidemic is more advanced. A census or major health survey provides an opportunity to generate data to aid in targeting.

Targeting also includes mapping the availability of key services to address such questions as: where are interventions already underway; how adequate are these interventions; and where is the mismatch greatest between problems and existing responses? Such data must also be tested by review on the ground and consultation with people in the communities where problems appear to be greatest.

The second stage of targeting depends even more heavily on people in the most affected areas who can say which of their many problems concern them the most. They are also in the best position to identify the children and households who are at greatest risk. The most vulnerable members of a community are the least able to make their needs known, and local residents generally understand much better than outsiders what factors indicate serious vulnerability. Through a participatory process, they can identify locally relevant indicators of vulnerability and use these to assess relative levels of need among children and households. For example, communities have identified such factors as the following:

- whether either or both parents are living and provide care,
- age and health of the guardian,
- whether there is an adult guardian,
- age and sex of the children,
- whether the children are in or out of school,
- household size,
- health problems,
- loss of home or possessions,
- separation of siblings,
- how frequently a cooking fire is seen at a household,
- quality and frequency of meals,

- past and current economic activity,
- receipt of external support, and
- access to arable land.

Local targeting is most effectively done by communities that are already mobilizing and using their own resources to address local needs: They are very careful to direct locally generated resources to the children and households they are most concerned about. Competition and other problems can arise, though, when external resources are offered and local residents are asked to decide how to distribute them. Community groups that have already begun to use local resources to assist those about whom they are most concerned are better able to channel external resources effectively.

Effective targeting also requires transparency. Local groups can best stimulate broad community participation and support when they are open about their aims and activities. Likewise, any external body that provides support for a local initiative is well advised to let the community at large know what resources it has provided and for what purpose, so residents and leaders can hold accountable those responsible for allocating and managing the resources provided.

MONITORING, EVALUATION, AND RESEARCH

The unprecedented characteristics of the HIV/AIDS pandemic necessitate ongoing monitoring of its impacts, evaluation of interventions, and research on strategic issues. To ensure that interventions actually make a difference in the lives of vulnerable children and families, their results must be measured. The findings, in turn, provide a basis for adjusting interventions to make them more effective and for deciding how best to use resources. These mechanisms should include participatory appraisal methods that community residents can use to measure the local impacts of HIV/AIDS and the effectiveness of their responses.

It is also important to identify within a country those NGO, university, and private-sector groups that can be called on to undertake short-term research and produce quick, practical reports on specific issues. Examples of possible strategic monitoring and research issues include the following:

- Develop child and community vulnerability indices to use in mapping and setting geographic priorities for interventions.
- Identify the processes, approaches, and models most suited to urban, periurban, or rural communities and different farming systems.
- Create ways that home-based care activities, especially those involving children and youth, can contribute to HIV prevention.
- Monitor impacts of HIV/AIDS on family and community economic coping strategies.

BUILDING POLITICAL, PUBLIC, AND DONOR SUPPORT

The safety, well-being, and development of a massive and growing number of African children are progressively being undermined by HIV/AIDS. Serious, concerted action is finally beginning to emerge in the most affected countries of that region. It is imperative that the countries in Asia, Central and Eastern Europe, the Caribbean, and Latin America do not make the mistake of most African countries by avoiding the issue until it reaches dramatic proportions. The UNGASS goals for orphans and vulnerable children have been agreed on by all countries and they call for serious, concerted action now. The only hope for an adequate and effective response lies in planned, collaborative action by all parties. Policymakers, community leaders, religious organizations, donors, the academic community, and the public all must play a role in each country to piece together and maintain an effective national response.

Generating increased awareness is essential but not sufficient; it will stimulate sympathy but probably little action. Awareness-raising must be linked with efforts to generate a broadly shared sense of responsibility to support and protect those affected by HIV/AIDS. It is important to convey a clear vision of how to help affected children and families and to identify the concrete steps necessary to make this happen.

A participatory national situation analysis, carried out jointly by key bodies in government and civil society, can be the first step in mobilizing action. This kind of process can generate information needed for broad social mobilization as well as for specific program and policy development. A campaign to sensitize the public should involve leaders and well-known individuals who can amplify and transmit key information and messages. This may include government leaders, representatives of the media, religious leaders, and popular sports and entertainment figures. In Zambia, for example, journalists formed the Media Network for Orphans and Vulnerable Children. National leaders must find the wisdom and courage to speak out clearly and often – not only about the threats posed by HIV/AIDS, but also about what is being done and what remains to be done.

CONCLUSION

Families and communities are the first line of response to children affected by HIV/AIDS. Millions of people struggle every day to survive and to provide whatever care they can to their vulnerable children and ill family members. But their resources are limited and many cannot by themselves provide adequate care, protection, and support. Families and communities cannot win this fight alone and many desperately need external assistance. Mobilizing communities and strengthening household economic and caring capacities can be the foundation of effective, sustained national responses. External assistance and capacity building can enable communities to expand their activities incrementally as their capacities grow. Significant programmatic and policy action and planning are also needed to piece together an adequate national response. Governments must fulfill the right of every child to attend school and to access basic services, and governments also have the ultimate responsibility to ensure children's protection. Approaches to HIV prevention, care, and treatment that have been shown to work must be expanded and replicated. Better forms of family and community-based care must be greatly expanded to ensure protection and nurturing care for any child who slips through family and community safety nets. Each of us must recognize the urgency of these tasks, find ways to work together, and do it now.

ACKNOWLEDGMENT

The Displaced Children and Orphans Fund of the United States Agency for International Development and the Orphan Project, New York City, supported the preparation of the original version of this chapter in 1998. It was updated by the author in 2004.

References

Adelski, E., P. Bourdeau, J. B. Doamba, T. Lairez, and J. P. Ouedraogo. 2001. *Final impact evaluation report on development activity proposal: 1997–2001*. Ouaggadougou: Catholic Relief Services/Burkina Faso, May 1.

Alden, J., J. Williamson, and G. Salole. 1991. Managing Uganda's orphans crisis. Report prepared for Displaced Children and Orphans Fund, USAID.

Allen, H. 2002. CARE International's Village Savings and Loan Programmes in Africa: Micro Finance for the Rural Poor that Works. CARE, Tanzania. http://www.kcenter.com/care/edu/CARE%20Publications.htm

Allen, H., P. Koegler, and J. Rushawa. 2002. End of term evaluation of Kupfuma Ishungu Rural Microfinance Project (RMFP), Zimbabwe. CARE Zimbabwe, Harare.

Barnes, C. (with E. Keogh, N. Nemarundwe, L. Nyikahadzoi, and E. Weiss). 2002. *Microfinance and households coping with HIV/AIDS in Zimbabwe: An exploratory study*. Horizons Final Report. Washington, DC: Population Council, September. http://www.eldis.org/static/DOC13059.htm

Donahue, J. 2002. Children, HIV/AIDS, and poverty in southern Africa. Paper presented at the Southern Africa Regional Poverty Network Conference, Pretoria, April 9–10.

Donahue, J., and J. Williamson. 1999. *Community mobilization to mitigate the impacts of HIV/AIDS*. Washington, DC: USAID Displaced Children and Orphans Fund, September 1. http://www.dec.org/pdf/_docs/pnacj024.pdf

The framework for the protection, care, and support of orphans and vulnerable children living in a world with HIV and AIDS. 2004. Prepared by The Global Partners Forum for Orphans and Vulnerable Children, convened and led by UNICEF, July. Available at http://www.unicef.org

Hepburn, A. 2001. Primary education in eastern and southern Africa: Increasing access for orphans and vulnerable children in AIDS-affected areas. Report prepared for the Displaced Children and Orphans Fund, USAID, Terry Sanford Institute of Public Policy, Duke University, June. Available at http://www.usaid.gov/

IFAD (International Fund for Agricultural Development). 2002. Mid-term review of the UWESO Development Programme (UDP): Implemented by Uganda Women's Effort to Save Orphans (UWESO), Financed by the Belgian Survival Fund (BSF) through the International Fund for Agricultural Development (IFAD). November–December.

Meintjes, H., D. Budlender, S. Giese, and L. Johnson. 2004. Social security for children in the context of AIDS: Questioning the State's response. *AIDS Bulletin of the Medical Research Council of South Africa* 13(2):1–9.

Nampanya-Serpell, N. 1999. Draft report for the Displaced Children and Orphans Fund, USAID, on cost-effectiveness of interventions to benefit orphans and other vulnerable children.

Phiri, S. N., G. Foster, and M. Nzima. 2001. *Expanding and strengthening community action: A study of ways to scale up community mobilization interventions to mitigate the effect of HIV/AIDS on children and families.* Washington, DC: Displaced Children and Orphans Fund, USAID. Available at http://www.usaid.gov/our_work/humanitarian_assistance/the_funds/pubs/ovc.html

Sikwibele, A., C. Mweetwa, and J. Williamson. 2001. A midterm review of the Scope-OVC program in Zambia: Conducted June 18–29, 2001. USAID, Lusaka, Zambia.

Tumushabe, J. 1999. UWESO Savings and Credit Scheme (USCS) evaluation report. Uganda Women's Effort to Save Orphans, May. (Confidential report.)

UNICEF. 2003. *Africa's orphaned generations.* New York: UNICEF, November. http://www.unicef.org/publications/africas_orphaned_generations.pdf

United Nations. 1989. *Convention on the rights of the child.* UN General Assembly Res. 44/25, UN GAOR, 44th sess., 41st plen. mtg., annex, UN Doc. A/RES/44/25 (December 12). Geneva: United Nations. http://www.unchr.ch/html/menu3/b/k2crc.htm

———. 2001. Declaration of Commitment on HIV/AIDS. UN GA 26th Special sess., UN Doc. A/Res/S-26/2 (2001), June 25–27. Available at http://www.un.org/ga/aids/coverage/FinalDeclarationHIVAIDS.html

USAID, UNICEF, and UNAIDS. 2002. *Children on the brink 2002: A joint report on orphan estimates and program strategies.* Washington, DC: TvT Associates/The Synergy Project, USAID. http://www.unicef.org/publications/pub_children_on_the_brink_en.pdf

———. 2004. *Children on the brink 2004: A joint report of new orphan estimates and a framework for action.* New York: USAID. Available at http://www.unicef.org

USAID, UNAIDS, WHO, UNICEF, and the Policy Project. 2004. *Coverage of selected services for HIV/AIDS prevention, care and support in low and middle income countries in 2003.* June, 84 pages. http://www.policyproject.com/pubs/generalreport/CoverageSurveyReport.pdf

Vermaak, K., N. Mavimbela, J. Chege, and E. Esu-Williams. 2004. *Challenges faced by households in caring for orphans and vulnerable children.* Research Update. Washington, DC: Population Council/Horizons and Frontiers.

Williamson, J., A. Cox, and B. Johnston. 2004. *Conducting a situation analysis of orphans and vulnerable children affected by HIV/AIDS: A framework and resource guide*. Washington, DC: Office of Sustainable Development, Bureau for Africa, USAID, February.

Williamson, J., and J. Donahue. 1996. Developing interventions to benefit children and families affected by HIV/AIDS: A review of the COPE program in Malawi for the Displaced Children and Orphans Fund. Washington, DC: Displaced Children and Orphans Fund, USAID.

Wright, G. A. N., D. Kasente, G. Ssemogerere, and L. Mutesasira. 1999. Vulnerability, risks, assets, and empowerment: The impact of microfinance on poverty alleviation. Commissioned in preparation for the *World Development Report 2001*, MicroSave-Africa and Uganda Women's Finance Trust, March. http://www.undp.org/sum/MicroSave/ftp_downloads/UWFTstudyFinal.pdf

Chronology of Important Events

Mid to late 1970s   Previously unknown disease emerges in Africa and other continents.

1981   U.S. Centers for Disease Control and Prevention (CDC) reports first cases in New York and Los Angeles.

1982   CDC names the disease acquired immune deficiency syndrome (AIDS).

1984   Virus later named human immune deficiency (HIV) is identified in Paris and Bethesda, MD.

Late 1980s   Programs for children orphaned by AIDS are developed in Rakai and Masaka Districts in Uganda and the Kagera Region of Tanzania.

1988   Six papers on orphans in Africa are presented at the Global AIDS Conference in London, including Christopher Beer, Ann Rose, and Ken Tout, "AIDS: The Grandmother's Burden," published in *The Global Impact of AIDS*, ed. Alan F. Fleming, Manuel Carballo, David W. FitzSimons, Michael R. Bailey, and Jonathan Mann, 171–74 (New York: Liss).

1989   Save the Children UK and the Uganda Ministry of Labour and Social Affairs conduct the first survey of orphan prevalence, quantifying the magnitude of the growing orphan population in areas seriously affected by HIV/AIDS.

1990   With support from UNICEF Uganda, the Uganda Community-Based Association for Child Welfare, a consortium of organizations and government departments, is established to improve collaboration and strengthen the capacity of the growing number of programs responding to children orphaned by AIDS.

Susan Hunter publishes "Orphans as a Window on the AIDS Epidemic in Sub-Saharan Africa: Initial Results and Implications of a Study in Uganda" in *Social Science and Medicine* 31 (6), based on her work with Save the Children UK. As the first published research article on orphans and AIDS in Africa, it begins to draw international attention to the issue.

Elizabeth Preble publishes "Women, Children, and AIDS in Africa: An Impending Disaster," *New York University Journal of International Law and Politics*, November 15, the first international estimate of orphaning.

1991 In June UNICEF convenes representatives from Africa and the international community at the Innocenti Research Centre in Florence for the first international consultation on children losing their parents to AIDS.

The First Lady of Uganda, Madame Janet Museveni, asks United States officials for help in assessing the situation of children orphaned by AIDS. In response, the U.S. Agency for International Development (USAID) sends a team from its Displaced Children and Orphans Fund (DCOF) in August. This group issues a report, "Managing Uganda's Orphans Crisis," endorsing the fundamental importance of strengthening family and community capacities to care for their orphaned children as a primary response to orphaning.

International and bilateral organizations begin to recognize the proliferation of grassroots efforts in AIDS-affected communities to respond to the needs of children orphaned by AIDS.

In Zambia, Family Health Trust establishes the Children in Distress Network (CINDI).

The Orphan Project, a private organization, is created in New York City to do research and policy analysis on children orphaned by AIDS in the United States.

In the United States, representatives of nongovernmental organizations (NGOs), the DCOF, and the World Bank form the AIDS Orphans Task Force for information exchange, collaboration, and advocacy.

1992 The first national conference in response to orphaning due to AIDS, "Managing Uganda's Orphans Crisis," is held in Kampala, Uganda, sponsored by the Ministry of Labour and Social Affairs and USAID Uganda.

The government of Malawi's Task Force on Orphans issues the first national policy statement on orphans.

Martha Ainsworth and A.A. Rwegarulira publish the first longitudinal findings concerning the economic impacts of AIDS on families in *Coping with the AIDS Epidemic in Tanzania: Survivor Assistance*, The World Bank, Africa Technical Department, Technical Working Paper No. 6, July 1992.

The Orphan Generation, a video showing some of the responses to orphans and vulnerable children in Uganda, is distributed by Strategies for Hope.

In December, David Michaels and Carol Levine of the Orphan Project publish the first estimate of the number of children left motherless as a result of the HIV/AIDS epidemic in the United States in the *Journal of the American Medical Association*.

1993 The Families, Orphans and Children Under Stress (FOCUS) orphan-visiting program is established by volunteers in a rural community near Mutare, Zimbabwe.

1994 The Lusaka Declaration is adopted at a workshop in Zambia. It stresses the magnitude of the problem, the place of institutional care, the need for material and financial support for affected families, and the right to basic education as well as survival skills and vocational training.

The World Health Organization and UNICEF jointly publish *Action for Children Affected by AIDS: Program Profiles and Lessons Learned*.

USAID/DCOF funds the Foundation for International Community Assistance to initiate a microfinance program targeting areas seriously affected by HIV/AIDS in Uganda.

The Orphan Project publishes "Orphans of the HIV Epidemic: Unmet Needs in Six U.S. Cities" (1994), still the only analysis of its kind in the U.S.

1994–95 The Thai Red Cross Society and the East–West Center with support from Save the Children UK carry out a national assessment of the impact of HIV/AIDS on children in Thailand, the first such effort in Asia and the Pacific.

1996 Save the Children US begins a systematic approach to mobilizing and strengthening community responses to HIV/AIDS and orphaning through the COPE program in Namwera, Malawi.

1997 USAID publishes *Children on the Brink: Strategies to Support Children Isolated by HIV/AIDS* written by Susan Hunter and John Williamson, which contains the first multicountry (twenty-three countries) estimates of orphaning (for children through age fourteen) and five basic strategies to respond to orphaning due to AIDS.

USAID, UNICEF, and other donors begin to meet at the international level to exchange information and collaborate in response to orphaning.

1998   The CINDI network in KwaZulu-Natal organizes the first African regional conference on orphans, "Raising the Orphan Generation," in Pietermaritzburg, South Africa, June. Graça Machel, a leading child advocate from Mozambique, was the guest of honor and an active participant.

Convened by The Orphan Project, New York City, international technical experts meet in October at the White Oak Conference Center in Yulee, Florida, to review practice and research and identify action needed for children affected by AIDS.

A UN General Discussion titled "Children Living in a World with AIDS" stresses the relevance of the UN Convention on the Rights of the Child to prevention and care efforts and urges an holistic approach to HIV/AIDS.

1998–99   Profiles of the impacts of AIDS on children are developed in 12 countries in Eastern and Southern Africa by Susan Hunter for UNICEF to mobilize national-level action.

1999   The first national situation analysis of orphans and vulnerable children is carried out in Zambia in cooperation with the national government with the joint support of USAID, UNICEF, the World Bank, and the Swedish International Development Agency.

2000   *The White Oak Report: Building International Support for Children Affected by AIDS,* by Carol Levine and Geoff Foster, is published in New York by The Orphan Project.

At the 13th International AIDS Conference in Durban, South Africa, USAID, UNAIDS, and UNICEF present draft principles to guide programming for orphans and other vulnerable children, beginning a global review process. For the first time in this conference's history a special track on orphans and vulnerable children is included.

Children on the Brink 2000: Updated Estimates and Recommendations for Intervention (executive summary) by Hunter and Williamson, presenting revised estimates of the number of orphans in thirty-four countries, is published by USAID.

Fourteen countries in Eastern and Southern Africa send delegations to a regional workshop in Lusaka in November and develop technical guidance and country action steps regarding orphans and vulnerable children.

2001   In June the UN General Assembly Special Session on HIV/AIDS (UNGASS) establishes specific goals for children orphaned and made vulnerable by HIV/AIDS.

2002 USAID, UNICEF, and UNAIDS publish *Children on the Brink 2002: A Joint Report on Orphan Estimates and Program Strategies* with estimates of orphaning in eighty-eight countries and twelve Principles for Programming that evolved from the global review process begun in 2000 at the Durban AIDS conference.

The UN Special Session on Children issues the *World Fit for Children Declaration*, which affirms the action for children called for in the UNGASS on HIV/AIDS.

In April delegations from twenty-one western and central African countries meet in Yamoussoukro, Côte d'Ivoire, for the first workshop on orphans and other vulnerable children in that region, and in November delegations from twenty eastern and southern African countries meet in Windhoek, Namibia, to assess progress toward meeting the UNGASS goals. Delegations at both workshops prepare country action plans that address five priorities for national action: situation analysis, policy, action plan, mechanism for coordination, and monitoring and evaluation.

The Regional Psychosocial Support Initiative is formed to advocate for and scale up psychosocial support for orphans and vulnerable children in Africa through technical support and capacity building.

In September a group of prominent African leaders participate in an Africa Leadership Consultation, "Urgent Action for Children on the Brink." It is convened in Johannesburg by Nelson Mandela and Graça Machel in collaboration with the UN Secretary-General's Special Envoy for HIV/AIDS in Africa, Stephen Lewis, with support from UNICEF and UNAIDS. Participants sought consensus on priorities for a scaled-up emergency response to the orphans and vulnerable children crisis in sub-Saharan Africa and proposed actions to mobilize the leadership, partnerships, and resources required to deliver on the promises made at the UNGASS to children affected by HIV/AIDS in Africa.

The first situation analysis concerning orphans and vulnerable children in the Caribbean region is carried out in Jamaica.

2003 The International HIV/AIDS Alliance issues Building Blocks: Africa-wide Briefing Notes, setting out five programming areas relevant to orphans and vulnerable children in January.

The Global Partners Forum for Orphaned and Other Children Made Vulnerable by HIV/AIDS is convened in Geneva in October and a global framework for action is reviewed and endorsed in principle by participants. The Global Network for Better Care is initiated.

2004 *The Framework for the Protection, Care, and Support of Orphans and Vulnerable Children Living in a World with HIV and AIDS* is published in

July with the endorsement of twenty-three international organizations and NGOs.

USAID, UNICEF, and UNAIDS publish *Children on the Brink 2004: A Joint Report of New Orphan Estimates and a Framework for Action* and present estimates of orphaning through age seventeen for ninety-three countries.

The Rapid Assessment, Analysis and Action Planning (RAAAP) process is carried out in seventeen countries in sub-Saharan Africa, with the support of UNAIDS, UNICEF, USAID and WFP, to produce national plans of action for orphans and vulnerable children.

Resource Guide

The literature on children and HIV/AIDS is vast and growing. There are many valuable publications in many different forms. Unfortunately these resources are not always easily accessible, even in university libraries. The Internet is a valuable resource, and throughout the book Web citations have been provided where feasible. Internet-based citations, however, are subject to change and disappearance. Many resources are available on more than one Web site; if the designated URL does not take you to the document, try a search on the title or author.

Each chapter contains many references on its specific subject. This resource guide repeats some of those references and adds others. It is a selective list, largely but not exclusively focused on publications that deal with international data and issues rather than single-country information.

Literature Reviews and Bibliographies

Busza, J. 1999. *Literature review: Challenging HIV-related stigma and discrimination in Southeast Asia; Past successes and future priorities.* New York: Population Council/ Horizons. http://www.popcouncil.org/pdfs/HORIZONS_paper.pdf

Foster, G., and J. Williamson. 2000. A review of current literature on the impact of HIV/AIDS on children in sub-Saharan Africa. *AIDS* 14 (supplement 3)· S275–84.

Richter, L., J. Manegold, and R. Pather. 2004. *Family and community interventions for children Affected by AIDS.* Cape Town: Human Sciences Research Council Publishers. 182 pages. Available at http://www.hsrcpublishers.ac.za/

Williamson, J. 2004. *A family is for a lifetime: Part I, A discussion of the need for family care for children impacted by HIV/AIDS; part II, An annotated bibliography.* Washington, DC: The Synergy Project, March. 85 pages. Available at http://www.synergyaids.com/resources.asp?id=5088

General Material on AIDS-Affected Children and Families

Association François-Xavier Bagnoud. 2000. *Orphan alert: International perspectives on children left behind by HIV/AIDS.* 28 pages.
http://www.albinasactionfororphans.org/learn/ORPHANALERT1.pdf

Drew, R. S., C. Makufa, and G. Foster. 1998. Strategies for providing care and support to children orphaned by AIDS. *AIDS Care* 10 (suppl.1): S9–15.

Forgotten families: Older people as carers of orphans and vulnerable children. 2003. Policy Report. HelpAge International and the International HIF/AIDS Alliance. 28 pages.
http://www.helpage.org/images/pdfs/HIVAIDS/ForgottenFamilieReport.pdf

Foster, G. 1998. Today's children: Challenges to child health promotion in countries with severe AIDS epidemics. *AIDS Care* 10 (suppl. 1): S17–23.

———. 2002. The capacity of the extended family safety net for orphans in Africa. *Psychology, Health, and Medicine* 5:55–62.

———. 2004. Understanding community responses to the situation of children affected by AIDS: Lessons for external agencies. In *One step further: Responses to HIV/AIDS,* ed. A. Sisask, 91–115. SIDA studies no. 7. Geneva: United Nations Research Institute in Social Development. 28 pages. Available at http://www.unrisd.org

Foster G., and S. Germann. 2002. The orphan crisis. Chapter 44 in *AIDS in Africa,* ed. M. Essex, S. Mboup, P. Kanki, R. J. Marlink, and S. D. Tlou, 664–775. New York: Kluwer Academic/Plenum.

Foster, G., C. Makufa, R. Drew, S. Kambeu, and K. Saurombe. 1996. Supporting children in need through a community-based orphan visiting programme. *AIDS Care* 8:389–403.

Foster, G., C. Makufa, R. Drew, and E. Kralovec. 1997. Factors leading to the establishment of child-headed households: The case of Zimbabwe. *Health Transition Review* 7 (suppl. 2): 155–68. http://htc.anu.edu.au/pdfs//Foster1.pdf

The framework for the protection, care, and support of orphans and vulnerable children living in a world with HIV and AIDS. 2004. Prepared by Partners Forum for Orphans and Vulnerable Children, convened and led by UNICEF, July. Available at http://www.unicef.org

Hunter, S. 2000. *Reshaping societies: HIV/AIDS and social change; A resource book for planning, programs, and policy making.* Glens Falls, NY: Hudson Run Press. 376 pages.

Levine, C., ed. 1993. *A death in the family: Orphans of the HIV epidemic.* New York: United Hospital Fund. 157 pages.

Levine, C., and G. Foster. 2000. *The White Oak report: Building international support for children affected by AIDS.* New York: The Orphan Project. 76 pages. Available at http://www.aidsinfonyc.org/orphan/

Monk, N. 2003. *Orphan alert 2: Children of the HIV/AIDS pandemic; The challenge of India.* Neil Monk, author and researcher. 64 pages.
http://www.albinasactionfororphans.org/learn/ORPHANALERT2.pdf

Subbarao, K., and D. Coury. 2003. *Orphans in sub-Saharan countries: A framework for public action.* Washington, DC: Human Development Network, World Bank, June. 111 pages. http://wbln0018.worldbank.org/HDNet/HDDocs.nsf/0/b67a743352b38f7685256e1a0078c414/$FILE/OrphansinSSA.pdf

Tobis, D. 2000. *Moving from residential institutions to community-based social services in Central and Eastern Europe and the former Soviet Union.* Washington, DC: World Bank. Available at http://www.worldbank.org

UNICEF. 2003. *Africa's orphaned generations.* New York: UNICEF, November. 52 pages. Available at http://www.unicef.org/publications/index_16271.html.

USAID, UNICEF, and UNAIDS. 2002. *Children on the brink 2002: A joint report on orphan estimates and program strategies.* Washington, DC: TvT Associates/The Synergy Project, USAID. http://www.unicef.org/publications/pub_children_on_the_brink_en.pdf

Williamson, J., G. Foster, and M. Lorey. 2002. Mechanisms for channeling resources to grassroots groups supporting orphans and other vulnerable children. http://www.synergyaids.com/resources.asp?id=3025

African Regional Workshops

Loudon, M. 2002. *Eastern and Southern Africa Regional Workshop on Children Affected by HIV/AIDS: Implementing the UNGASS goals for orphans and other children made vulnerable by HIV/AIDS.* Report on a workshop convened by the UNICEF Eastern and Southern Africa Regional Office in Windhoek, Namibia, November 25–29. 163 pages. Available at http://www.sarpn.org.za/documents/d0000458/index.php

UNICEF, USAID, Family Health International, International Save the Children Alliance, and UNAIDS. 2002. Report on West and Central Africa Regional Workshop on Orphans and Other Vulnerable Children, Yamoussoukro, Côte d'Ivoire, April 7–12. 60 pages. Available at http://www.fhi.org/

Guidance Documents and Toolkits

Child Protection Society of Zimbabwe. 1999. *How can we help? Approaches to community-based care: A guide for groups and organisations wishing to assist orphans and other children in distress.* Edited by Sandra Morreira. Child Protection Society of Zimbabwe. 68 pages. http://www.womenchildrenhiv.org/pdf/p09-of/of-03-05.pdf

Grainger, C., D. Webb, and L. Elliot. 2001. *Children affected by HIV/AIDS: Rights and responsibilities in the developing world.* Knowledge Working Paper no. 23. London: Save the Children. 132 pages.

International HIV/AIDS Alliance. 2003. Building blocks: Africa wide briefing notes. Locally adaptable resources for communities working with orphans and vulnerable children. Includes six booklets: Overview, 24 pages; Education, 20 pages; Health and nutrition, 24 pages; Psychosocial support, 28 pages; Economic strengthening, 24 pages; and Social inclusion, 20 pages. Available at http://www.aidsalliance.org/building_blocks.htm

Situation Analysis

DeMarco, R. 2005. *Conducting a participatory situation analysis of orphans and vulnerable children affected by HIV/AIDS: Guidelines and tools, A framework and resource guide.* Arlington, VA, Family Health International with USAID and Implementing

AIDS Prevention and Care Project. 210 pages. *http://www.fhi.org/en/HIVAIDS/ pub/guide/ovcguide.htm*

Foster, G., C. Makufa, R. Drew, S. Mashumba, and S. Kambeu. 1995. Perceptions of children and community members concerning the circumstances of orphans in rural Zimbabwe. *AIDS Care* 9: 391–406.

Foster, G., R. Shakespeare, F. Chinemana, H. Jackson, S. Gregson, C. Marange, and S. Mashumba. 1995. Orphan prevalence and extended family care in a peri-urban community in Zimbabwe. *AIDS Care* 7:3–17.

Manda, K. D., M. J. Kelly, and M. Loudon. 1999. *Orphans and vulnerable children: A situation analysis, 1999.* Joint USAID/UNICEF/SIDA/Study Fund project, Government of Zambia. 399 pages. Available at http:www.harare.unesco.org

Wakhweya, A., C. Kateregga, J. Konde-Lule, R. Mukyala, L. Sabin, M. Williams, and H. K. Heggenhougen. 2002. *A situation analysis of orphans in Uganda, orphans, and their households: Caring for their future – today.* Ministry of Gender, Labour, and Social Development, Government of Uganda; Uganda AIDS Commission, November. 316 pages.
http://www.bumc.bu.edu/www/sph/cih/Images/s_afinal.pdf

Williamson, J., A. Cox, and B. Johnston. 2004. *Conducting a situation analysis of orphans and vulnerable children affected by HIV/AIDS: A framework and resource guide,* February. Washington, DC: Office of Sustainable Development, Bureau for Africa, USAID. 55 pages. Available at http://www.synergyaids.com/

Assessments and Evaluations

Foster, G., and L. Jiwli. 2001. Psychosocial support of children affected by AIDS: An evaluation and review of Masiye Camp. Bulawayo, Zimbabwe, June. http://www.harare.unesco.org/hivaids/view_absract.asp?id=240.doc

Lee, T., G. Foster, C. Makufa, and S. Hinton. 2002. Care and support of children and women: Families, orphans, and children under stress in Zimbabwe. *Evaluation and Program Planning* 25:59–70.

McDermott, P., J. Brakarsh, P. Chigara, L. Cogswell, C. Coombe, T. Himmelfarb, M. Loudon, and J. Williamson. 2003. Report on the mid-term review of the STRIVE Project. Submitted to Catholic Relief Services, Zimbabwe, and USAID Zimbabwe, July 10. 179 pages. http://www.sara.aed.org/tech_areas/ovc/strive-report.pdf

Nyamukapa, C. A., G. Foster, and S. Gregson. 2003. Orphans' household circumstances and access to education in a maturing HIV epidemic in eastern Zimbabwe. *Journal of Social Development in Africa* 18(2): 7–32.

Socioeconomic Impacts of HIV/AIDS and Microeconomic Responses

Donahue, J., K. Kabuccho, and S. Osinde. 2001. *HIV/AIDS: Responding to a silent crisis among microfinance clients in Kenya and Uganda.* Nairobi, Kenya: MicroSave-Africa, September. 36 pages. Available at http://www.alternative-finance.org.uk/

Muwanga, F. T. 2002. *Impact of HIV/AIDS on agriculture and the private sector in Swaziland: The demographic, social, and economic impact on subsistence agriculture, commercial agriculture, Ministry of Agriculture, and co-operatives and business.* Swaziland, August. 80 pages. http://www.gdnet.org/fulltext/muwanga2.pdf

Parker, J., I. Singh, and K. Hattel. 2000. *The role of microfinance in the fight against HIV/AIDS*. A report to The Joint United Nations Programme on HIV/AIDS (UNAIDS). Bethesda, MD: Development Alternatives, Inc., September 15. 24 pages. Available at
http://www.dai.com/pdfs/UNAIDS_policy_Paper_on_Microfinance.pdf

United Nations Food and Agriculture Organization (FAO). 2002. HIV/AIDS, food security, and rural livelihood. FAO HIV/AIDS Programme. 4 pages. http://www.fao.org/hivaids/publications/hivaids.pdf

White, J., ed. 2002. *Facing the challenge: NGO experiences of mitigating the impacts of HIV/AIDS in sub-Saharan Africa*. Natural Resources Institute, University of Greenwich, UK, November. 76 pages.
http://www.nri.org/news/pdfaidsreportnov2002.pdf

Community Mobilization and Capacity Building

Donahue, J., S. Hunter, L. Sussman, and J. Williamson. 1999. A supplemental report on community mobilization and microfinance services as HIV/AIDS mitigation tools. Produced in conjunction with the combined USAID/UNICEF assessment *Children affected by HIV/AIDS in Kenya: An overview of issues and action to strengthen community care and support.* 24 pages.
http://www.dec.org/pdf_docs/pnacg780.pdf.

Donahue, J., and J. Williamson. 1999. *Community mobilization to mitigate the impacts of HIV/AIDS*. Washington, DC: Displaced Children and Orphans Fund, USAID, September. 9 pages. http://www.dec.org/pdf_docs/pnacjo24.pdf

Foster, G. 2002. Supporting community efforts to assist orphans in Africa. *New England Journal of Medicine* 346 (24): 1907–9.

Phiri, S. N., G. Foster, and M. Nzima. 2001. *Expanding and strengthening community action: A study of ways to scale up community mobilization interventions to mitigate the effect of HIV/AIDS on children and families*. Washington, DC: Displaced Children and Orphans Fund, USAID. Available at http://www.usaid.gov/our_work/humanitarian_assistance/the_funds/pubs/ovc.html

Care for Children without Adequate Family Care

Human Rights Watch. 2001. In the shadow of death: HIV/AIDS and children's rights in Kenya. *Kenya* 13(4A).1–35. Available from
http://www.hrw.org/reports/2001/kenya

International Save the Children Alliance. 2003. *A last resort: The growing concern about children in residential care; Save the Children's position on residential care*. London: Save the Children UK. 23 pages. Available at
http://www.savethechildren.net/homepage/

Tolfree, D. K. 2003. *Community-based care for separated children*. Stockholm: Save the Children Sweden. 16 pages. Available at http://www.rb.se/www/eng/Programme/Childrenandfamilies/withoutfamily/

———. 2003. *Whose children? Separated children's protection and participation in emergencies*. Stockholm: Save the Children Sweden.

Education

Ainsworth, M., and D. Filmer. 2002. Poverty, AIDS, and children's schooling: A targeting dilemma. World Bank Policy Research Working Paper 2885. Operations Evaluation Department and Development Research Group, World Bank, September. 44 pages. Available at http://www.worldbank.org/

Coombe, C. 2002. Mitigating the impact of HIV/AIDS on education supply, demand, and quality. Chapter 12 of *AIDS, public policy, and child well-being*, ed. Giovanni Andrea Cornia. Florence: UNICEF-Innocenti Research Center, June. 52 pages. Available at http://www.unicef-icdc.org/siteguide/indexsearch.html

Hepburn, A. 2001. Primary education in eastern and southern Africa: Increasing access for orphans and vulnerable children in AIDS-affected areas. Report prepared for the Displaced Children and Orphans Fund, USAID, Terry Sanford Institute of Public Policy, Duke University, April. 70 pages. Available at http://www.usaid.gov/our_work/humanitarian_assistance/the_funds/pubs/ovc.html

Scaling Up

Foster, G., and J. Sherman. 2001. *Expanding support to orphans and vulnerable children*: Workshop Report. Harare: Oak Foundation. Available at http://www.synergyaids.com/resources.asp?id=220/.

Responses of Religious Bodies

Foster, G. 2004. *Study of the response by faith-based organizations to orphans and vulnerable children*. New York: World Conference of Religions for Peace and UNICEF. 34 pages. http://www.unicef.org/aids/FBO_OVC_study_summary.pdf

Children with HIV/AIDS

Care for children infected and those affected by HIV/AIDS: A handbook for community health workers. 2003. Kampala, Uganda: Save the Children UK. 123 pages. http://www.savethechildren.org.uk/temp/scuk/cache/cmsattach/1099_HIVCareHandbook.pdf

HIV/AIDS and Armed Conflict

International Save the Children HIV/AIDS Co-ordinating Group. 2002. *HIV and conflict: A double emergency*. London: Save the Children UK. 32 pages. http://www.savethechildren.org.uk/temp/scuk/cache/cmsattach/212/hivconflict.pdf

Law and Policy

Smart, R. 2003. *Policies for orphans and vulnerable children: A framework for moving ahead*. The Policy Project, USAID, July. 27 pages.
http://www.policyproject.com/pubs/generalreport/OVC_policies.pdf

Psychosocial Issues

Cook, M. 1998. *Starting from strengths: Community care for orphaned children*. Facilitator's Guide. Victoria: University of Victoria; Zomba, Malawi: Chancellor College, July. 149 pages plus appendices. Available at http://web.uvic.ca/icrd/pub_resources.html#manuals

Humuliza Project: Manual. n.d. A training manual enabling teachers and other adults to counsel orphans or children of terminally sick parents. Basel, Switzerland: Humuliza/Terre des Hommes. Available at www.terredeshommes.ch/humuliza/humuliza.html

E-mail Listservs

Children Affected by AIDS (CABA). To subscribe to the CABA forum, send a message to: listserv@list.s-3.com with the following in the body SUBSCRIBE CABA.

Orphans and Vulnerable Children Task Force. http://groups.yahoo.com/group/ovctaskforce/ This is an online forum and information exchange.

The Psychosocial Support E-Forum. This forum is a project of the Regional Psychosocial Support Initiative for Children Affected by AIDS (REPSSI), which was created by the Salvation Army and Terre des Hommes, Switzerland. To register, send an e-mail message to forum.admin@repssi.org or go to http://www.repssi.org/cgi-bin/ultimatebb.cgi

Basic information about REPSSI is available at http://www.repssi.org/

Web Sites

Association François-Xavier Bagnoud (AFXB). http://www.afxb.org/en
Founded in 1989 by Albina du Boisvouvray, AFXB is an international nongovernmental association whose mission is to advocate for and provide direct support to families and communities affected by HIV/AIDS. The Web site describes AFXB programs in eleven countries as well as the AFXB Center on Health and Human Rights, Harvard University, and the International Pediatric HIV Training Program at the University of Medicine and Dentistry of New Jersey.

Children in Distress Network (CINDI). http://www.cindi.org.za/
CINDI is a consortium of over seventy nongovernmental organizations, government departments, and individuals that network in the interests of children affected by HIV/AIDS in the KwaZulu-Natal Midlands Region of South Africa. Among the working groups described on the Web site are Children Helping Children and Home-Based Care.

Children's Rights Network. http://www.crin.org
This Web site has updates on children's rights issues and links to reports and publications. Viewers can also sign up for e-mail information and a listserv.

Community Response to the HIV/AIDS Epidemic (CORE) Initiative. http://www.coreinitiative.org/

The CORE Initiative is a USAID-funded global program that aims to strengthen the capacity of community-based and faith-based organizations to respond. CARE International is the lead organization, in partnership with many others. The Web site contains technical resources, information about grants, and links to other resources.

Displaced Children and Orphans Fund, USAID. http://www.usaid.gov/our_work/humanitarian_assistance/thefunds/dcof/index.html
The Web site describes the Displaced Children and Orphans Fund (DCOF) programs in nineteen countries and the Peace Corp. It has links to its publications. For more general information on USAID's HIV/AIDS programs, see http://www.usaid.gov/our_work/global_health/aids/

The Firelight Foundation http://www.firelightfoundation.org/
The Firelight Foundation is a charity based in Santa Cruz, CA, that makes small grants to grassroots, community-based organizations for direct support to meet the needs and rights of orphans and vulnerable children affected by HIV/AIDS in sub-Saharan Africa. The Web site has information about its programs.

Hope for African Children Initiative. http://www.hopeforafricanchildren.org/
The Hope for African Children Initiative brings together six organizations concerned with HIV/AIDS: CARE, Plan International, Save the Children, Society of Women and AIDS in Africa, World Conference on Religion and Peace, and World Vision. Established with seed money from the Bill and Melinda Gates Foundation, it now has programs operating in Kenya, Malawi, and Uganda.

Human Rights Watch. http://www.hrw.org
Includes reports on failures to fulfil the rights of children affected by AIDS in Kenya, sexual abuse of girls in Zambia, abuses against children affected by AIDS in India, and others.

Interagency Coalition on AIDS and Development http://www.icad.org
This Canadian coalition of more than one hundred organizations focuses on both global and domestic responses to the HIV/AIDS epidemic. The Web site has fact sheets, publications, and other information.

InSite http://hivinsite.ucsf.edu/InSite
Sponsored by the University of California San Francisco School of Medicine HIV/AIDS information center, this site has updated information about treatment, prevention, and policies.

The International HIV/AIDS Alliance http://www.aidsalliance.org/eng/
The International HIV/AIDS Alliance is a British charity that supports community action on HIV/AIDS in developing countries. The Web site has descriptions of programs, toolkits, and publications.

Orphans and Other Vulnerable Children Support Toolkit. http://www.ovcsupport.net/sw505.asp
Jointly established by the International HIV/AIDS Alliance and Family Health International, this Web site makes available many key documents relevant to children affected by HIV/AIDS.

The Synergy Project http://www.synergyaids.com
The Synergy Project provides technical assistance and services to USAID to design, evaluate, and coordinate HIV/AIDS programs and to disseminate lessons learned. The Web site contains information about program evaluation and links to publications.

UNAIDS http://www.unaids.org/en/default.asp
The Joint UN Programme on AIDS (UNAIDS) is a consortium of nine UN organizations concerned with HIV/AIDS, including UNICEF, the World Health Organization, and the World Bank Group. The Web site has extensive resources.

UNICEF http://www.unicef.org/
 The major UN organization concerned with children, UNICEF has offices and
 programs around the world. The Web site has links to publications and other
 resources.
U.S. Centers for Disease Control and Prevention (CDC) http://www.cdc.gov/
 The CDC is the primary U.S. governmental agency for collecting and dissem-
 inating data on HIV/AIDS in the United States. It includes several centers, of
 which the primary one for HIV/AIDS is the National Center for HIV, STD, and
 TB Prevention. The Web site contains information on the Global AIDS Program
 as well as on the epidemic in the United States.
Women, Children, and HIV http://www.womenchildrenhiv.org
 This Web site is a project of the Association François-Xavier Bagnoud and the
 HIV Information Center of the University of California, San Francisco, School
 of Medicine. It contains links to many of the articles and reports cited in this
 volume.
World Bank Group, Early Childhood Development
 http://www.worldbank.org/children/aidsgroup.html
 The World Bank Group is the largest source of funding for education and
 HIV/AIDS programs. This Web site contains information on governmental agencies and other resources. Other sections of the World Bank Group's Web site contain research reports on HIV/AIDS and economic development and education.

Videos

Everyone's Child. 1996. VHS, 16 mm and 35 mm. Directed by Tsitsi Dangarembga.
 Produced in Zimbabwe by Media for Development Trust. 90 minutes. There
 is also a 20-minute training video drawn from the film with written material.
 http://www.mfd.co.zw/index.cfm
General information available at: http://www.newsreel.org/films/everyone.htm
 The Orphan Generation. 1992. Produced by Small World Productions. 10-
 and 40-minute segments. Can be ordered through the UNICEF Web site
 http://www.unicef.org/

Index

abuse
  in residential care, 12
  sexual, 3, 67–8, 188, 189–91
Accumulating Savings and Credits
    Associations. *See* ASCAs
ACS (Administration for Children's
    Services), 218
Administration for Children's Services. *See*
    ACS
adolescent sexual behavior
  HIV prevalence studies and, 236
  in New Zealand, 236
  in Uganda, 235–6
  in US, 236
  values-based belief systems and, 169
adoptions, 11, 29–30
  in CRC, 142
  intercountry, 30
  legal parameters of, 25
  nontraditional families and, 29
  restrictions for, 29–30
  in South Africa, 29
Africa
  CABA in, 5, 11, 96
  child development in, 111
  community "safety nets" in, 112, 164
  "extended-extended families" in, 16, 17,
    163, 178
  FBOs in, 160, 178
  HIV/AIDS affliction rates in, 4, 168
  HIV/AIDS disclosure in, 105
  institutional care in, 12
  oral traditions in, 164–5
  orphan rates in, 1
  orphan support programs in, 124–7
  religion's influence in, 159–60, 163
  situation analyses in, 270
  social discrimination in, 106
African Summit on HIV/AIDS,
    Tuberculosis, and Other Related
    Diseases, 141
African Union Ministerial Conference on
    Human Rights in Africa, 141
African Americans
  churches and, 218–19
  health care and, 221
  HIV/AIDS and, 216
"age of consent," 148
"age of majority," 148
AIDS (acquired immune deficiency
    syndrome), *See also* HIV/AIDS
  economic toll of, 37
  medical definitions of, 1
"AIDS babies," 216
"AIDS generation," 68
"AIDS orphan," 3
alcohol abuse, 192
Annan, Kofi, 81
antiretroviral therapy (short course), 201
  child mortality rates and, 203
  efficacy of, 197
  perinatal HIV transmission and, 197
ASCAs (Accumulating Savings and Credits
    Associations), 51–2
  ROSCAs v., 51
  terms of agreement for, 51
ASEAN Heads of Government Summit,
    205
Asian Red Cross/Red Crescent Aid Task
    Force, 194, 196

Printed in the United States
By Bookmasters